PSYCHOSOCIAL ISSUES
NEAR
THE END OF LIFE

PSYCHOSOCIAL ISSUES NEAR THE END OF LIFE

A Resource for Professional Care Providers

Edited by

JAMES L. WERTH JR.

AND

DEAN BLEVINS

American Psychological Association
Washington, DC

Published by
American Psychological Association
750 First Street, NE
Washington, DC 20002
www.apa.org

To order
APA Order Department
P.O. Box 92984
Washington, DC 20090-2984
Tel: (800) 374-2721; Direct: (202) 336-5510
Fax: (202) 336-5502; TDD/TTY: (202) 336-6123
Online: www.apa.org/books/
E-mail: order@apa.org

In the U.K., Europe, Africa, and the Middle East, copies may be ordered from
American Psychological Association
3 Henrietta Street
Covent Garden, London
WC2E 8LU England

Typeset in Goudy by Stephen McDougal, Mechanicsville, MD

Printer: Data Reproductions, Auburn Hills, MI
Cover Designer: Cassandra Chu Design, San Francisco, CA
Technical/Production Editors: Gail B. Munroe and Tiffany L. Klaff

The opinions and statements published are the responsibility of the authors, and such opinions and statements do not necessarily represent the policies of the American Psychological Association.

Library of Congress Cataloging-in-Publication Data

Psychosocial issues near the end of life : a resource for professional care providers / edited by James L. Werth, Jr. and Dean Blevins.— 1st ed.
    p. cm.
    Includes bibliographical references and index.
    ISBN 1-59147-236-9
    1. Terminal care. 2. Sick—Psychology. 3. Death—Psychological aspects.
I. Werth, James L. II. Blevins, Dean.

    R726.8.P796 2005
    362.17'5—dc22   2005002346

British Library Cataloguing-in-Publication Data
A CIP record is available from the British Library.

Printed in the United States of America
First Edition

The editors dedicate this book to Becky and her family and friends for showing us how to live life fully and with dignity to the very end; care for, and then let go of, those we love; and share deep loss in meaningful ways.

Jim Werth especially wants to express his appreciation to Linda for making the hardest decision a sibling should never have to make, even though it was the right one.

CONTENTS

CONTRIBUTORS

Jennifer Abbey, MA, Fordham University, Bronx, NY

Rebecca S. Allen, PhD, University of Alabama, Tuscaloosa

Elizabeth J. Bergman, MA, University of South Florida, Tampa

Dean Blevins, PhD, Center for Mental Healthcare and Outcomes Research (CeMHOR) & South Central Mental Illness Research, Education, and Clinical Care (MIRECC), Central Arkansas Veterans Healthcare System, North Little Rock; Department of Psychiatry, College of Medicine, University of Arkansas for Medical Sciences, Little Rock

William Breitbart, MD, Memorial Sloan-Kettering Cancer Center, New York

Stephen R. Connor, PhD, National Hospice and Palliative Care Organization, Fairfax Station, VA

Peter H. Ditto, PhD, University of California, Irvine

Christopher A. Gibson, PhD, Memorial Sloan-Kettering Cancer Center, New York

William E. Haley, PhD, University of South Florida, Tampa

Karen Orloff Kaplan, MSW, MPH, ScD, former President and CEO, Last Acts Partnership, Washington, DC

Kevin P. Kaut, PhD, University of Akron, OH

Phillip M. Kleespies, PhD, Department of Veterans Affairs Boston Healthcare System, West Roxbury, MA

Anne Kosinski, BS, Memorial Sloan-Kettering Cancer Center, New York

Jeffrey Lycan, RN, BS, Ohio Hospice and Palliative Care Organization, Columbus

Christian J. Nelson, PhD, Memorial Sloan-Kettering Cancer Center, New York

Danai Papadatou, PhD, University of Athens, Greece

Hayley Pessin, PhD, Memorial Sloan-Kettering Cancer Center, New York

Lucinda L. Roff, PhD, University of Alabama, Tuscaloosa

Barry Rosenfeld, PhD, Fordham University, Bronx, NY

Bettina Schmid, MS, University of Alabama, Tuscaloosa

J. Donald Schumacher, PsyD, National Hospice and Palliative Care Organization, Alexandria, VA

Judith M. Stillion, PhD, Center for Active Retirement Education, Kennesaw, GA

Alexis Tomarken, CSW, Memorial Sloan-Kettering Cancer Center, New York

James L. Werth Jr., PhD, University of Akron, Ohio

FOREWORD:
TRANSFORMING DYING IN AMERICA

KAREN ORLOFF KAPLAN

My grandparents died at home. The family gathered around the bed-side. There were tears, laughter, and, of course, food and stories, stories, sto-ries. The physician offered what comfort measures were available many years ago, and each of my grandparents died unafraid, in the arms of loved ones, in peace, and with great dignity. My children's grandparents died in the hospi-tal, in intensive care units. No children were allowed, no food, no noise, no stories, little peace, even less dignity, but sadly, much pain. As recently as 10 years ago, many, if not most, people died exactly this way.

What happened in a single generation? What transformed death from a natural part of a full life cycle into a medical event? What robbed it of dignity and compassion and filled it with isolation, fear, pain, and loss of precious control? The answers tell a story of the scientific miracles of recent decades and underscore the countless triumphs of modern medicine. They also tell of some of the abject failures of this nation's health care system.

One of the most significant among the many ways our health care sys-tem fails is the relative lack of attention clinicians pay to the psychosocial needs of patients who are dying and of these patients' families. Although quality palliative care involves treating the bio-psycho-socio-spiritual issues facing dying patients (see Kaut, chap. 5), psychologists have been late com-ing to the bedside of these patients (see Connor, Lycan, & Schumacher, chap. 9; see also Haley, Larson, Kasl-Godley, Neimeyer, & Kwilosz, 2003). In many settings, their absence leaves a gaping hole in the care provided. The chapters in this book speak to the issues psychologists and other health and mental health care providers must address more vigorously and to some of the interventions needed. The book is an essential tool for psychology students and practitioners—a tool to enhance understanding and provide a road map to compassionate and effective treatment of dying patients and their loved ones. In this foreword, I give the reader a brief overview of the historical influences that have led to the current practice of neglecting psychosocial issues near the end of life and to contemporary developments that have created an environment in which practitioners have great need for the information presented in the chapters of this book.

HISTORICAL INFLUENCES

To understand some of the reasons psychologists have not been sufficiently present at the bedside of dying people, it is necessary to consider what happened to the dying process in the Untied States over the past several decades. As Stillion discusses in chapter 1, in the 40 years or so between the 1950s when my grandparents died and the 1990s when my children's grandparents passed away, the era of powerful antibiotics was born. Dialysis, transplants, and laser surgery were developed. Life support machinery and techniques became commonplace, as did diagnostic procedures that identified serious illness at its onset and tracked it throughout its course. Ecstatic at the marvels that were routinely brought about in physicians' offices and hospitals, the medical profession and the public began to see death as a failure—a failure of the medical profession to find the right intervention to stave off death and of the patient who did not live on, much less get better.

As death became an increasingly repugnant enemy, we moved it further from our sight. Death became a taboo subject in homes and hospitals and, sadly, in medical schools. We taught our medical students and other health care professionals little, if anything, about using the increasingly superb technology to ease a dying person's symptoms or compassionate communication to ease spiritual pain and family suffering.

Slightly more than a decade ago, a cultural revolution began—quietly, slowly—but tenaciously (see also Connor et al., chap. 9). A small group of visionary leaders embarked on multifaceted efforts to improve the care—and caring—that people received as they neared the end of their lives and that provided for their families. These efforts and the changes that accompanied them came about for many reasons; among them, two were, in different ways, vitally important and highly visible.

One significant phenomenon that prompted change was the shift of the media spotlight to issues concerning dying and death. The media covered several groundbreaking legal cases during the 1990s, substantially raising awareness of end-of-life issues (see Stillion, chap. 1). For example, the U.S. Supreme Court, in *Cruzan v. Director, Missouri Department of Health*

(1990), reaffirmed an individual's (or his or her surrogate decision maker's) rights to refuse treatment, whereas in *Vacco v. Quill* (1997) and *Washington v. Glucksberg* (1997) the Court addressed the issue of a state's authority over matters of legalizing physician-assisted suicide.

At the same time, the media was paying rapt attention to Jack Kevorkian and the patients in whose suicides he so publicly assisted. Both careful and sensational reporting of the court cases and Kevorkian's activity focused the nation's attention on two important facts: Not everyone wanted to prolong his or her dying process with technologic interventions, and far too many people suffered needlessly atrocious deaths. Widespread print news, television, and radio coverage made it permissible to discuss, and even encouraged discussing, death with one's family, friends, and colleagues. Increasing recognition emerged that everyone had a story about a bad death experienced by a friend or family member. And most, when asked, admitted fear that such horrific endings would be their lot as well.

Another event driving the nascent cultural revolution was the publication of a landmark study, *SUPPORT* (SUPPORT Principal Investigators, 1995). This was the first major study documenting serious deficiencies in physical and psychosocial care for dying patients and their families. Its appearance in the professional and lay press and the subsequent publication of an Institute of Medicine (IOM) report, *Approaching Death: Improving Care at the End of Life* (Field & Cassel, 1997) resulted in initiatives that collectively are bringing about welcome changes in the way people die in America. Further, as several recognized experts noted, "Considering the deep-seated antipathy of Americans to facing death and dying, change is occurring relatively quickly in end-of-life care" (Metzger & Kaplan, 2001, p. 1).

The SUPPORT study, IOM report, and associated research examined many areas of concern, one of which was the range of legal, organizational, and economic obstacles that routinely impede delivery of reliably excellent care near the end of life. For example, as Ditto discusses in chapter 4 of this volume, advance directives (living wills and medical powers of attorney) are not living up to their promise for a variety of regulatory and psychosocial reasons, and as Allen and colleagues review in chapter 8, loved ones have difficulty getting their needs met. It is also difficult to access quality end-of-life care because, with the exception of the Medicare hospice benefit (see Connor et al., chap. 9), there is minimal insurance coverage for holistic care. Further, the nation's health care system fails to provide a seamless continuum of care for people as they move along the frequently lengthy trajectory from diagnosis of a serious, life-limiting illness to death.

An analysis conducted by Last Acts (2002) titled *Means to a Better End: A Report on Dying in America Today* also discussed the problems in care near the end of life. This study rated end-of-life care in each state according to eight criteria and conveyed sobering findings:

Despite many recent improvements in end-of-life care and greater public awareness about it, this report shows that Americans at best have no better than a fair chance of finding good care for their loved ones or for themselves when facing a life-threatening illness. (p. 3)

Although the study documented pockets of outstanding end-of-life care, particularly that provided by many hospices, several of the findings (summarized in the list that follows) highlight failures that have profound psychosocial implications:

1. Despite federal legislation (Patient Self Determination Act, 1990) requiring that health care providers tell patients about advance directives, surprisingly few Americans actually complete them (less than 25% overall).
2. Only 24.9% of Americans die at home, although more than 70% say that is their wish.
3. The average length of stay in hospice has dropped from 70 days in 1983 to 36 days more recently. In 1998, 28% of hospice patients were enrolled for 1 week or less before dying.
4. In 2000, only 42% of U.S. hospitals offered a formal pain management program; only 23% offered formal hospice programs, and only 14% offered palliative care programs.
5. Only 16 states received a grade of A or B for the strength of their pain policies.
6. Although end-of-life spiritual concerns rank high among those listed by the public, only hospice programs consistently provide this type of care.
7. Although America is a nation of multiple racial, ethnic, and economic communities, little attention is paid to the unique ways in which different communities regard the dying process and whether they have sufficient access to care that is acceptable to them.
8. Among the recommendations contained in *Means to a Better End*, four stand out as basic requirements for sustaining positive change in end-of-life care: making quality end-of-life care a national health policy priority; making end-of-life care a special priority in aging policy; supporting public and private initiatives to meet the needs of family caregivers; and encouraging policies to enhance consumers' knowledge of the options for quality care near the end of life.

On the professional side, setting training and practice standards and encouraging requirements for continuing professional education—for physicians, nurses, psychologists, social workers, and clergy—about end-of-life care constitute the backbone of quality service delivery. Given these findings and recommendations, I am pleased that this book is available, for its contents address these problem areas and provide direction for improving care near the end of life. The results of the SUPPORT study, conclusions of the IOM report, findings presented in *Means to a Better End,* and the extensive media coverage of issues concerning death and dying occurred in an environment in which the elderly were a growing segment of the population and consumer choice was increasingly highly valued. Together, these factors stimulated a still growing movement to improve the way people die in America. As this movement continues to gather momentum, change is taking place along two parallel tracks: the first involving the public and individual consumers; the second, care-providing professionals. A combination of generous foundation funding and sustained, creative leadership in the field have nurtured change in each sector.[1]

CONTEMPORARY DEVELOPMENTS

This book adds to the momentum for change by providing a much needed resource for psychologists, psychiatrists, and other mental health professionals. It will assist them in addressing the neglected area of psychosocial issues for those near the end of life. It is the first comprehensive book on the topic for psychologists and other professionals providing psychosocial care to dying people and their loved ones. The importance of the psychological, spiritual, interpersonal, and societal issues is highlighted in the *Precepts of Palliative Care* (*Precepts,* Last Acts, 1997), which most experts broadly accept and consider to be the gold standard for care near the end of life. The five components constituting quality end-of-life care are as follows:

1. Pain and other physical and psychological symptoms should be alleviated and comfort maximized by medical care that conforms to best-practice standards and that is consistent with the person's values and preferences.
2. The physical and emotional environment should be as pleasant and supportive as possible and include time spent with loved ones and other people of choice.
3. Dying persons and their families should be cared for in a manner that respects inherent dignity.
4. Dying persons should be able to exercise personal autonomy (control) to the extent desired and feasible.

---

[1]The Robert Wood Johnson Foundation led the nurturing of the movement to improve care near the end of life by infusing more than $160 million into these efforts with the Soros-funded Open Society Institute's Project on Death in America and the Nathan Cummings Foundation also contributing significant funds.

5. Dying persons should be able to explore issues of meaning and spirituality, with support from others as desired.

All of these areas focus on the need to address psychosocial issues, and all are addressed in this book. The chapters by Kaut (chap. 5), Gibson's team (chap. 6), and Rosenfeld and colleagues (chap. 7) address the identification and treatment of the primary psychological symptoms that may negatively affect dying people's quality of life. Similarly, Allen and her coauthors (chap. 8) review the roles of personal caregivers and their needs. Both Blevins and Papadatou, in their chapter on culture (chap. 2), and Werth and Kleespies, in their chapter on ethics (chap. 3), address issues of dignity and autonomy in end-of-life situations. Addressing spirituality and meaning is infused throughout the chapters but is most readily apparent in Kaut's chapter.

Thus, in discussing how mental health professionals can foster the highest quality care near the end of life, each of the chapters in this book respects these principles. A particular strength across the chapters is the integration of issues that are directly relevant to researchers, practitioners, educators, and policymakers. In fact, in the concluding chapter, the editors summarize these discussions and provide top priorities for each of these groups to continue moving the field forward.

Although noteworthy programs have been developed to provide end-of-life treatment education for practicing medical clinicians, unfortunately no such training is available for psychologists. Education for Physicians in End-of-Life Care (EPEC) and End-of-Life Nursing Education Consortium (ELNEC) are comprehensive, modular-based, train-the-trainer programs that have reached hundreds of thousands of physicians and nurses. Social workers have developed programs through the Project on Death in America, and clergy have developed several major programs. These are but a few of the many successful programs that, during the past decade, have provided already practicing clinicians with new competency in end-of-life care and have begun training a new generation of health care professionals to provide technically excellent, compassionate, and comprehensive care to those nearing the end of life.

A void exists in the psychological realm, however. This volume begins to fill the educational gap for psychology students and practitioners. Because psychosocial issues have been widely accepted as a primary source of distress in persons near the end of life, it is only natural that psychologists should be a part of treatment teams—but before they can be involved, they need training and resources, and this book is a significant contribution to the still small list of available books on the topic. The chapters by Kaut (chap. 5) and Blevins and Papadatou (chap. 2) provide insights into how mental health providers can respect individual differences in faith and spirituality in their own practice, in addition to manners of approaching such existential concerns by collaborating with leaders in the faith-based community.

Yet however well-trained the health care professional, to be successful in providing quality care near the end of life, he or she must be working with a patient relatively well prepared to approach the subject. Thus, the parallel track of the movement to improve end-of-life care focuses on the consumer. Here again, the media has made an enormous difference in the willingness of Americans to address issues of death. Although clearly not a subject that the American public is likely to relish, media attention to studies such as SUPPORT, debacles such as Kevorkian's assisted suicides, and the tragedy played out between family members, the state legislature, courts, and health care providers regarding Terri Schiavo in Florida have all made end-of-life care a "front-burner" issue in the public's mind.

Television has played a particularly important role in raising public awareness about end-of-life issues. Millions of Americans viewed the Judith and Bill Moyers PBS special *On Our Own Terms: Moyers on Dying,* which succeeded in engaging hundreds of community coalitions in local activities to focus attention on the lessons the program provided. Now, in response to other media attention and Hollywood's Last Acts Writers Project, it is not uncommon to see prime-time medical and legal television series (e.g., *ER, Scrubs, Law and Order, The West Wing*) dealing with end-of-life issues in poignant, compelling stories.

Just as the Last Acts campaign addressed professional and public matters relating to end-of-life care through organizations, another long-time player focused on a person-by-person level. Partnership for Caring, a 67-year-old nonprofit organization dedicated to improving the care people receive near the end of life, helped to develop the concept and fact of advance directives and the state and federal laws supporting them. The only national organization that provided state-specific directives and a 24/7 hotline to respond to consumer questions, concerns, and crises around end-of-life care, Partnership for Caring provided education about planning in advance for end-of-life care to millions of people during the past decade. Nonetheless, there is still work to be done in this area, and Ditto's chapter (chap. 4) provides cogent food for thought about the use of advance directives.

I have pointed out only some of the more prominent initiatives to improve care of dying individuals on a professional level and have touched on only a few of the initiatives geared to the public and individual consumers. Nevertheless, it is essential to underscore, as noted in *Transforming Death in America: A State of the Nation Report* (Metzger & Kaplan, 2001), the following:

> We've seen important changes during the past ten years. There is increased interest in end-of-life care and the process of death and dying as the baby boomers face the deaths of their parents and grandparents. And when they begin to face their own mortality, their interest in this subject is reinforced. (p. 29)

In summary, during the past decade we have witnessed, and many have participated in, the generation of a cultural revolution to reinstate dying and death as an acknowledged, respected, and well treated part of the life cycle. There has been significant progress, but not nearly enough. Looking back, we have come a long way. Looking forward, there is a long way yet to travel. The present book undoubtedly will contribute to this journey.

As part of the movement to improve care near the end of life, this book, with its comprehensive focus on the psychosocial issues near the end of life, is an essential tool for both students and teachers of end-of-life care. My children's experience with their grandparents' deaths was the epitome of what the movement seeks to change. The purpose of this book is to help ensure that their children's experience with grandparents' final days—our final days—is significantly improved.

REFERENCES

Cruzan v. Director, Missouri Department of Health, 497 U.S. 261 (1990).

Field, M. J., & Cassel, C. K. (Eds.). (1997). *Approaching death: Improving care at the end of life*. Washington, DC: National Academy Press.

Haley, W. E., Larson, D. G., Kasl-Godley, J., Neimeyer, R. A., & Kwilosz, D. M. (2003). Roles for psychologists in end-of-life care: Emerging models of practice. *Professional Psychology: Research and Practice, 34*, 626–633.

Last Acts. (1997). *Precepts of palliative care*. Retrieved January 21, 2004, from http://www.lastacts.org/docs/profprecepts.pdf

Last Acts. (2002). *Means to a better end: A report on dying in America today*. Washington, DC: Author.

Metzger, M. A., & Kaplan, K. O. (2001). *Transforming death in America: A state of the nation report*. Washington, DC: Last Acts.

Patient Self-Determination Act of 1990, Publ. L. No. 101–508, 4206, 4751 of the Omnibus Reconciliation Act of 1990.

SUPPORT Principal Investigators. (1995). A controlled trial to improve care for seriously ill hospitalized patients: The Study to Understand Prognoses and Preferences of Outcomes and Risks of Treatment (SUPPORT). *Journal of the American Medical Association, 274*, 1591–1598.

Vacco v. Quill, 117 U.S. 2293 (1997).

Washington v. Glucksberg, 177 U.S. 2258 (1997).

ACKNOWLEDGMENTS

We express our gratitude to many people who contributed in one way or another to this book's coming to fruition. First are the executive board members of the Society for the Psychological Study of Social Issues (SPSSI, Division 9 of the American Psychological Association [APA]), who provided funding for the international conference held in February 2002 that was the impetus for this book. Most of the chapters are modifications of presentations made during the meeting. Donna Kwilosz, Robert Neimeyer, Steven Passik, Margaret Stroebe, and Sharon Valente also spoke but were unable to participate in this end product, so we thank them here. In addition, John Anderson and Camille Preston were instrumental in securing the grant and in planning and implementing the conference.

We also want to thank three people at APA Books: Susan Reynolds for her support as the book went through its transformations, Phuong Huynh for her thorough editing and assistance with the revision process, and Emily Leonard for her willingness to jump in at the end of the revision process. Two anonymous reviewers also provided helpful feedback and strengthened the final product. Finally, we thank the contributors for their stellar writing and for adhering to our timelines. Their research and applied work are making significant differences in the lives of dying people and their loved ones.

PSYCHOSOCIAL ISSUES
NEAR
THE END OF LIFE

INTRODUCTION

JAMES L. WERTH JR. AND DEAN BLEVINS

The overall purpose of this book is to inform psychologists and other mental health professionals about the possibilities and potential issues associated with providing services to people who are dying and their loved ones. Our hope is that this book will give clinicians a foundational source for information regarding the psychological, spiritual, interpersonal, and societal (i.e., psychosocial) aspects of the dying process so that they can provide effective services to people who are facing this situation themselves or through someone they know.

A strong impetus for developing this book was our perceptions, based on empirical evidence (e.g., Working Group on Assisted Suicide and End-of-Life Decisions, 2000) and clinical experience, that (a) physical symptoms can usually be effectively controlled near the end of life and, once they are, psychosocial issues rise to the fore but they are less well recognized and treated; and (b) one of the primary reasons for this lack of recognition and treatment is the lack of attention that has been given to the psychosocial aspects of dying by everyone involved in the health care system, including psychologists (see Werth, 2002a). Of course, there are exceptions to these broad statements, but, essentially, psychologists have been few and far between in writing about the end of life or participating in visible national committees (see Working Group on Assisted Suicide and End-of-Life Decisions, 2000).

On one hand, the relative lack of involvement of psychologists may be a good thing because it is likely that few of us have received training in end-of-life issues during graduate training or continuing education (CE) and therefore may not be professionally competent to provide care. On the other hand, this means that dying individuals and their loved ones rarely benefit from all that we have to offer. It therefore should not be surprising that when there are discussions of the need for services and lists of professionals who can provide services near the end of life, psychologists are not mentioned (e.g., Field & Cassel, 1997).

With the publication of this book, however, along with two other recent titles (Kleespies, 2004; Rosenfeld, 2004), the American Psychological Association (APA) has sprinted to the forefront of the national mental health organizations in attending to psychosocial issues—better late than never. In fact, in a relatively short period of time, the APA has gone from the professional organization with the least involvement in end-of-life issues to that with the largest commitment to them. In less than a decade, it has convened three working groups (and one subgroup on children and adolescents) focusing on end-of-life issues, all of which have been involved in the development of notable publications. The Assisted Suicide Statement Work Group met once and provided the structure for the APA's first publication on end-of-life issues: *Terminal Illness and Hastened Death Requests: The Important Role of the Mental Health Professional* (see Farberman, 1997). This led to the Working Group on Assisted Suicide and End-of-Life Decisions, which met several times from 1998 to 2000, wrote a substantial and comprehensive report to the APA Board of Directors (Working Group on Assisted Suicide and End-of-Life Decisions, 2000), and drafted resolutions on assisted suicide and on end-of-life care for adults. These resolutions were modified and approved by the APA Council of Representatives in 2001 (they can be found at http://www.apa.org/pi/eol/activities.html).

The most recent group is the Ad Hoc Committee on End-of-Life Issues, which has been in existence since 2001. The members of this group (William Haley, Donna Kwilosz, Robert Neimeyer, Judith Stillion, and Sharon Valente, along with James Werth) and its APA staff liaison (John Anderson from the APA Office on AIDS) have been working on various end-of-life initiatives, including developing online CE modules.

CONTENTS

Although no book can be truly comprehensive, we believe we have addressed most of the major areas associated with psychosocial issues near the end of life. The Foreword is written by Dr. Karen Kaplan, the former executive director of probably the most important national organization focused on public awareness and education of end-of-life issues, Last Acts Partnership (which evolved from a merger of Last Acts and Partnership for Caring). She provides a foundation for the book by discussing recent developments in caring near the end of life.

In chapter 1, Stillion integrates data revealing how the end-of-life environment has changed over the years. Her discussion expands on some of the ideas set forth by Kaplan in the Foreword while laying a foundation for understanding how and why people are faced with the decisions and why the psychosocial issues described in this book arise. Although it may not be made evident by the authors of the subsequent chapters, it is important that the psychologist understand the developments Stillion describes to have a sense of the changes that have occurred, and will likely continue to happen, that complicate the dying process. The APA Working Group on Assisted Suicide and End-of-Life Decisions (2000) provides additional information on these issues, as does Field and Cassel (1997).

Blevins and Papadatou capitalize on the fact that the first author was born and raised in the United States whereas Papadatou is a native of Greece. Thus, their chapter goes beyond the traditional analysis of cultural issues found in many discussions of this topic in the end-of-life literature and brings in a model for explaining and understanding some of the results that have emerged in the research thus far while also providing some help in care provision. As with Stillion's chapter, the other authors discuss cultural considerations to varying degrees, but readers who keep Blevins and Papadatou's review in mind will clearly see how culture can affect the analyses the authors offer. The APA Working Group on Assisted Suicide and End-of-Life Decisions (2000; see also APA "fact sheet" at http://www.apa.org/pi/eol/factsheets.html) covered these issues; other recent sources are Braun, Pietsch, and Blanchette (2000) and Morgan and Laungani (2002).

Werth and Kleespies, in the third chapter, hone in on issues of special interest to psychologists who are service providers. They excerpt parts of the recent APA (2002) *Ethical Principles of Psychologists and Code of Conduct* and discuss the relationship with, and implications for, working with clients and their families on end-of-life issues. They also review some of the decisions that dying individuals and their loved ones, as well as the involved health care providers, may have to make that involve ethical considerations. The therapist who integrates this material into her or his clinical decision making will be more likely to practice up to the standard of care. Because this is a more specialized area, there are fewer resources available, but the reader can find additional discussions in Kleespies (2004) and Werth (1999, 2002b).

Ditto's chapter discusses issues that affect the legal processes associated with end-of-life decision making. He provides a compelling argument that the best ideas in theory are not necessarily the best ideas in practice and highlights how important it is to explore things empirically instead of relying on assumptions, demonstrating how the good *idea* of advance directives (living wills and durable powers of attorney) does not always translate into the good *practice* of implementing care directives. As disturbing as his conclusions may seem at first glance, his chapter also points to the possibility that psychological science may provide answers regarding how to use advance directives to get people the care they want and not to provide care they do not desire. Aside from Ditto's own work, another good source of information about advance directives is Doukas and McCullough (1991).

Kaut's chapter shifts the focus directly to clinical care by offering a comprehensive framework for assessment. In doing so, he adopts a multidimensional approach that highlights the importance of triangulating information from numerous sources and in one way or another touches on the content of other chapters. Because he has a neuropsychology background, his framework includes more attention to the cognitive issues that may arise near the end of life than previous models. There have been other sets of assessment guidelines suggested (e.g., Werth, Benjamin, & Farrenkopf, 2000; Working Group on Assisted Suicide and End-of-Life Decisions, 2000), but Kaut's model is less of a list of questions to ask or specific issues to consider than a way of thinking about assessment and working with the unique issues of the dying person and her or his loved ones.

Gibson, Breitbart, Tomarken, Kosinski, and Nelson actually surprised us with their chapter because we did not think they could include both a review of the major psychosocial issues and suggestions for state-of-the-art care in a single chapter; they did so, however, drawing heavily on their own and their colleagues' decades of experience at Memorial Sloan-Kettering Cancer Center. They also offer the reader a sense of some of the more medical aspects of dying and the interface between the person's physical and psychological needs, given their work in a hospital setting. Because the authors have also been involved in some of the key research in this area, the chapter incorporates a necessary empirical piece to the discussion. Other thorough sources include Chochinov and Breitbart (2000); Kleespies (2004); Steinberg and Youngner (1998); and Werth, Gordon, and Johnson (2002).

Rosenfeld, Abbey, and Pessin focus on two issues that are of vital importance in end-of-life care and decision making: clinical depression and hopelessness. Significant misunderstanding and misinformation exist about the prevalence and effect of major depression among dying individuals; this chapter goes a long way toward dispelling the myths. In addition, the authors emphasize the importance of hopelessness and that it is not a normal state of mind for people with terminal conditions. The authors offer the reader a comprehensive perspective by examining both assessment and treatment of these conditions. Interested readers may want to examine Block (2000) and Wilson, Chochniov, de Faye, and Breitbart (2000) for additional information.

Allen, Haley, Roff, Schmid, and Bergman focus our attention on the people providing care for their loved ones during the dying process. As anyone who has been a caregiver knows, there is the potential for both benefit and burden in the caregiving role, and the authors highlight this in their chapter. These authors are scientists and practitioners and therefore bring empirical and practical ideas to the chapter, thereby providing the reader with a sense of what is established and what is on the cutting edge in terms of helping the helpers. The authors also integrate material related to Ditto's earlier chapter on advance directives because of the familial roles of creating or implementing them. Additional sources of information about families and caregivers near the end of life can be found in Rosen (1998); Nadeau (1998); and Haley, Allen, Reynolds, Chen, Burton, and Gallagher-Thompson (2002).

Connor, Lycan, and Schumacher bring extensive experience to their chapter on hospice and psychologists. The authors all have some background in hospice administration, and two are psychologists. Thus, they are in a somewhat unique position to discuss why psychologists have not traditionally been involved with hospices and offer suggestions for how we can become more involved in the future. The interdisciplinary model that is the hallmark of hospice is certainly the gold standard for end-of-life care; psychologists need to figure out how to become more involved in teams—in hospices or elsewhere. Other recent articles that specifically address psychologists and teamwork include Connor, Egan, Kwilosz, Larson, and Reese (2002) and Haley, Larson, Kasl-Godley, Neimeyer, and Kwilosz (2003).

We wrote the final chapter in an effort to bring together ideas and recommendations set forth by the authors of the Foreword and of the other nine chapters. We wanted to provide a blueprint for future research, care, education, and policy that we believe would help to substantially improve psychosocial care near the end of life.

We were unable to cover a few areas in as much detail as we may have liked, but here we refer interested readers to other sources. First, although various authors mention grief and loss, for more comprehensive coverage, we point the reader to Stroebe, Hansson, Stroebe, and Schut's (2001) compendium on bereavement research, Neimeyer's (2001) work on finding meaning in the wake of loss, and Rando's (2000) discussion of anticipatory mourning. Second, the issues that surround caring for children and adolescents near the end of life present many unique challenges for mental health professionals. Although Stillion (chap. 1) discusses this topic most extensively in this volume, much is left unaddressed. APA is currently completing work on a report addressing end-of-life issues for children and adolescents (check http://www.apa.org/pi/eol/). Third, those who want to delve into the controversial issue of assisted death can read all about it in Rosenfeld (2004). Fourth, the financial issues that surround dying and end-of-life care are significant, both in terms of their potential influence on decision making and access to care as well as their influence on how and whether psychologists become more prominent participants in end-of-life caregiving. Werth and Kleespies (chap. 3) and Connor and colleagues (chap. 9) briefly acknowledge these issues, but space constraints preclude a full exploration. The reader interested in finances and end-of-life care should begin by consulting Buntin and Huskamp (2002); Campbell, Lynn, Louis, and Shugarman (2004); Mitchell (2003); and Payne, Coyne, and Smith (2002). Finally, those who want a self-help resource for clients can review Lynn and Harrold (1999). The reader may also wish to consult classic texts including Garfield's (1978) collection and Weisman's (1972) work. Finally, a comprehensive series of articles can be found in two issues of the *American Behavioral Scientist* on end-of-life care and decisions (October and November 2002, volume 46, issues 2 and 3).

CONCLUSION

We hope that this book provides readers with direction when providing care for people who are dying and for their loved ones while also encouraging researchers, educators, and policymakers to focus attention on the psychosocial issues near the end of life. We all need to work together to maximize the chances that people will die in a way that is most consistent with their own and their loved ones' wishes.

REFERENCES

American Psychological Association. (2002). Ethical principles of psychologists and code of conduct. *American Psychologist, 57,* 1060–1073.

Block, S. D. (2000). Assessing and managing depression in the terminally ill patient. *Annals of Internal Medicine, 132,* 209–218.

Braun, K. L., Pietsch, J. H., & Blanchette, P. L. (2000). *Cultural issues in end-of-life decision making.* Thousand Oaks, CA: Sage.

Buntin, M. B., & Huskamp, H. (2002). What is known about the economics of end-of-life care for Medicare Beneficiaries? *The Gerontologist, 42*(Special Issue III), 40–48.

Campbell, D. E., Lynn, J., Louis, T. A., & Shugarman, L. R. (2004). Medicare program expenditures associated with hospice use. *Annals of Internal Medicine, 140,* 267–277.

Chochinov, H. M., & Breitbart, W. (2000). *Handbook of psychiatry in palliative medicine.* New York: Oxford University Press.

Connor, S. R., Egan, K. A., Kwilosz, D. M., Larson, D. G., & Reese, D. J. (2002). Interdisciplinary approaches to assisting when end-of-life care and decision-making. *American Behavioral Scientist, 46,* 340–356.

Doukas, D. J., & McCullough, L. B. (1991). The values history: The evaluation of the patient's values and advance directives. *Journal of Family Practice, 32,* 145–153.

Farberman, R. K. (1997). Terminal illness and hastened death requests: The important role of the mental health professional. *Professional Psychology: Research and Practice, 28,* 544–547.

Field, M. J., & Cassel, C. K. (Eds.). (1997). *Approaching death: Improving care at the end of life.* Washington, DC: National Academy Press.

Garfield, C. A. (Ed.). (1978). *Psychosocial care of the dying patient.* New York: McGraw-Hill.

Haley, W. E., Allen, R. S., Reynolds, S., Chen, H., Burton, A., & Gallagher-Thompson, D. (2002). Family issues in end-of-life decision making and end-of-life care. *American Behavioral Scientist, 46*, 284–298.

Haley, W. E., Larson, D. G., Kasl-Godley, J., Neimeyer, R. A., & Kwilosz, D. M. (2003). Roles for psychologists in end-of-life care: Emerging models of practice. *Professional Psychology: Research and Practice, 34*, 626–633.

Kleespies, P. M. (2004). *Life and death decisions: Psychological and ethical considerations in end-of-life care.* Washington, DC: American Psychological Association.

Lynn, J., & Harrold, J. (1999). *Handbook for mortals: Guidance for people facing serious illness.* New York: Oxford University Press.

Mitchell, S. L. (2003). Financial incentives for placing feeding tubes in nursing home residents with advanced dementia. *Journal of the American Geriatrics Society, 51*, 129–131.

Morgan, J. D., & Laungani, P. (Eds.). (2002). *Death and bereavement around the world* (Vols. 1–5). Amityville, NY: Baywood.

Nadeau, J. W. (1998). *Families making sense of death.* Thousand Oaks, CA: Sage.

Neimeyer, R. A. (Ed.). (2001). *Meaning reconstruction and the experience of loss.* Washington, DC: American Psychological Association.

Payne, S. K., Coyne, P., & Smith, T. J. (2002). The health economics of palliative care. *Oncology, 16*, 801–808.

Rando, T. A. (Ed.). (2000). *Clinical dimensions of anticipatory mourning.* Champaign, IL: Research Press.

Rosen, E. J. (1998). *Families facing death* (rev. ed.). San Francisco: Jossey-Bass.

Rosenfeld, B. (2004). *Assisted suicide and the right to die: The interface of social science, public policy, and medical ethics.* Washington, DC: American Psychological Association.

Steinberg, M. D., & Youngner, S. J. (Eds.). (1998). *End-of-life decisions: A psychosocial perspective.* Washington, DC: American Psychiatric Press.

Stroebe, M. S., Hansson, R. O., Stroebe, W., & Schut, H. (Eds.). (2001). *Handbook of bereavement research: Consequences, coping, and care.* Washington, DC: American Psychological Association.

Weisman, A. D. (1972). *On dying and denying: A psychiatric study of terminality.* New York: Behavioral Publications.

Werth, J. L., Jr. (1999). Mental health professionals and assisted death: Perceived ethical obligations and proposed guidelines for practice. *Ethics and Behavior, 9*, 159–183.

Werth, J. L., Jr. (2002a). Introduction: Behavioral science and the end of life. *American Behavioral Scientist, 46*, 195–203.

Werth, J. L., Jr. (2002b). Legal and ethical considerations for mental health professionals related to end-of-life care and decision-making. *American Behavioral Scientist, 46*, 373–388.

Werth, J. L., Jr., Benjamin, G. A. H., & Farrenkopf, T. (2000). Requests for physician assisted death: Guidelines for assessing mental capacity and impaired judgment. *Psychology, Public Policy, and Law, 6*, 348–372.

Werth, J. L., Jr., Gordon, J. R., & Johnson, R. R. (2002). Psychosocial issues near the end of life. *Aging and Mental Health, 6,* 402–412.

Wilson, K. G., Chochinov, H. M., de Faye, B. J., & Breitbart, W. (2000). Diagnosis and management of depression in palliative care. In H. M. Chochinov & W. Breitbart (Eds.), *Handbook of psychiatry in palliative medicine* (pp. 25–49). New York: Oxford University Press.

Working Group on Assisted Suicide and End-of-Life Decisions. (2000). *Report to the Board of Directors.* Washington, DC: American Psychological Association. Retrieved January 25, 2004, from http://www.apa.org/pi/aseolf.html

1

UNDERSTANDING THE END OF LIFE: AN OVERVIEW

JUDITH M. STILLION

Dying, death, and end-of-life decision-making became salient issues for professionals in a variety of medical and health related fields during the last century. This chapter reviews the factors that have led to increasing interest in the subject as well as the sweeping changes that have taken place over the last 100 years in the location and conditions associated with dying. It also examines the ways in which these changes affect the psychosocial aspects of the dying process. Finally, it introduces the concepts of child and adolescent development and cohort membership as integral psychosocial factors to be considered when working with dying persons and their families.

DEMOGRAPHIC CHANGES IN LIFE EXPECTANCY

During the 20th century, life expectancy increased dramatically in most developed countries. A few examples illustrate this point. In the decade 1900–1910, Japan had a life expectancy of approximately 40 years. By 1995–2000, life expectancy had increased to almost 80 years (American Association of Retired Persons, 2001). Sweden's comparative figures showed an increase in life expectancy from around 60 years to a little over 80 years in that same time period. In the United States, life expectancy increased from about 45 in 1900 to an all-time high of 77.2 years in 2001, a gain of more than 32 years in one century (National Center for Health Statistics [NCHS], 2002).

Increasing life expectancy brought with it a natural increase in the number of older adults in most developed countries. By the end of the 20th century, between 12 and 18 of every 100 persons in the population of many developed countries were over 65. This is only part of the story, however. If we include persons aged 60 and older, the percentage of older adults increases substantially. For example, in 2000, the percentage of residents aged 60 and over in Germany was 21%; in Italy, 22%; in Japan, 21%; in the United Kingdom, 20%; and in the United States, 16% (Markson, 2003).

By 2000, there were 35 million persons over age 65 in the United States. Moreover, the older adult population is expected to double between now and the year 2030, resulting in a ratio of one elderly person to five nonelderly persons (Administration on Aging, 2002). The "old old," those 85 and over, are the most rapidly growing sector of the aged. The latest available statistics show that the total number of years persons aged 65 can expect to live is 17.9, whereas persons aged 85 can expect another 8.6 years of life (Arias, 2002). By the year 2050, people over 85 are expected to make up 24% of elderly Americans and 5% of all Americans, numbering more than 19 million. People over the age of 100 numbered approximately 50,500 in 2000, a 35% increase from the figure of 37,300 in 1990 (NCHS, 2002).

Implications of Increasing Life Expectancy

The graying of the U.S. population and of other developed countries has very real implications for those working in the end-of-life field. Inherent in the aging process is an understanding that each year makes death a more imminent certainty. Although young persons may die, older adults must. This realization permits time to prepare for death. Many older persons are living with chronic, life-threatening illnesses over longer and longer periods of time, a situation that has dramatic implications for families and friends as well as for the health care and insurance industries.

In 2000, the U.S. Medicare program, which enrolls all persons over 65 as well as some younger qualified persons, had 40 million enrollees and expenditures of $222 billion (NCHS, 2002). More than 95% of persons age 65 and older report having expenses for health services compared with 82% of those under 65. An estimated 27% of Medicare costs are for the last year of life (Hogan, Lunney, Gabel, & Lynn, 2001). One study showed that Medicare program payments of people who had died were approximately 6 times higher than those for people still alive (Hogan et al., 2001). Increased life expectancy and health care costs are inextricably linked.

TABLE 1.1
International Comparison of Life Expectancy at Birth
by Sex and Year of Reporting

	Year	Male	Female
France	1999	75.00	82.50
Germany	1997–1999	74.44	80.57
Italy	1999	75.00	82.50
Japan	2001	78.07	84.93
Sweden	2000	77.38	82.03
United Kingdom	1998–2000	75.13	79.98
United States	2001	78.07	84.93

Note. Data from Ministry of Health, Labour, and Welfare (2002).

Direct costs of health care during the final year of life are only one measure of the total cost. The stress of caring for a dying person takes a toll on all caregivers. As persons become ever more involved in caring for an individual who has a terminal illness, their lives can become increasingly narrow. They may neglect their own health through lack of proper nutrition, exercise, or socializing. If employed, they may find that their performance on the job is negatively affected. Many find they must leave their jobs prematurely to devote full time to caretaking duties, which negatively affects their financial status. Depression, loneliness, and stress-related illnesses find fertile ground in even the most devoted caregivers (see Allen et al., chap. 8, for further discussion of stress and caregiving).

These realities call for a new approach to working with chronically ill older adults. The knowledge and skills of persons who work in areas such as pain control, anxiety reduction, situational counseling, treatment of depression, and existential psychology are needed. Several chapters in this volume address these issues (Kaut, chap. 5; Gibson, Breitbart, Tomarken, Kosinski, & Nelson, chap. 6; Rosenfeld, Abbey, & Pessin, chap. 7). On the societal level, the need is urgent for more professionals in all human service fields to study the gerontology literature.

Life Expectancy and Gender

The overall figures on life expectancy may be misleading. Gender differences exist in nearly every country that reports mortality statistics. Table 1.1 shows the gender differential in life expectancy for seven developed countries by year of reporting. It demonstrates that women in the countries reporting live an average of 4 to 6 years longer than men in the same country. In the United States, female infants born in 2001 could expect to live to 79.8 compared with 74.3 years for their male counterparts. This represents a decrease in the differential between men and women from a high of 7.8 years in the 1970s to the current figure of 5.5 years (Minimo, Arias, Kochanek,

Murphy, & Smith, 2002). Increased mortality from lung cancer and other diseases associated with increased cigarette smoking among women coupled with a decrease in mortality among men from cardiac disease may be the two major factors involved in the decreasing gender differential in death.

A majority of older adults are women, and the gender differential in death increases with increasing age. The Administration on Aging predicts that by 2050, "women aged 85 and over will outnumber men aged 85 and over by more than 4 million, or nearly 60 percent, and women will make up 61 percent of the population ages 85 and over" (Siegel, 1996, p. 45).

Greater longevity of women carries with it some special challenges. For example, women aged 65 years are much more likely to be unmarried or widowed than are their male age peers (Stroebe & Stroebe, 1993; Stillion, 1984). By age 75, only a minority of women remain married, and most are widowed. In contrast, among men aged 75 years and older, a majority are married and a minority are widowed (Schaie & Willis, 1996). Older widows are also less likely to remarry than older widowers (Stroebe & Stroebe, 1993) and are far more likely to live alone than are older men. In 1998, more than 31% of women aged 65 to 74 years were living alone compared with only 13.9% of men. Among persons aged 75 and older, almost 53% of the population of women were living alone compared with just over 22% of men of the same age (Spraggins, 2000). In addition, women absorb the bulk of caregiving duties (see Allen et al., chap. 8).

Economic inequities also have a negative impact on older women. Although women have made great strides toward equality in education, the same has not been true in earnings, with women bringing in only a fraction of their male counterparts' median earnings. Such continuing inequities coupled with greater longevity contribute to the fact that older women are more likely than older men to exhaust their financial resources, are less likely to have private insurance coverage, and are more likely to have to depend on Medicare and Medicaid than are men (Canetto, 2001). The implications of these facts are clear. When working in the field of end of life, mental health professionals should be prepared to explore financial and psychological burdens of caregiving in addition to helping caregivers, the majority of whom are women, to cope with grief and loss. They also should understand the effects of male and female socialization on help-seeking behavior, dependency, autonomy, and acceptance of authority.

Life Expectancy and Ethnicity

Because chapter 2 (by Blevins & Papadatou) deals in depth with ethnic differences, this chapter merely introduces the topic. There were increases in life expectancy across the 20th century for all ethnic groups. Inequities still exist, however. The National Vital Statistics Reports published by the NCHS of the Centers for Disease Control and Prevention (CDC) give life expectancy only for Blacks and Whites. In 2000, White female infants had the highest life expectancy at birth (80.0 years), whereas Black female infants could expect to live only 74.9 years. White males at birth had a life expectancy of 74.8 compared with Black males, whose life expectancy was 68.2 years (Arias, 2002). Updated figures for other ethnic groups are harder to obtain because the United States is in the process of redefining ethnicity; however, Hispanics and Asians appear to live longer than other ethnic groups (Guend, Swallen, & Kindig, 2002).

By 2030, the ethnic minority population is projected to represent 25.4% of the elderly population. Although the increase in older Whites will equal 81%, Hispanics will increase by 328%; African American elders will increase by 131%; American Indians, Eskimos, and Aleuts will increase by 147%; and Asian and Pacific Islanders will increase by 285% (Administration on Aging, 2002).

Ethnic disparities in life expectancy carry with them additional imperatives for those who work with dying persons to recognize the existence of basic inequities and to respect different cultural traditions and rituals surrounding aging, sickness and death.

Changes in the Causes of Death

Changes in the causes of death across the 20th century have major implications for social scientists interested in the end of life. In 1900, the 10 leading causes of death were influenza and pneumonia; tuberculosis; heart disease, diarrhea, and enteritis (under 2 years of age); nephritis; accidental unspecified causes; cerebral hemorrhage, thrombosis, and embolism; cancer and malignant tumors; diphtheria, typhoid, and paratyphoid fever (Centers for Disease Control and Prevention, 1999). Clearly, most people died from infectious illnesses or accidents that caused death with certainty and relative rapidity. In 2001, the leading causes were heart disease; malignant neoplasm (cancer); cerebrovascular diseases (stroke); chronic lower respiratory diseases; accidents (unintentional injuries); diabetes mellitus; influenza and pneumonia; Alzheimer's disease; nephritis, nephrotic syndrome, and nephrosis (kidney disease); and septicemia (NCHS, 2002). The contemporary list of the 10 most common causes includes only one (accidents) that typically results in a quick death. Nearly three of every four deaths in persons over age 25 in the United States are caused by chronic disease. It has been estimated that 70% to 80% of people in advanced industrial nations face death later in life from diseases with long, downhill deterioriative declines (Lunney, Lynn, Foley, Lipson, & Guralnik, 2003). Within one century, then, death evolved from a sudden event to one that occurs after a prolonged illness for the majority of people. This change has created a situation in which seriously ill individuals have time to address multiple decisions concerning the course of treatments they will pursue as well as time to contemplate the meaning of their lives and deaths. Moreover, families and friends of persons with terminal prognoses have both the opportunity and the awesome responsibility of supporting dying persons for months or even for years.

CHANGES IN HEALTH CARE

During the 20th century, major developments occurred in medical knowledge and practice. In the mid-1900s, the discovery of penicillin began a new era during which formerly deadly illnesses could be attacked with antibiotics. New techniques in blood storage, transfusions, and kidney dialysis made it possible for people to survive accidents and to live for a prolonged period with life-threatening kidney disease. Complex surgical procedures aided by ever-expanding technological innovations that permitted hitherto impossible surgeries, such as heart bypasses, prolonged both the quantity and quality of life for millions. Developments in radiation and chemotherapy permitted additional millions to live as survivors rather than victims of cancer. New treatments for AIDS, once called the new plague of the 20th century, changed that disease from a certain death sentence to a life-threatening chronic disease. Transplantation of organs and replacement of knees, hips, and other parts of the body offered a new promise of prolonged active life. These and many other innovations stemming from hard work and research have fed into the increases in life expectancy and longevity.

Although universally applauded, these increases have presented new and challenging problems. Foremost among these is the question, "Is life at any cost always a blessing?" Economists, philosophers, lawmakers, educators, ethicists, and citizen groups have attempted to address this question in many ways. In the early 1990s, three English neurologists put the matter before the medical community in this way (Mitchell, Kerridge, & Lovat, 1993):

> Why do we persist in the relentless pursuit of artificial nourishment and other treatments to maintain unconscious existence? Will they [patients] be treated because of our ethical commitment to their humanity, or because of an ethical paralysis in the face of biotechnical progress? (p. 75)

CHANGES IN LOCATION AND TIMING OF DEATH

Increasing sophistication of medical treatment brought with it important changes in both the location and timing of death. In the earliest years of the 20th century, the United States was primarily a nation of small family farms. Persons lived closer to the land, and the events of birth and death were experienced firsthand from early childhood. Infant mortality and deaths in childhood were also more numerous, so death was accepted (albeit reluctantly) as an integral part of life. As life expectancy increased and as both medical and technological achievements grew, death gradually became more of an institutionalized affair. Instead of dying a relatively quick death at home attended by family, friends, and perhaps the family doctor, people typically died after a lengthy period in an institutional setting, frequently hooked to futile machines dedicated to preserving the quantity, if not the quality, of life.

By 1992, approximately 57% of deaths occurred in hospitals or medical centers, 20% in homes, 17% in nursing homes, and 6% in other places (Field & Cassel, 1997). The new technologies enabled the medical community to prolong life almost indefinitely. As a result, the American Hospital Association estimated that in the 1990s, 70% of the 6,000 or so daily deaths are "somehow timed or negotiated, with all concerned parties privately concurring on withdrawal of some death-delaying technology" (Webb, 1997, quoting Meisel, 1992, p. 335).

SOCIAL MOVEMENTS IN THE 20TH CENTURY

Partially in reaction to the new technological way of dying and partly as a result of the changing demographics mentioned earlier, a new movement was born. Called by various names, it is perhaps best considered the death awareness movement. Spurred on by the now-classic Kubler-Ross (1969) book *On Death and Dying,* the most visible component of these activities is the remarkably rapid spread of the hospice philosophy in the United States and other countries.

The development of the modern hospice (see Kaplan, Foreword; Connor, Lycan, & Schumacher, chap. 9), founded in England by Dr. Cicely Saunders in 1967, is the most impressive innovation in care for dying persons in the 20th century. The underlying principle of hospice was, and is, an emphasis on care, rather than cure; pain control; and a dedication to the family, in addition to the patient, as the unit for care. Self-determined life closure, safe and comfortable dying, and effective grieving were desired outcomes of hospice (National Hospice Organization, Standards and Accreditation Committee, 1997). Unlike British freestanding hospices, as the hospice philosophy was adopted in the United States, the American hospice movement emphasized care in a "homelike" atmosphere and thus avoided building new edifices, opting to bring hospice programs into homes or nursing homes within a community (Miller, Mor, Gage, & Coppola, 2001). By 1982, the movement had gained wide acceptance and, with the passage of the Tax Equity and Fiscal Responsibility Act (TEFRA), a hospice benefit was introduced into Medicare, thus assuring the future of the hospice movement (Miller et al., 2001). By 2002, the National Hospice and Palliative Care Organization (2004) estimated that there were 3,200 operational hospice programs in the United States, including the District of Columbia, the Commonwealth of Puerto Rico, and the Territory of Guam, serving nearly 900,000 people.

As the growth of the hospice movement proceeded, so did an emphasis on palliative care. Today, palliative care occurs within hospice but may also be practiced outside of a traditional hospice setting or organization. Palliative care is a broader type of treatment because although it emphasizes relief of both physical pain and psychological suffering, it is not necessarily limited to the last few months of life, and one does not need to forgo curative interventions. Regardless of when it occurs, many health care professionals practicing palliative care emphasize that the end-of-life period can be one of continuing development (e.g., Byock, 1996). On the other hand, although community-based hospice programs are having an impact on the place of death, dying and death remain hidden from the everyday lives of people who are not personally involved with dying persons. In addition, families are not necessarily as knowledgeable about the end of life or as intimately involved in vital caregiving as was the case in earlier centuries. Therefore, even though home care may be increasing, it is a different type of care, buttressed by health care professionals as well as by trained volunteers from hospices, which may not provide the same opportunities for growth and development as existed previously.

Another aspect of the death awareness movement included a series of lawsuits beginning in the mid-1970s and culminating in a U.S. Supreme Court decision in 1990. Kaplan (in the Foreword) highlights these high-profile cases as a factor in the public's growing recognition of end-of-life issues. The case of Karen Quinlan (*In re Quinlan*, 1976) established a patient's rights, and by extension the rights of parents or guardian, to refuse treatment. The importance of competency and quality-of-life issues was established in a 1977 case of Joseph Saikewicz, a 67-year-old mentally retarded man with leukemia (*Superintendent of Belchertown State School v. Saikewicz*, 1977). The court held that Saikewicz did not have to be moved from his home to receive life-prolonging treatments. The case of Paul Brophy (*Brophy v. New England Sinai Hospital, Inc.*, 1986), settled in 1986, led to the decision that the right to refuse medical treatment, which was established in the Karen Quinlan case, applies to all medical treatments including the withdrawal of food and water. Another widely publicized case was that of Nancy Cruzan, a 23-year-old woman who was in a persistent vegetative state and required the use of a feeding tube (*Cruzan v. Director, Missouri Department of Health*, 1990). The U.S. Supreme Court upheld the right to refuse treatment and found that artificial feeding could not be distinguished from other forms of medical treatment (Stillion & McDowell, 1996). Every state has specific legislation that protects medical doctors from legal action if they do not give treatment to dying persons who had expressed wishes to end life-sustaining measures (Meisel, Snyder, & Quill, 2000).

Another crucial development during this period was the publication of the initial findings from the Study to Understand Prognoses and Preferences for Outcomes and Risks of Treatments (SUPPORT Principal Investigators,

1995). This widely publicized study showed that dying in the United States was more painful and lonelier than it needed to be, that physicians did not understand what patients wanted, and that the cost of dying was exorbitant. Following the publication of that report, the Robert Wood Johnson Foundation funded Last Acts, which described itself as "a campaign to improve end-of-life care by a coalition of professional and consumer organizations" (Last Acts, n.d., ¶ 1). Last Acts was a coalition made up of almost 1,200 organizations that had a stake in improving end-of-life care. In 2004, Last Acts merged with the Partnership for Caring (renamed as Last Acts Partnership) but has continued efforts sponsoring conferences, maintaining a newsletter, and forming committees that produce guidance for others. By seeking and obtaining the support of professional and consumer organizations, this project raises public awareness and furthers the dialogue about the quality of care near the end of life (see Kaplan's Foreword for additional discussion of these developments).

PERSONAL CONTROL INITIATIVES

As public awareness was raised concerning typical medical treatment near the end of life, individuals and groups attempted to regain some personal control over the dying process with the development and promotion of advance directives. Advance directives include the medical power of attorney and the living will (see Ditto, chap. 4, for additional discussion of these documents). Attempts to publicize the need for this type of documentation were so successful that by the end of the 20th century, advance directives regarding treatment of dying individuals had become legally recognized documents in all states. Education about the need for such documents and research into the effectiveness with which they are honored has been widespread. Materials such as those represented by Project Grace in Florida or Critical Conditions in Georgia have been distributed widely.

These documents highlight the fact that decision points exist along the complete dying trajectory, beginning with the diagnosis and prognosis and ending with the decision concerning resuscitation attempts when death occurs. Because of these changes, persons near the end of life, and those who care about them, are often confronted with multiple decisions concerning where they want to die, how much technological and medical support they prefer, and at what point they prefer to stop aggressive treatments. The patient and family members may need the direct counseling of social workers or psychologists to reach consensus about the optimal conditions surrounding dying. This is especially true when the dying person has not expressed his or her wishes, may no longer be able to make them known, or where family members are in disagreement concerning life-prolonging measures. Connor and colleagues (chap. 9) discuss the roles of psychologists in various settings at the end of life, and Werth and Kleespies (chap. 3) address competency and ethical issues in such work.

In addition, advance directives encourage individuals to think through their personal preferences for treatment. Two patients faced with metastatic cancer who are given the same diagnosis and prognosis may react very differently. One may decide to endure the most comprehensive and aggressive course of treatment despite side effects, and the other may decide to "let nature take its course." One may decide to enlist the help and support of family and friends, and another may decide to keep silent and not "bother" those whom he or she loves with the news. If the disease progresses, both will have to decide where they wish to be as they grow weaker. One may decide on home care with or without the services of community hospice. Another may decide to forgo hospice and rely on the primary physician and hospitalizations during critical periods. Questions concerning pain control also arise, including levels of analgesics or narcotics and the method of administering them (e.g., by mouth, intravenously, by pump). Instructions on withholding or withdrawing fluids when death is imminent and resuscitation when breathing stops are also among the myriad decisions facing terminally ill people. Well-designed materials (e.g., Veterans Health Administration, 2001; see generally, Growthhouse, http://www.growthhouse.org) are available to help people examine the full array of end-of-life decisions and address them from their own values and preferences. Nevertheless, the promise of the concept of advance directives has not necessarily carried through to actual implementation (see Allen et al., chap. 8; Ditto, chap. 4).

SPECIAL ISSUES FOR CHILDREN NEAR THE END OF LIFE

Although the earlier focus of this chapter discussed dying mainly in terms of older people, it is important to recognize that death occurs to people of all ages. Deaths among children and adolescents have decreased dramatically across the past century, but they still occur with heartbreaking regularity. Approximately 53,000 children die in the United States each year, half from chronic extended illnesses (National Hospice and Palliative Care Organization, 2002). Because this is true, an understanding of the normal developmental literature and how it is changed by serious, life-threatening illness is important to those working in end of life (Stillion & Papadatou, 2002). Beginning in the mid–20th century, researchers focused on children's understanding of death (see Wass, 1989, for a review). Such research highlighted the need to apply what is known about child development concerning the age and developmental level of dying children and adolescents as well as their well siblings and friends.

Cognitive understanding of the meaning of death generally follows the stages laid out by Piaget and culminates in a mature understanding of death: that death is irreversible, final, inevitable, and caused by specific external or internal forces (Speece & Brent, 1984). To reach that understanding, children pass through a sensorimotor stage (ages 0–2) in which there is little or no real understanding of death, and death is equated with separation. Death anxiety is separation anxiety for very young children. Children then move into a preoperational stage in which the concept of death is tied with the magical thinking so characteristic of that age. Preoperational children often believe death is reversible and that sick people can be made well again through wishing or magic. When children reach school age (ages 6–12), they enter a stage of concrete operations. During this period, they collect a great number of facts regarding illness and death and become capable of experiencing true death anxiety. In the final stage, older children and adolescents are capable of asking deeper philosophical questions about the nature of illness and death.

Evidence suggests that the experience of a life-threatening illness may change the pace at which children attain a mature understanding of death (Schonfeld, 1999). Bluebond-Langner's (1978) classic work, *The Private Worlds of Dying Children*, showed that seriously ill children's concepts of self change predictably as their disease process moves along. Such children begin by seeing themselves as sick but expect a return to health with treatment. As the disease continues, children gather information about the disease through many avenues, including parents, friends, medical staff, and books (and, more recently, the Internet). They grow to believe that they are seriously ill but cling to the hope of a normal life in the future. With ongoing illness, many children accept the fact that their disease will be constant but expect to continue with the help of medical treatments. Their self-concepts change to reflect such knowledge, and they come to see themselves as different from "normal" kids. Finally, even young children living with chronic illness come to the realization that medicine may fail and that the end of their illness may result in death.

Recognition that terminally ill children and adolescents continue to have the same psychosocial needs as their well peers is also important. For example, the need of a 2-year-old to assert his or her growing autonomy does not disappear because of illness, nor does the need for the 10-year-old to avoid a sense of inferiority by working industriously, or the 15-year-old to develop his or her identity and dream about or experience intimacy. A thorough understanding of Erikson's (1950) theory of psychosocial development and the work it has generated is an invaluable aid in working with dying children and adolescents and their siblings. The special needs of children who are dying or who have parents or siblings who are dying are complex and deserve book-length attention in their own right.

UNDERSTANDING THE END OF LIFE FROM
A GENERATIONAL PERSPECTIVE

Another tool that is helpful to mental health professionals working in end-of-life care is familiarity with the diversity that is inherent in different generations (see Blevins & Papadatou, chap. 2). Because "cohort" means any group that has shared experiences based on time and place, social scientists refer to this as the cohort effect. Although recognized for years, especially by life-span psychologists (e.g., Schaie, 1965; Schaie & Strother, 1968), this effect received more attention after the publication of *Generations* (Strauss & Howe, 1991), which suggested that there is a "peer personality" within every living cohort (however, the degree to which these "cohorts" reflect the experiences and beliefs of non-ethnic-majority individuals is open to question). Strauss and Howe suggested that understanding the values and attitudes contained within the peer personality can be an aid to meeting cohort members' needs and understanding their life views. Much of the lack of awareness and sensitivity in communication between persons of different cohorts may lie in misunderstandings based on one group's experiences and shaped values of persons born at or about the same time in history who have experienced coming of age crises that give them a shared personality profile compared with the experiences and beliefs of a different cohort.

Strauss and Howe pointed out, for example, that members of the GI generation, born between 1901 and 1924, differ significantly in the way they face crisis situations from the silent generation, born between 1925 and 1942, and the baby boom generation, born between 1943 and 1960. Understanding the nature of each generation may help to promote better psychosocial care at the end of life. It should also be noted, however, that cohort differences are not solely between the "generations" defined as GI, silent, and baby boom. This conceptualization is only one manner of looking at differences between age cohorts and is not supported by everyone in the field. In addition, the generalization to the end of life is only speculative and certainly will not apply to everyone in each "generation."

Members of the GI cohort were between ages 82 and 102+ in 2005. They came of age during World War II and are a civic generation, who believe in working together within society's structures to solve problems. They led the developments in technology, chemistry, and medicine that fed into the increase in life expectancy in the 20th century. As we have seen, they are the first generation to profit in large numbers from this lengthened life and have a history of facing crises with courage. They are veterans of life, well acquainted with death, and, as a group, they bring to end of life the strength and courage typical of their generation.

The silent generation, ranging in age between 63 and 80 in 2005, has been called an "adaptive" cohort. Their gift to society has been to stress fairness, and they have been leaders and mediators in the great debates of civil rights and the women's movement of the 20th century. As a group, they are likely to continue to value fair treatment in end-of-life discussions and to face the end of life with equanimity and courage.

The baby boom generation was aged 45 to 62 in 2005. Their central peer personality is one of activism, protest, and idealism. They are not easily accepting of the concept of aging and are already bringing their energies to end-of-life-related subjects, demanding better care for their aged parents in nursing homes and working hard to improve Medicare and Medicaid programs. It is almost as though their youthful slogan, "Hell no, we won't go!" is now being directed toward aging and death. They also have come of age in a psychologically oriented media culture, are accustomed to seeking help for psychological problems, and are relatively sophisticated in the use of professionals as consultants in complicated problems of adult living. Therefore, they are more likely to seek help with end-of-life decision making than previous cohorts have been.

The next generation, the Xers, were labeled a "reactive" group by Strauss and Howe (1991). People in this generation, aged 24 to 44 in 2005, are quite realistic in their view of death. Their cohort saw a much higher risk of dying from accidents, murder, and suicide than did earlier generations. This group also came of age among images of violent death, both fictionalized and real. Reports of two wars in the Persian Gulf and daily carnage in cities around the globe fed their perceptions of the world. Characterized as a "streetwise" generation, large numbers of this cohort have diminished expectations as they follow in the wake of the large baby boom generation. As a group, they are likely to have realistic, even cynically acceptant, attitudes toward death.

The youngest generation, the Millennials, are still being born. The oldest were just 23 in 2005. According to Strauss and Howe (1991), they are likely to represent a new civic generation and work together to improve society in many ways. Perhaps their efforts will result in greater equity and higher quality of care for all people near the end of life.

SUMMARY

Various changes throughout the 20th century have led to the need for psychology to be involved in end-of-life decision making. Life expectancy at birth increased, almost doubling across the period. This resulted in growing numbers of elderly persons, who have time to consider the way in which they wish to die. Causes of death also changed as medicine and technology developed to address acute illnesses. As people lived longer with life-threatening illnesses, a new awareness grew concerning the need for quality care near the end of life. Groups and individuals mobilized to address this need. The hospice movement grew, as did discussions concerning who should control the conditions and timing of death. The growing literature in gerontology, child and adolescent development, and generational or cohort differences added value to understanding the quality of care needed near the end of life. Increasing involvement of mental health professionals in the field promises to extend that value exponentially in the future.

REFERENCES

Administration on Aging. (2002). *A profile of older Americans, 2002.* Washington, DC: U.S. Department of Health and Human Services. Retrieved March 10, 2004, from http://www.aoa.dhhs.gov/prof/Statistics/profile/2002profile.pdf

American Association of Retired Persons. (2001). *Global aging, achieving its potential.* Washington, DC: Author.

Arias, E. (2002). United States life tables, 2000. *National Vital Statistics Reports, 51*(3). Hyattsville, MD: National Center for Health Statistics. Retrieved March 10, 2004, from http://www.cdc.gov/nchs/data/nvsr/nvsr51/nvsr51_03.pdf

Bluebond-Langner, M. (1978). *The private worlds of dying children.* Princeton, NJ: Princeton University Press.

Brophy v. New England Sinai Hospital, Inc., 497 N.E.2d 626 (1986).

Byock, I. R. (1996). The nature of suffering and the nature of opportunity at the end of life. *Clinics in Geriatric Medicine, 12,* 237–251.

Canetto, S. (2001). Older adult women: Issues, resources and challenges. In R. K. Unger (Ed.), *Handbook of the psychology of women and gender* (pp. 183–197). New York: Wiley.

Centers for Disease Control and Prevention. (1999, July 30). Control of infectious diseases. *Morbidity and Mortality Weekly Report, 48*(29), 621–629.

Cruzan v. Director, Missouri Department of Health, 497 U.S. 261 (1990).

Erikson, E. (1950). *Childhood and society.* New York: Norton.

Field, M. J., & Cassel, C. K. (Eds.). (1997). *Approaching death: Improving care at the end of life.* Washington, DC: National Academy Press.

Guend, H., Swallen, K. C., & Kindig, D. (2002). *Exploring the racial/ethnic gap in healthy life expectancy: United States 1989–1991* (Center for Demography and Ecology Working Paper No. 2002–02). Madison: University of Wisconsin.

Hogan, C., Lunney, J. R., Gabel, J., & Lynn, J. (2001). Medicare beneficiaries' costs of care in the last year of life. *Health Affairs, 20,* 188–195.

In re Quinlan, A.2d 647, 664 (1976).

Kubler-Ross, E. (1969). *On death and dying.* New York: Macmillan.

Last Acts. (n.d.). Retrieved March 10, 2004, from http://www.lastacts.org/

Lunney, J. R., Lynn, J., Foley, D. J., Lipson, S., & Guralnik, J. M. (2003). Patterns of functional decline at the end of life. *Journal of the American Medical Association, 289,* 2387–2392.

Markson, E. W. (2003). *Social gerontology today: An introduction.* Los Angeles: Roxbury.

Meisel, A., Snyder, L., & Quill, T. E. (2000). Seven legal barriers to end-of-life care. *Journal of the American Medical Association, 284,* 2495–2501.

Miller, S. C., Mor, V., Gage, B., & Coppola, K. M. (2001) Hospice and its role in improving end-of-life care. In M. P. Lawton (Ed.), *Annual review of gerontology and geriatrics, Volume 20. Focus on the end of life: Scientific and social issues* (pp. 193–223). New York: Springer Publishing Company.

Minimo, A. M., Arias, E., Kochanek, K. D., Murphy, S. L., & Smith, B. L. (2002). Deaths: Final data for 2000. *National Vital Statistics Reports, 50*(15). Hyattsville, MD: National Center for Health Statistics. Retrieved March 10, 2004, from http://www.cdc.gov/nchs/data/nvsr/nvsr50/nvsr50_15.pdf

Ministry of Health, Labour and Welfare. (2002). *Abridged life table.* Tokyo: Statistics and Information Department, Minister's Secretariat. Retrieved March 10, 2004, from http://www.jinjapan.org/stat/stats/02VIT25.html

Mitchell K., Kerridge I., & Lovat, T. (1993). Medical futility, treatment withdrawal and the persistent vegetative state. *Journal of Medical Ethics, 19*(2), 71–76.

National Center for Health Statistics. (2002). *Health, United States, 2002, with chartbook on trends in the health of Americans.* Hyattsville, MD: Author.

National Hospice Organization, Standards and Accreditation Committee. (1997). *A pathway for patients and families facing terminal illness.* Alexandria, VA: Author.

National Hospice and Palliative Care Organization. (2002). *A call for change: Recommendations to improve the care of children living with life-threatening conditions.* Alexandria, VA: Author.

National Hospice and Palliative Care Organization. (2004). *NHPCO facts and figures.* Retrieved March 8, 2004, from http://www.nhpco.org/i4a/pages/index.cfm?pageid=3362

Schaie, K. W. (1965). A general model for the study of developmental problems. *Psychological Bulletin, 64,* 92–107.

Schaie, K. W., & Strother, C. R. (1968). The effect of time and cohort differences on the interpretation of age changes in cognitive behavior. *Multivariate Behavioral Research, 3,* 259–293.

Schaie, K. W., & Willis, S. L. (1996). *Adult development and aging* (4th ed.). New York: HarperCollins.

Schonfeld, D. J. (1999). Children, terminal illness, and death. *Home Health Care Consultant, 6*(2), 27–29.

Siegel, J. (1996). *Aging into the 21st century.* Washington, DC: Administration on Aging.

Spraggins, R. E. (2000). Census brief: Women in the United States: A profile. *Current Populations Report, CENBR/00-1.* Washington, DC: U.S. Census Bureau. Retrieved March 10, 2004, from http://www.census.gov/prod/2000pubs/cenbr001.pdf

Speece, M. W., & Brent, S. B. (1984). Children's understanding of death: A review of three components of a death concept. *Child Development, 55,* 1671–1686.

Stillion, J. M. (1984). Women and widowhood: The suffering beyond grief. In J. Freeman (Ed.), *Women: A feminist perspective* (pp. 282–296). Palo Alto, CA: Mayfield.

Stillion, J. M., & McDowell, E. E. (1996). *Suicide across the lifespan: Premature exits* (2nd ed.). Washington, DC: Taylor & Francis.

Stillion, J. M., & Papadatou, D. (2002). Suffer the children: An examination of psychosocial issues in children and adolescents with terminal illness. *American Behavioral Scientist, 46,* 299–315.

Stroebe, M. S., & Stroebe, W. (1993) The mortality of bereavement: A review. In M. S. Stroebe, W. Stroebe, & R. O. Hansson (Eds.), *Handbook of bereavement* (pp. 175–195). New York: Cambridge University Press.

Strauss, W., & Howe, N. (1991). *Generations: The history of America's future, 1584–2069.* New York: Morrow.

Superintendent of Belchertown State School v. Saikewicz, 370 N.E.2d 417 (1977).

SUPPORT Principal Investigators. (1995). A controlled trial to improve care for seriously ill patients. *Journal of the American Medical Association, 274,* 1591–1598.

Veterans Health Administration. (2001). *Your life, your choices.* Washington, DC: Author. Retrieved March 10, 2004, from http://www.hsrd.research.va.gov/publications/internal/ylyc.pdf

Wass, H. (1989). Children and death. In R. Kastenbaum & B. Kastenbaum (Eds.), *Encyclopedia of death* (pp. 49–54). Phoenix, AZ: Oryx.

Webb, M. (1997). *The good death.* New York: Bantam.

2

THE EFFECTS OF CULTURE IN END-OF-LIFE SITUATIONS

DEAN BLEVINS AND DANAI PAPADATOU

In many ways, attention to end-of-life care began light-years ahead of other domains of health care. With such seminal works as Glaser and Strauss (1965, 1968), Kubler-Ross (1969), and Saunders (1969), the individuality of patients and their significant others, as well as health care providers, received explicit recognition. Persons who work with terminally ill individuals often recognize the importance that both medical and psychosocial issues assume in providing quality end-of-life care (Steinberg & Youngner, 1998; Steinhauser et al., 2000). The recognition of psychosocial issues has been in large part because of the traditionally holistic focus of disciplines such as nursing and social work, which were instrumental to the foundation of the modern end-of-life movement. Psychology has only recently begun to assume an active role in end-of-life care. With the exception of thanatology and gerontology journals, issues related to death and dying are rarely addressed in the literature. Many professionals still perceive death and dying as a medical phenomenon because most were trained under and operate within the much larger health care systems of the modern world that are dominated by a medical model of care.

Attending to psychosocial issues requires a consideration of the influence of culture on the needs and preferences of persons near the end of life, in addition to the implications cultural diversity has on the services available and provided to them. No health care provider can be expected to have a complete knowledge of all possible direct, indirect, and interaction effects on end-of-life care that result from the numerous facets of cultural diversity. Even if this could be assumed, such information has only begun to be collected and assembled into books (e.g., Braun, Pietsch, & Blanchette, 2000; Morgan & Laungani, 2002) and journal articles (e.g., Werth, Blevins, Toussaint, & Durham, 2002). These efforts have been and will continue to contribute to the education of professionals. This chapter aims to provide an overview of the literature, highlighting the state of the field in terms of research and care delivery. Because the vast majority of the related literature, however, has been focused on specific geographic regions (e.g., countries, U.S. states, or groups of countries or states), ethnicities, or religions, we wish to first extend this scope and provide a generalizable framework to understand how to provide culturally sensitive care. For a theoretical framework to be generalizable across the many facets of culture, it must focus on the core principles that underlie the differences that have been empirically identified, rather than trying to approach cultural diversity by only looking at one small component of culture in isolation (i.e., age, ethnicity/race, gender, disability status, sexual orientation). In this chapter, explicit attention is devoted to the complexity of cultural influences on end-of-life care and how understanding this fact can lead to clinical practice that is maximally meaningful and helpful for the dying and the bereaved. We hope that tables and an extensive reference list will serve as a resource for readers who are interested in pursuing specific topics in greater detail because space constraints prevent a detailed discussion of all of the relevant literature.

DEFINING CULTURE

This chapter adopts the broadest possible definition of culture. Culture is specifically defined as any shared system of beliefs and behavioral norms that provide an understanding of the world and influence behavior (see Last Acts, 2001). In research, this has most often been operationalized as ethnicity, religious affiliation, or geographic region. Research, albeit limited, has also identified the importance of a number of other characteristics in end-of-life care, including age, gender, sexual orientation, and disability or health status. These characteristics may influence a person's social reality, care preferences, decisions, and behaviors in the face of death. We focus on the core values that characterize a culture to provide a flexible framework that may help the professional to understand better and interact more effectively with people from different cultures, regardless of whether she or he has any functional knowledge of that culture. Literature that has used the traditional approach to considering cultural diversity in end-of-life care is only briefly summarized because numerous reviews are available.

CULTURAL CORE VALUES

A majority of the professional literature on cultural issues in end-of-life situations has been conducted in the United States, England, and Australia. This may largely be the result of the growing influence of hospice or palliative care in these countries, which has spurred many discussions ranging from funding health care services to the educational curricula of medical schools (Rhymes, 1996). In the limited literature addressing transcultural issues, cultures are often classified as "Eastern" or "Western." Such a dichotomous approach may lead to rigid, arbitrary categorizations when in reality people rarely fit into these opposite categories. Most contemporary work on culture includes some type of qualifier cautioning readers not to stereotype particular segments of society because differences within a group are usually greater than differences between groups (for examples, see Braun, Onaka, & Horiuchi, 2000; Braun, Tanji, & Heck, 2001; Hern, Koenig, Moore, & Marshall, 1998). It therefore seems more appropriate to understand people in relation to a number of core values that affect how they perceive, experience, and cope with life and death within their social context.

Laungani (1994, 1999a, 1999b, 2002; see also Parkes, Laungani, & Young, 1997) referred to four core values when he analyzed how death and bereavement is perceived and dealt with in different cultures: (a) individualism–collectivism/communalism; (b) free will–determinism; (c) materialism–spiritualism; and (d) cognitivism–emotionalism. These core values are not discrete or dichotomous categories, but each extends along a continuum between extreme poles, and varies over time. This dimensional approach has the advantage of allowing us to examine attitudes and behaviors between and within cultural groups (Laungani, 1999a), which may change positions whenever a culture undergoes changes.

Individualism–Collectivism/Communalism

Societies and families vary in the emphasis placed on autonomous or collective decision making. Individualism refers to a person's ability to be self-sufficient, to remain autonomous, independent, and in control over her or his life. As Triandis (1994) suggested, individualism is concerned with giving priority to one's personal goals over the goals of one's ingroup. Collectivism, on the other hand, is the perspective in which the community's and family's goals are given priority over one's personal goals. Laungani (1999b), however, preferred to use the term "communalism" because he argues that collectivism refers to a vague impression of large, amorphous crowds of people gathered together responding to collectivistic values. The term communalism suggests that people live within a community and abide by the norms and values of their community and yet live side by side with a variety of other communities. Such is the reality of people living in countries such as India, Sri Lanka, Indonesia, and many others (including those with large immigrant populations) where different communities with different values coexist within the same nation or society. Communalistic cultures tend to value interdependence, interconnectedness, and mutual consideration, often leading members of a given community to abide strictly by the norms and values of their social context.

Free Will–Determinism

Cultures that value free will assume that each person has full responsibility and control over her or his actions, whereas cultures that value determinism perceive that an individual's life is controlled by higher forces such as the Law of Karma, God, or a divine spirit. Such beliefs have a direct influence on how decisions are made near the end of life or whether patients, families, or care providers should make certain decisions. Research relevant to this dimension includes studies concerning differing religious traditions, as well as certain ethnic groups.

Materialism–Spiritualism

In materialistic cultures, there is a prevailing belief in the existence of a material world in which phenomena are explained in a pragmatic and object-oriented way; abstract, spiritual or nonmaterial explanations are viewed with great skepticism. By contrast, cultures that value spiritualism entertain both material as well as supernatural explanations, which are not perceived as contradictory. Death, for example, may be accepted as the result of a disease but also explained in terms of sorcery, evil eye, or evil spirits. The traditional cross-cultural research between industrialized and agrarian countries, which is inextricably intertwined with dominant spiritual practices, provides the best example of this dimension.

Cognitivism–Emotionalism

Cultures high on cognitivism are work- and activity-oriented, focusing on task and goal achievement through rationality, logic, objectivity, and control. Time is precious for achieving goals, solving problems, and "working through" conflicts. By contrast, societies high on emotionalism are more relation-oriented, supporting the open expression of feelings, which are not considered a sign of vulnerability or weakness. The influence from the dominance of the scientific approach in the health care and social mentality of industrialized countries has resulted in distinctly different views from agrarian or semi-industrialized nations.

We believe that the core values of emotionalism and cognitivism proposed by Laungani (1999b) risk stereotyping individuals from different cultures by discriminating between those who "feel" and those who "think," when in reality they have different ways of coping with life tasks. We therefore suggest the consideration of referring to "task-orientation" versus "relation-orientation" approaches in life. A task-orientation approach is goal directed and cognitivism is highly prized to ensure one's achievements, whereas a relation-orientation aims primarily at the development of bonds through mutual exchange of feelings, thoughts, and shared experiences.

Idealogism–Pragmatism

Triandis (1994) referred to an additional set of core values, ideologism, and pragmatism that affect how people in a given culture perceive and cope with life and death. In ideological cultures, a religious, political, or philosophical ideology usually dominates the way people perceive reality, behave, and communicate with each other. In cultures that value pragmatism, people focus on what is concrete, precise, detailed, and works in a given situation. Theoretical and abstract or general values and principles tend to be perceived as vague and ineffective in daily communications and negotiations.

These core values can help us reflect and better understand the social context within which the modern palliative care movement was born and developed in North America and England—a time when such countries were undergoing significant social changes. Each of these dimensions crosscuts the traditional manner of defining culture as ethnicity, religion, age, and so forth, which are not only limited in generalizability, but also may mask the complex interactions of the sociocultural influences on people's beliefs and behaviors. To understand the importance of these core values and the constraints to considering them in end-of-life care, we expand on the discussions in this volume by Kaplan (Foreword) and Stillion (chap. 1), considering how dominant attitudes in end-of-life care have evolved over time.

CHANGING CARE FOCI OVER TIME

The dramatic progress and achievements of Western medicine throughout the 20th century affected not only survival and quality of life, but also the way people experienced the dying process. Most people continue to die in high-tech institutions under the care of "experts," rather than at home among family and loved ones. Values of conquest and control produced an ethic of "saving life at all costs." This medical ethic led to the provision of impersonal care and to the institutionalization and medicalization of the dying patient. The "expert" caregiver possessed power and authority over the patient's body and course of life. The focus of care became the *quest for solving the riddle of each disease*, which involved specifying a diagnosis, formulating an accurate prognosis, and offering an effective treatment that would lead to cure (Nuland, 1994). The patient and her or his death had no place in this professional quest.

In response to these social changes and emerging values that affected the care of the dying, a few sensitive health care professionals in North America (e.g., Benoliel, 1993; Feifel, 1959; Glaser & Strauss, 1965, 1968; Kubler-Ross, 1969; Martinson et al., 1978) and England (e.g., Dominica, 1985; Saunders, 1969) proposed an alternative, *personalized approach* to the care of the dying (see also Conner, Lycan, & Schumacher, chap. 9). This approach, according to Benoliel (1993)—a pioneer of the palliative care movement—comprised the opportunity for each patient to (a) know what is happening and have the ability to talk about it with concerned others, (b) participate in decisions affecting how she or he will live with an illness and die, and (c) experience loss and grief instead of hiding these emotions and deal with existential questions and concerns that all humans face at the end of life.

A closer examination of this individualized, personal, and caring approach for those who are dying reveals some major underlying values that characterize the current practice of palliative care in most Western countries: (a) openness in communication and truth telling, (b) patient participation in decision making and the promotion of autonomy, and (c) expressivism in feelings, concerns, and needs, and a promotion of self as well as death awareness.

In the early development of the palliative care movement, the dying and the bereaved were expected to move quietly and stoically through stages and phases before coming to terms with impending or actual death. The recent literature, however, presents a somewhat different expectation: Patients and family members should be honestly informed and actively participate in decisions and openly express their concerns, needs, and grief. This is reflected in Last Acts' *Precepts of Palliative Care* (Last Acts, 1997), as is discussed in Kaplan's Foreword, which hold that such openness is necessary to work through unfinished business and come to some sort of resolution that will increase the chances of a "good death" for the dying and a "positive adjustment" to loss for the bereaved (see, however, Center for the Advancement of Health, 2004).

It is not by chance that today some of the most popular models adopted in palliative care and bereavement support focus on "tasks" that need to be accomplished (Corr, Nabe, & Corr, 2001). Doka (1993) and Corr (1992), for example, presented models discussing tasks with which patients and families may choose to cope through the dying process. Others (e.g., Worden,

2001) focus on the postterminal phase of grief and adjusting to the loss of a loved one. The concept of *coping with tasks*, which clearly reflects individual-istic and self-deterministic values, gives the dying and the bereaved an orien-tation of control over their lives and provides them with a script. This script is, in reality, a *heroic script* because patients are expected to display courage by being aware that they are dying and by being expressive, which subsequently allows them to make health care decisions while caregivers display care and concern. According to Seale (1998), such a script suits the conditions of late modernity, which promotes awareness and self-determinism. Ditto (chap. 4) and Allen and colleagues (chap. 8) make this orientation explicit in discus-sions of advance directives and surrogate decision making.

The critical question, however, is how do these values, which are rel-evant primarily in the provision of palliative care services in North America and North Europe, fit in other cultures? Are they generalizable or appropri-ate? Are the concerns and needs of dying patients universal or different? How can they be met effectively in different cultural settings?

SIMILARITIES AND DIFFERENCES IN THE NEEDS OF DYING PEOPLE

There are extremely few cross-cultural studies illuminating the needs of dying patients and of their families; the majority of research has been con-ducted within a single culture and, most often, on a single dimension of that culture. Furthermore, researchers have not attempted to compare and con-trast different cultures with the framework just presented. Thus, although the literature reviewed in the following two sections uses the traditional dis-tinctions between specific cultures to present extant research findings, we hold that there is a need to consider core values, rather than cultural labels, across groups. For example, in a recent study of patients receiving palliative services in the United States, Kutner, Steiner, Corbett, Jahnigen, and Barton (1999) found that the needs of dying patients were extremely diverse and could not be predicted based on the individual's characteristics. Such find-ings highlight and reinforce our call to avoid pigeonholing people into spe-cific subgroups. Psychosocial needs and decisions must be assessed on a case-by-case basis, according to underlying values. Work by Braun and colleagues (Braun et al., 2000, 2001) and Hern et al. (1998) have illustrated problems associated with the overgeneralization of cultural labels.

Despite this diversity, we hold that all humans share some common, universal needs in the face of death. It is unfortunate that professionals often tend to overemphasize the differences among people from different cultures and, consequently, cover or disguise the essential similarities in the dying process, which is a human and universal phenomenon. We next describe some of these common needs along with the differences they present in the

TABLE 2.1
Similarities and Differences Between Cultures

Similarities	Differences
Need for information	Patterns of communication
Need to attribute meaning to suffering, life, dying, and death	Systems of meanings attributed to suffering, life, dying, and death
Need to maintain a sense of "dignity" and ensure a good or appropriate death	Definition of "dying with dignity" and of "good" or "appropriate" death
Need for care and support	Nature and site of care and support

way they are experienced, communicated, and met by different individuals and across cultures (see Table 2.1).

Need for Information

Empirical data (Fielding & Hung, 1996) have challenged the belief that patients from Eastern cultures want less information than patients and their families from Western cultures. Information about one's health situation helps both the patient and her or his family to avoid uncertainty, maximize control, bring order to chaos, and make sense of the illness and their experience in the face of impending death (Fallowfield, Jenkins, & Beveridge, 2001).

Significant differences exist across cultures, however, in how such information is communicated to seriously ill and dying patients. In an interesting transcultural study conducted by Bruera et al. (2000), the attitudes and beliefs of palliative care specialists toward communication with terminally ill patients were examined in South America, Canada, and in the French-speaking countries of Europe. Even though the physicians who participated in the study reported that they would like to be told the truth if they were terminally ill, when asked about the needs of their patients, only 18% of South American and 26% of the European physicians, compared with 93% of the Canadian physicians, thought that the majority of their patients would wish to know.

In another study conducted by the International Psycho-Oncology Society (Koinuma, 1995), oncologists from 28 countries were asked whether they disclosed the diagnosis and prognosis of cancer to their patients. The rates varied among countries, particularly if the prognosis was unfavorable. The lowest prevalence of disclosure was Greece (24%), and the highest were Finland (89%) and the United States (87%). Among Asian countries, Japan presented a prevalence of 30%, China 41%, and the Philippines 60%.

These findings suggest that the context in which information is shared, and the patterns by which it is communicated, vary greatly. Dying within the Greek culture, for example, as in many other communal or context-dependent societies, is a family affair, and communication issues related to dying occur at a family level, leaving much unsaid and implicit. "How" something is said becomes more important than "what" is said, because what matters is maintaining a sense of balance and unity among those involved in the dying process. The lack of open verbal exchange does not imply lack of communication. Both the patient and family engage in behaviors, practices, and rituals that may symbolically acknowledge the impending separation, but concurrently maintain a facade of mutual pretence that allows them to function in their prescribed roles. In a study with Greek mothers of children who died from cancer, Papadatou and her colleagues found that all were aware of their child's impending death and believed that their child—who was never openly informed of the diagnosis—knew she or he was dying and indirectly exchanged good-byes without ever breaking the rule of silence (Papadatou, Yfantopoulos, & Kosmidis, 1996).

Need to Attribute Meaning

Another universal need is to attribute meaning to one's experiences in the face of death. In some cultures, the dominant religion or philosophy provides a context within which the dying patient is integrated into the world of the living, and a story with meaning and coherence is created about the person's birth, life, and death. This integration and meaning-making process is important not only for the dying and the bereaved, but for society that maintains the thread linking its past, present, and future—in other words, its history (Walter, 1999).

Attributing meaning to one's life and death affects how patients and family members are likely to experience and respond to the dying process and death. Take, for example, the Hindu belief in the Law of Karma. It suggests that events in life are not determined by individuals, but are *destined* to happen and explained in relation to one's moral actions in one's present or past lives. Such beliefs may reduce some of the death-related fears, help the patient and family sustain much of the suffering throughout the dying process, and empower them with the hope in an afterlife (Laungani, 2002). This does not mean that Hindus do not occasionally hope for a miracle and rely on medicine to save a patient's life, but those endorsing this belief system sustain and cope with ambiguity and controversy differently from those relying on more Western-derived religions.

By contrast, in cultures in which religious beliefs have become secular, the process of attributing meaning to life and death becomes a private affair that is often initiated whenever one's life is threatened or death is impending. One function of Western palliative care that is not fully recognized is to help the patient and family to edit a personal story that is invested with meaning. In many ways, in secular societies, it becomes the responsibility of a multidisciplinary team to develop an appropriate context and even improvise rituals that will help the dying patient and family to create a personal story and mark the passage from life to death. An example of such an approach is the Legacy intervention described by Allen and colleagues (chap. 8).

Need to Maintain a Sense of Dignity

Every "good" life story has a beginning, middle, and end that includes what an individual believes would be a "good death." But how do individuals define a "good" death in different cultures? Within several Western countries, a "good" death, which may more accurately be portrayed as an "appropriate" or "dignified" death (see Chochinov, 2002), is mostly characterized by two values, which may seem paradoxical when in reality they are not: autonomy and social belonging. Autonomy refers to the opportunity given to the dying person to choose how she or he wishes to live her or his remaining life, as well as how she or he wishes to die. Social belonging refers to the integration of the dying with loved ones or care providers into a nurturing and accepting environment. In such a context, "social death" (through isolation or abandonment) does not precede "physical death." Thus, an important goal of palliative care is to attend to psychosocial issues, as opposed to only medical concerns, as a means of enhancing one's quality of life near the end of life (Walter, 1999).

Each culture offers its own definitions and means by which a "good death" should be achieved. In some communalistic cultures, for example, the dying conditions are not primarily determined by the patient, but by the family. So the patient's true autonomy lies in her or his freedom to delegate to the physician or loved ones the responsibility to make all decisions for her or him near the end of life. This delegation of authority is culturally implicit and ensures that a "good death" becomes a *collective affair*, assumed by a community of loved ones and providers.

Take, for example, the Jewish ethnic identity, which is tightly interwoven with Jewish religious traditions. According to the dominant ethnic and religious cultural beliefs in Israel, even though the sanctity of life should be preserved as long as possible, unnecessary prolongation of life is not required (Bodell & Weng, 2000). Research findings indicate that decisions aiming to ensure a good death result from a negotiated process among the patient and family members who, despite their personal preferences, are nonetheless affected by cultural traditions or mores that may constrain care delivery options; cultural mores may be reflected in the dominant practice patterns of the medical community, codified in legal statutes, or both (Leichtentritt & Rettig, 2000, 2002).

Need for Care and Support

The nature of palliative care services, as well as the site in which these are provided, need to be culturally appropriate. As mentioned earlier, in societies that are family and community oriented, the role of the extended family is paramount in the process of caring and supporting the dying and the bereaved. The extended family can include several generations, in addition to the person's friends and significant others. Her or his individuality is submerged into the collective ego of the family and one's community. As a result, when a serious illness or dying process affects an individual's life, it also affects the entire family, which mobilizes its resources to offer and receive support and decide about the nature and site of care. Although personal preferences and decisions are central to an individualistic society, these are virtually nonexistent in a communalistic society. A person's life, to a large extent, centers round the extended family, which assumes an active and defined role near and at the end of life (Laungani, 1999a).

In many ways, use of hospices and nursing homes in the United States and other Western countries reflects the gradual dissolution of stable and extended-family structures. This creates a growing need to ensure comfort and support in the caring environment of an appropriate institution at the end of a person's life. It is only recently that increasing attention has been directed to the psychosocial needs of persons dying in long-term care facilities and the care provided mostly by health care providers (e.g., Allen et al., chap. 8, this volume; Blevins & Deason-Howell, 2002; Kayser-Jones, 2002).

RESEARCH ON SPECIFIC CULTURES

Although this chapter is primarily concerned with presenting a framework that can be used across the traditionally researched divisions of culture, it would do the literature a great disservice not to acknowledge what has been learned about specific cultures to date. In this section, an overview of the most commonly discussed topics in recent years is presented with special consideration of the extant research pertaining to age and cohort, ethnicity, gender, disability and health status, religion, and sexual orientation.

Most of the literature on cultural issues in end-of-life care can be divided in two major categories: (a) general discussions or review articles on one or more particular cultural dimension(s) and (b) empirical studies investigating one or more cultural dimension(s). Tables 2.2 and 2.3 highlight only a few recent publications across these alternatives and can serve as a resource to pursue particular questions in more detail. Specifically, Table 2.2 summarizes literature (reviews, research, and commentaries) on a single cultural dimension, separated by topic area. Table 2.3 summarizes material that has spanned more than one of the traditional cultural dimensions.

Before presenting a brief discussion of these various cultural dimensions, we address the issue of nationality, which is critical in cross-cultural research. Although there is often a national identity, which is a conglomeration of all of the characteristics of diversity, studies conducted with entire

TABLE 2.2
Direct Effects of the Characteristics of Culture

Topics	General	Age and cohort	Disability status	Ethnicity	Religion and spirituality	Gender	Sexual orientation	Geographic region
General (coping, death attitudes, etc.)	Kagawa-Singer & Blackhall (2001); Pacquiao (2001); Werth et al. (2000)	Berger, Pereira, Baker, O'Mara, & Bolle (2002); Cicirelli (2001); Hines, Babrow, Badzek, & Moss (2001); Lockhart et al. (2001)		Barrett & Heller (2002); Bonura et al. (2001); Braun, Pietsch, et al. (2000); Sullivan (2001); Yick & Gupta (2002)	Driscoll (2001); Idler et al. (2001); O'Gorman (2002); Puchalski (2002); Shannon & Tatum (2002); Sulmasy (2002)	Depaola et al. (2003)	Campbell (2000); Catania et al. (1992); Deevey (2000); Nord (1998)	Campbell (1999); Mak (2001); Mola & Crisci (2001)
Service Utilization		Baggs (2002); Blevins & Deason-Howell (2002); Eng (2002); Iwashyna et al. (2002); Kayser-Jones (2002); Temkin-Greener & Mukamel (2002)		Frayne et al. (2002); Krakauer et al. (2002)	Clark (2001)	Bird et al. (2002); Cintron et al. (2003)		Hansen et al. (2002)

Ethics and legal concerns	Hallenbeck & Goldstein (1999)	Gordon (2002)	Batavia (2002)	Carrese & Rhodes (1995)				Nunez Olarte & Guillen (2001)
Particular treatments and decision making	Douglas & Brown (2002); Ersek et al. (1998)	Houts et al. (2002); Mills & Wilmoth (2002)	O'Brien et al. (1995)	Bodell & Weng (2000); Hopp & Duffy (2000); Murphy et al. (1996)		Perkins et al. (2004)	Stein & Bonuck (2001)	Braun, Onaka, et al. (2000); Esteban et al. (2001)
Family issues and relationships			Cooke et al. (1998)	Koffman & Higginson (2001)	Walsh et al. (1999)	Young et al. (1999)		Adamolekun (2001); Leichtentritt & Rettig (2002); Murray et al. (2003)
Professional caregivers			Curtis et al. (1999); Hoare & Nashman (1994); Kovacs & Rodgers (1995)	Cornelison (2001); McKinley & Blackford (2001)	Daaleman, & VandeCreek (2000); Lo et al. (2002); Siegel et al. (2002)	Mortier et al. (2003)		Dickenson (2000); Papadatou et al. (2001); Rebagliato et al. (2000); Richter et al. (2001)
Mental health					Breitbart (2002)			Goggin et al. (2000); Ruiz (2000); Shernoff (1998)

TABLE 2.3

Interaction Effects of the Characteristics of Culture

Topics	Age/region	Disability/region	Disability/religion	Disability/ethnicity	Religion/region	Religion/ethnicity	Religion/age	Age/ethnicity/region
General (coping, death attitudes, etc.)	Leichtentritt & Rettig (2000)		Lyon et al. (2001)			Koffman & Higginson (2002)		Becker (2002); Holt (2001); Leichtentritt & Rettig (2002)
Service utilization		Ngalula et al. (2002)		Sambamoorthi et al. (2000)				
Particular treatments and decision making	Marchand et al. (2001)			McKinley et al. (1996)	Tanida (2000)			Kiely et al. (2001)
Family issues and relationships				Owen et al. (2001)				
Professional Caregivers		Hinkka et al. (2002)			Strang et al. (2002)			Andresen (2001)
Mental Health							Van Ness & Larson (2002)	

countries rarely have sample sizes that would do justice to the vast diversity within national boundaries. Thus, these studies are often reporting the views pertinent to the dominant majority (i.e., the most common mix of the cultural dimensions). Because of this, we have included a separate column in Tables 2.2 and 2.3 noting when nationality (i.e., a politically defined geographic region) is used as a distinct cultural identity. Truly representative national samples have the potential to be interesting in the comparative sense because they not only represent a blending of all the dimensions of culture, but also include national perspectives on health care. Research conducted in the United States has often focused on a particular state (e.g., Hawaii, New York) or some other geographic region (east, north, south, west). Moreover, some researchers have equated ethnicity with nationality. This is not an acceptable practice, as few, if any, countries can claim to possess a single ethnic tradition.

Age and Cohort

Most frequently, age- or cohort-specific articles are concerned with older adults (i.e., those over 65 years) or focus on comparing older and younger adults who are dying. Limited research has touched on the issues particular to children and adolescents near or at the end of life (see Stillion & Papadatou, 2002). There are many ways to explore the concept of age (e.g., biological, chronological, social), a topic that is beyond the scope of this chapter. It is necessary to distinguish between cohort and age, however (see Stillion, chap. 1). A cohort is a group of individuals who are socialized and mature through a particular period in time and geographic region. Whereas all individuals will "age" similarly chronologically, every generation will differ in values as society continuously changes. A person who is 70 years old today will not necessarily have the same beliefs and values as a 70-year-old 20 years from now. Thus, any research discussing the effects of age on end-of-life issues is necessarily limited to a particular cohort of individuals. There has been no research exploring the importance of various age cohorts in end-of-life care.

Numerous publications discuss end-of-life issues for older adults in general, although some also address specific concerns with regard to access and utilization of particular services and decision making (i.e., accepting, rejecting, or withdrawing treatments). A small literature describes issues related to caregiving and decision making that family and friends of older dying adults with chronic progressive illnesses, such as dementia, encounter. Almost no attention has been given to the mental health issues that different age groups experience near the end of life.

Ethnicity

Ethnicity has been the most commonly discussed dimension of culture. Several reviews are available summarizing what has been gleaned from research to date (e.g., Braun, Pietsch, & Blanchette, 2000; Werth et al., 2002). Although most empirical research on ethnic differences has been conducted with groups in the United States, a growing body of literature has begun to consider the similarities and differences between ethnic groups in a number of other countries as well, including Britain, China, Greece, Israel, Italy, Japan, Nigeria, and Spain.

Within the United States, Americans from African, Asian/Pacific Islander, European, Hispanic, Indian, and Jewish descent have received the most attention in research. In other countries, ethnicity has most often been examined indirectly as nationality and should be considered with caution because of the issues noted earlier. Migration and the effects that traditional and acculturated values have on end-of-life care and decisions have also begun receiving attention. Becker (2002), for example, explored how Cambodian and Filipino immigrants in the United States viewed death and dying, with significant discussion of the frequent desire (despite their inability) to return to their homelands to die.

Disability and Health Status

Few studies have addressed concerns surrounding disability at the end of life, yet a growing number have focused on particular health conditions (e.g., dementia, cancer, HIV disease). Few studies have highlighted the specific similarities and differences that exist between patients with different disabilities and health conditions. Health status and disability are most often incidental to the research questions or used as a control variable. Topics that have received the most attention focus on decision making (especially in regard to cognitive impairment), the trajectories of the terminal illness, service utilization, and grief.

Religion and Spirituality

Similar to ethnicity, religion and spirituality have also been commonly addressed in the end-of-life literature. Unlike ethnicity, however, most of the attention has been isolated to general discussions of religion or spirituality or on the practices of professional caregivers. Research has also explored the relationships among religion, ethnicity, geographic region, age, and disability or health status near the end of life. Although extensively researched, the operationalization of religion is either unclear (as in review articles and discussions) or the concepts are poorly measured. If one asks people what their religion is, most will respond with one of the dominant belief systems of a region; this, however, may have little or no relationship to the actual importance a spiritual or religious belief system may hold near the end of life. The personal importance or commitment to a belief system is rarely considered in cultural research (see Kaut, chap. 5).

Gender

Little research has been conducted on the influence of gender on end-of-life issues, beyond the area of physician-assisted suicide, for which the degree of support among men and women has often been compared. Because gender (or more commonly, sex) is often measured in national data sets common in the United States, health services research frequently considers it with respect to service utilization, caregiving, and mental health, which may or may not be directly related to the end of life. Given the large number of psychological studies documenting similarities and differences in the belief systems, attitudes, and behaviors between men and women, greater attention in research is warranted.

Sexual Orientation

The literature addressing sexual orientation and the end of life, for more than a decade, has almost exclusively focused on gay men who are living or dying with HIV/AIDS. Issues pertinent to lesbians, transsexuals, and bisexuals have been woefully neglected. The majority of work relevant to the end of life considers issues of grief and bereavement, decision making (especially in the use of advance directives), and mental health and counseling. Increasing attention has been directed toward issues of age, sexual orientation, and the end of life, yet research remains in its infancy (see Blevins & Werth, in press).

Interactions of Cultural Identities

As illustrated in Table 2.3, a number of studies have explored interactions among the various traditional cultural dimensions (i.e., age or cohort, disability and health status, ethnicity, gender, religion, sexual orientation, and geographic region). This literature, however, is more sparse than attempts to discuss or empirically investigate the importance of a single dimension. These studies highlight that research findings frequently attest to the need to qualify conclusions presented in single-dimension studies, reflecting the complexity of how the traditional dimensions of culture interact with each other. It is partly for this reason that we have attempted to present a framework that crosscuts these dimensions, considering universally underlying core values of individuals and whole cultures.

APPLICATION OF PALLIATIVE PRINCIPLES IN HEALTH CARE SETTINGS

To discuss cultural issues in the absence of their application to health care systems assumes that knowledge of different cultures is sufficient to ensure quality end-of-life care. It is well known that knowledge alone is insufficient to have an impact on the provision of health care. Thus, a more complex approach is required for successful and sustainable interventions to improve end-of-life care.

Although health care systems have their own unique cultural identities, they are a product of the larger historical and sociopolitical context. Kleinman (1980) recognized this in his classic writings on culture and medicine, stating, "Studies of our own society, and comparative research, must start with an appreciation of health care as a *system* that is social and cultural in origin, structure, function, and significance" (p. 27, emphasis in original). Thus, efforts to improve the sensitivity to cultural diversity in health care require consideration of the context within which care is being provided. In the United States, the Institute of Medicine (2001) published a report on impacting health care that highlighted the need to consider the influence of all major stakeholders to care provision: patients and families, providers, support systems for providers, and regulatory influences from the federal or central government. Neglecting any of these stakeholders will most certainly lead to frustration, if not failure, of interventions. In other nations, the relevant stakeholders may be different and should be explored by research. Some exemplary initiatives in different countries around the world aim at developing culturally appropriate services for dying and bereaved persons. We must not presume that the well-developed services from some Western countries are transferable to other parts of the globe.

RECOMMENDATIONS

Based on this review of the literature we can offer several recommendations that would contribute to advancing understanding of cultural issues near the end of life. We specifically discuss theory development, training and education, collaboration in practice, and transcultural research.

Theory Development

We are progressively entering a new era in which traditional theories and models on dying and bereavement are being challenged, as Western societies evolve and change. Academics question and reconsider the classification of human responses in terms of symptoms, stages, phases, or tasks to be achieved. An emerging theoretical revolution, which is perhaps more evident in the field of bereavement than in palliation, highlights the importance of diversity and acknowledges different ways of experiencing the dying and grieving processes. It disputes the necessity of "grief work," or "task achievement" and avoids judging whether containing or expressing feelings or forgetting or remembering the dead person is healthy or pathological; rather, it emphasizes that everyone is different and unique (Center for the Advancement of Health, 2004).

Models on suffering, loss, and grief, such as those proposed by Toombs (1993), Frank (1995); Neimeyer (2001); Klass, Silverman, and Nickman (1996); and Stroebe and Schut (2001) provide a wider theoretical context for understanding individuality and focus on the processes by which the dying and the bereaved construct their private and social worlds and attribute meaning to their experiences. These new models and theories will become useful if their foci move beyond the exploration of intrapsychic processes to understand human responses to death and dying within the social and cultural context in which they occur.

Training and Education

Communicating effectively with dying patients is considered critical to ensure quality of care near the end of life. Nevertheless, research findings conducted in various cultural settings suggest that such communication is perceived by nurses and physicians as the most difficult and stressful aspect of care (e.g., Jarrett & Payne, 1995; McGrath, Yates, Clinton, & Hart, 1999; Papadatou, Martinson, & Chung, 2001). In a world that is becoming increasingly diverse, if health care professionals do not receive training in culturally appropriate interpersonal relations and communication skills, they will continue to distance themselves and spend less time with patients, especially when they have different beliefs, attitudes, and values because of their cultural background.

Even though an increasing number of educational programs on adult and pediatric palliative care underscore the importance of communicating effectively with dying individuals and of being sensitive to their culture, few of these programs use innovative educational methods to train providers, and even fewer evaluate the effectiveness of their training methods. Ongoing training is imperative because the practice of palliative care requires a broad spectrum of knowledge and skills along with openness to various approaches of care in contrast to traditional biomedical care that promotes a more specialized and focused education. Innovative educational programs at the end of life, such as that being promoted by Education for Physicians on End-of-Life Care (http://www.epec.net), End-of-Life Nursing Education Consortium (http://www.aacn.nche.edu/ELNEC), and the National Hospice and Palliative Care Organization (http://www.nhpco.org), in addition to less well-known efforts by the U.S. Department of Veterans Affairs Training and Program Assessment for Palliative Care (Office of Academic Affiliations, 2002), need to be created, tested, and implemented in different cultural settings around the world.

Collaboration in Practice

Meeting the needs of dying persons in a culturally sensitive way is a major challenge that requires the collaboration of families, care providers, community, and political leaders. There are some exemplary initiatives among palliative care specialists who are cooperating in developing culturally appropriate services for dying and bereaved individuals in different countries. A fascinating project and demonstration of cross-cultural collaboration is the Asian-Pacific Hospice Palliative Care Network (http://www.aphn.org/), developed among Australian palliative care workers and Asian experts who work alongside each other to promote professional and public education and to develop palliative care programs in diverse Asian cultures. They build on the strengths that characterize each country and concurrently work around the weaknesses to provide services that are relevant to the needs of Asian populations and to the budgets of their nations. In the process of this enriching collaboration, both Australian and Asian pioneers are learning and benefiting from each other. Funding agencies, researchers, practitioners, and policymakers should not neglect the great potential that transcultural efforts in end-of-life education and practice can have for patients and for the field.

Transcultural Research

The greatest challenge, and perhaps the greatest hope, in palliative and bereavement care, is for those of us who live and work in various cultural settings to find effective ways to communicate, cooperate, and conduct research. Transcultural research is urgently needed to help us develop appropriate services for dying and bereaved persons that will meet their needs in a culturally sensitive way. We believe that such research needs to balance carefully quantitative and qualitative methodologies, both of which will be necessary to generate theories that better explain how individuals experience, respond, and cope with death and dying across cultures, in addition to developing innovative care delivery models that respect the goals of palliative care.

CONCLUSIONS

We have much to learn from each other. Greater attention to transcultural research and practice would represent a significant advance to the theoretical and empirical research in end-of-life care. Caring for dying and bereaved people who live in different cultures provides us with the privilege of learning from them. Our similarities may bring us closer, and our differences may expand horizons, urging us to think more broadly about what it is like to be human.

REFERENCES

Adamolekun, K. (2001). Survivors' motives for extravagant funerals among the Yorubas of western Nigeria. *Death Studies, 25*, 609–619.

Andresen, J. (2001). Cultural competence and health care: Japanese, Korean, and Indian patients in the United States. *Journal of Cultural Diversity, 8*, 109–121.

Baggs, J. G. (2002). End-of-life care for older adults in ICUs. *Annual Review of Nursing Research, 20*, 181–229.

Barrett, R. K., & Heller, K. S. (2002). Death and dying in the Black experience. *Journal of Palliative Medicine, 5*, 793–799.

Batavia, A. I. (2002). Disability versus futility in rationing health care services: Defining medical futility based on permanent unconsciousness—PVS, coma, and anencephaly. *Behavioral Sciences and the Law, 20*, 219–233.

Becker, G. (2002). Dying away from home: Quandaries of migration for elders in two ethnic groups. *Journal of Gerontology: Social Sciences, 57B*, S79–S95.

Benoliel, J. Q. (1993). Personal care in an impersonal world. In J. D. Morgan (Ed.), *Personal care in an impersonal world* (pp. 3–14). Amityville, NY: Baywood.

Berger, A., Pereira, D., Baker, K., O'Mara, A., & Bolle, J. (2002). A commentary: Social and cultural determinants of end-of-life care for elderly persons. *The Gerontologist, 42*(Special Issue III), 49–53.

Bird, C. E., Shugarman, L. R., & Lynn, J. (2002). Age and gender differences in health care utilization and spending for Medicare beneficiaries in their last years of life. *Journal of Palliative Medicine, 5*, 705–712.

Blevins, D., & Deason-Howell, L. M. (2002). End-of-life care in nursing homes: The interface of policy, research, and practice. *Behavioral Sciences and the Law, 20*, 271–286.

Blevins, D., & Werth, J. L., Jr. (in press). End-of-life issues for lesbian, gay, bisexual, and transgendered older adults. In D. Kimmel & S. David (Eds.), *Handbook of lesbian, gay, bisexual, and transgender aging*. New York: Columbia University Press.

Bodell, J., & Weng, M.-A. (2000). The Jewish patient and terminal dehydration: A hospice ethical dilemma. *American Journal of Hospice and Palliative Care, 17*, 185–188.

Bonura, D., Fender, M., Roesler, M., & Pacquiao, D. F. (2001). Culturally congruent end-of-life care for Jewish patients and their families. *Journal of Transcultural Nursing, 12*, 211–220.

Braun, K. L., Onaka, A. T., & Horiuchi, B. Y. (2000). Advance directive completion rates and end-of-life preferences in Hawaii. *Journal of the American Geriatrics Society, 49*, 1708–1713.

Braun, K. L., Pietsch, J. H., & Blanchette, P. L. (2000). *Cultural issues in end-of-life decision making*. Thousand Oaks, CA: Sage.

Braun, K. L., Tanji, V. M., & Heck, R. (2001). Support for physician-assisted suicide: Exploring the impact of ethnicity and attitudes toward planning for death. *Gerontologist, 41*, 51–60.

Breitbart, W. (2002). Spirituality and meaning in supportive care: Spirituality- and meaning-centered group psychotherapy interventions in advanced cancer. *Supportive Care in Cancer, 10*, 272–280.

Bruera, E., Neumann, C. M., Mazzocato, C., Stiefel, F. C., & Sala, R. (2000). Attitudes and beliefs of palliative care physicians regarding communication with terminally ill patients. *Palliative Medicine, 14*, 287–298.

Campbell, D. A. (2001). Hope and harm: A delicate balance. Death and dying in multicultural Australia. *Medical Journal of Australia, 175*, 540–541.

Campbell, T. (1999). AIDS-related death: A review of how bereaved gay men are affected. *Counselling Psychology Quarterly, 12*, 245–252.

Carrese, J. A., & Rhodes, L. A. (1995). Western bioethics on the Navajo reservation. *Journal of the American Medical Association, 274*, 826–829.

Catania, J. A., Turner, H. A., Kyung-hee, C., & Coates, T. J. (1992). Coping with death anxiety: Help-seeking and social support among gay men with various HIV diagnoses. *AIDS, 6*, 999–1005.

Center for the Advancement of Health. (2004). Report on bereavement and grief research. *Death Studies, 28*, 491–575.

Chochinov, H. M. (2002). Dignity-conserving care—A new model for palliative care: Helping the patient feel valued. *Journal of the American Medical Association, 287*, 2253–2260.

Cicirelli, V. G. (2001). Personal meanings of death in older adults and younger adults in relation to their fears of death. *Death Studies, 25*, 663–683.

Cintron, A., Hamel, M. B., Davis, R. B., Burns, R. B., Phillips, R. S., & McCarthy, E. P. (2003). Hospitalization of hospice patients with cancer. *Journal of Palliative Medicine, 6*, 757–768.

Clark, D. (2001). Religion, medicine, and community in the early origins of St. Christopher's Hospice. *Journal of Palliative Medicine, 4*, 353–360.

Cooke, M., Gourlay, L., Collette, L., Boccellari, A., Chesney, M. A., & Folkman, S. (1998). Informal care givers and the intention to hasten AIDS-related death. *Archives of Internal Medicine, 158*, 69–75.

Cornelison, A. H. (2001). Cultural barriers to compassionate care—patients' and health professionals' perspectives. *Bioethics Forum, 17*, 7–14.

Corr, C. A. (1992). A task-based approach to coping with dying. *Omega, 24*, 81–94.

Corr, C. A., Nabe, C. M., & Corr, D. (2001). *Death and dying, life and living* (3rd ed.). Pacific Grove, CA: Brooks/Cole.

Curtis, J. R., Patrick, D. L., Caldwell, E., Greenlee, H., & Collier, A. C. (1999). The quality of patient-doctor communication about end-of-life care: A study of patients with advanced AIDS and their primary care clinicians. *AIDS, 13*, 1123–1131.

Daaleman, T. P., & VandeCreek, L. (2000). Placing religion and spirituality in end-of-life care. *Journal of the American Medical Association, 284*, 2514–2517.

Deevey, S. (2000). Cultural variation in lesbian bereavement experiences in Ohio. *Journal of the Gay & Lesbian Medical Association, 4*, 9–17.

Depaola, S. J., Griffin, M., Young, J. R., & Neimeyer, R. A. (2003). Death anxiety and attitudes toward the elderly among older adults: The role of gender and ethnicity. *Death Studies, 27,* 335–354.

Dickenson, D. L. (2000). Are medical ethicists out of touch? Practitioner attitudes in the US and UK toward decisions at the end of life. *Journal of Medical Ethics, 26,* 254–260.

Doka, K. J. (1993). *Living with life-threatening illness: A guide for patients, families and caregivers.* Lexington, MA: Lexington Books.

Dominica, F. (1985). Helen House: A hospice for children. In C. A. Corr & D. M. Corr (Eds.), *Hospice approaches to pediatric care* (pp. 107–125). New York: Springer Publishing Company.

Douglas, R., & Brown, H. N. (2002). Patients' attitudes toward advance directives. *Journal of Nursing Scholarship, 34,* 61–65.

Driscoll, J. (2001). Spirituality and religion in end-of-life care. *Journal of Palliative Medicine, 4,* 333–335.

Eng, C. (2002). Future consideration for improving end-of-life care for older persons: Program of All-Inclusive Care for the Elderly (PACE). *Journal of Palliative Medicine, 5,* 305–309.

Ersek, M., Kagawa-Singer, M., Barnes, D., Blackhall, L. J., & Koenig, B. A. (1998). Multicultural considerations in the use of advance directives. *Oncology Nursing Forum, 25,* 1683–1690.

Esteban, A., Gordo, F., Solsona, J. F., Alia, I., Caballero, J., Bouza C., et al. (2001). Withdrawing and withholding life support in the intensive care unit: A Spanish prospective multi-centre observational study. *Intensive Care Medicine, 27,* 1744–1749.

Fallowfield, L., Jenkins, V., & Beveridge, H. (2001, September). *Truth may hurt but deceit hurts more: Communication in palliative care.* Paper presented at the 6th Australian Palliative Care Conference, Hobart, Tasmania.

Feifel, H. (1959). *The meanings of death.* New York: McGraw-Hill.

Fielding, R. G., & Hung, J. (1996). Preferences for information and involvement in decisions during cancer care among a Hong Kong Chinese population. *Psycho-oncology, 5,* 321–329.

Frank, A. W. (1995). *The wounded story teller.* Chicago: University of Chicago Press.

Frayne, S. M., Crawford, S. L., McGraw, S. A., Smith, K. W., & McKinlay, J. B. (2002). Help-seeking behaviors of Blacks and Whites dying from coronary heart disease. *Ethnicity and Health, 7,* 77–86.

Glaser, B. G., & Strauss, A. (1965). *Awareness of dying.* Chicago: Aldine.

Glaser, B. G., & Strauss, A. (1968). *Time for dying.* Chicago: Aldine.

Goggin, K., Sewell, M., Ferrando, S., Evans, S., Fishman, B., & Rabkin, J. G. (2000). Plans to hasten death among gay men with HIV/AIDS: Relationship to psychological adjustment. *AIDS Care, 12,* 125–136.

Gordon, M. (2002). Ethical challenges in end-of-life therapies in the elderly. *Drugs and Aging, 19,* 321–329.

Hallenbeck, J., & Goldstein, M. K. (1999). Decisions at the end of life: Cultural considerations beyond medical ethics. *Generations, 23,* 24–29.

Hansen, S. M., Tolle, S. W., & Martin, D. P. (2002). Factors associated with lower rates of in-hospital death. *Journal of Palliative Medicine, 5,* 677–685.

Hern, E. H., Jr., Koenig, B. A., Moore, L. J., & Marshall, P. A. (1998). The difference that culture can make in end-of-life decision-making. *Cambridge Quarterly of Healthcare Ethics, 7,* 27–40.

Hines, S. C., Babrow, A. S., Badzek, L., & Moss, A. (2001). From coping with life to coping with death: Problematic integration for the seriously ill elderly. *Health Communication, 13,* 327–342.

Hinkka, H., Kosunen, E., Lammi, U.-K., Metsanoja, R., Puustelli, A., & Kellokumpu-Lehtinen, P. (2002). Decision making in terminal care: A survey of Finnish doctors' treatment decisions in end-of-life scenarios involving a cancer and a dementia patient. *Palliative Medicine, 16,* 195–204.

Hoare, C. H., & Nashman, H. W. (1994). AIDS care in six Washington, D.C. area hospices: Satisfaction and stresses among professional caregivers. *International Journal of Stress Management, 1,* 185–204.

Holt, L. L. (2001). End of life customs among immigrants from Eritrea. *Journal of Transcultural Nursing, 12,* 146–154.

Hopp, F. P., & Duffy, S. A. (2000). Racial variations in end-of-life care. *Journal of the American Geriatrics Society, 48,* 658–663.

Houts, R. M., Smucker, W. D., Jacobson, J. A., Ditto, P. H., & Danks, J. H. (2002). Predicting elderly outpatients' life-sustaining treatment preferences over time: The majority rules. *Medical Decision Making, 22,* 39–52.

Idler, E. L., Kasl, S. V., & Hays, J. C. (2001). Patterns of religious practice and belief in the last year of life. *Journal of Gerontology: Social Sciences, 56B,* S326–S334.

Institute of Medicine. (2001). *Crossing the quality chasm: A new health system for the 21st century.* Washington, DC: National Academy Press.

Iwashyna, T. J., Zhang, J. X., & Christakis, N. A. (2002). Disease-specific patterns of hospice and related healthcare use in the incidence cohort of seriously ill elderly patients. *Journal of Palliative Medicine, 5,* 531–538.

Jarrett, N., & Payne, S. (1995). A selective review of the literature on nurse–patient communication: Has the patient's contribution been neglected? *Journal of Advanced Nursing, 22,* 72–78.

Kagawa-Singer, M., & Blackhall, L. J. (2001). Negotiating cross-cultural issues at the end of life. *Journal of the American Medical Association, 286,* 2993–3001.

Kayser-Jones, J. (2002). The experience of dying: An ethnographic nursing home study. *The Gerontologist, 42,* 11–19.

Kiely, D. K., Mitchell, S. L., Marlow, A., Murphy, K. M., & Morris, J. N. (2001). Racial and state differences in the designation of advance directives in nursing home residents. *Journal of the American Geriatrics Society, 49,* 1346–1352.

Klass, D., Silverman, P. R., & Nickman, S. L. (Eds.). (1996). *Continuing bonds: New understandings of grief*. Washington, DC: Taylor & Francis.

Kleinman, A. (1980). *Patients and healers in the context of culture: An exploration of the borderland between anthropology, medicine, and psychiatry*. Berkeley: University of California Press.

Koffman, J., & Higginson, I. J. (2001). Accounts of carers' satisfaction with health care at the end of life: A comparison of first generation Black Caribbeans and White patients with advanced disease. *Palliative Medicine, 15*, 337–345.

Koffman, J., & Higginson, I. J. (2002). Religious faith and support at the end of life: A comparison of first generation Black Caribbean and White populations. *Palliative Medicine, 16*, 540–541.

Koinuma, N. (1995, October). An international perspective on full discourse. *Full Texts and Abstracts of the 2nd International Congress of Psycho-Oncology*. Kobe, Japan: International Congress of Psycho-Oncology.

Kovacs, P. J., & Rodgers, A. Y. (1995). Meeting the social service needs of persons with AIDS: Hospices' response. *The Hospice Journal, 10*, 49–65.

Krakauer, E. L., Crenner, C., & Fox, K. (2002). Barriers to optimum end-of-life care for minority patients. *Journal of the American Geriatrics Society, 50*, 182–190.

Kubler-Ross, E. (1969). *On death and dying*. New York: Macmillan.

Kutner, J. S., Steiner, J. F., Corbett, K. K., Jahnigen, D. W., & Barton, P. L. (1999). Information needs in terminal illness. *Social Science and Medicine, 48*, 1341–1352.

Last Acts. (1997). *Precepts of palliative care*. Retrieved January 21, 2004, from http://www.lastacts.org/docs/profprecepts.pdf

Last Acts. (2001). *Diversity and end-of-life care: Literature review/annotated bibliography*. Washington, DC: Author.

Laungani, P. (1994). Cultural differences in stress: India and England. *Counselling Psychology Review, 9*(4), 25–37.

Laungani, P. (1999a). Death among Hindus in India and England. *International Journal of Group Tensions, 28*, 85–114.

Laungani, P. (1999b). Cultural influences on identity and behavior: India and Britain. In Y. T. Lee, C. R. McCauley, & J. G. Draguns (Eds.), *Personality and perception across culture* (pp. 191–212). Mahwah, NJ: Erlbaum.

Laungani, P. (2002). Hindu spirituality in life, death, and bereavement. In J. D. Morgan & P. Laungani (Eds.), *Death and Bereavement around the world* (Vol. 1, pp. 9–38). Amityville, NY: Baywood.

Leichtentritt, R. D., & Rettig, K. D. (2000). The good death: Reaching an inductive understanding. *Omega, 41*, 221–248.

Leichtentritt, R. D., & Rettig, K. D. (2002). Family beliefs about end-of-life decisions: An interpersonal perspective. *Death Studies, 26*, 567–594.

Lo, B., Ruston, D., Kates, L. W., Arnold, R. M., Cohen, C. B., Faber-Langendoen, K., et al. (2002). Discussing religious and spiritual issues at the end of life: A practical guide for physicians. *Journal of the American Medical Association, 287,* 749–754.

Lockhart, L. K., Bookwala, J., Fagerlin, A., Coppola, K. M., Ditto, P. H., Danks, J. H., et al. (2001). Older adults' attitudes toward death: Links to perceptions of health and concerns about end-of-life issues. *Omega, 43,* 331–347.

Lyon, M. E., Townsend-Akpan, C., & Thompson, A. (2001). Spirituality and end-of-life care for an adolescent with AIDS. *AIDS Patient Care and STDs, 15,* 555–560.

Mak, J. H. J. (2001). Awareness of dying: An experience of Chinese patients with terminal cancer. *Omega, 43,* 259–279.

Marchand, L., Cloutier, V. M., Gjerde, C., & Haq, C. (2001). Factors influencing rural Wisconsin elders in completing advance directives. *Wisconsin Medical Journal, 100*(9), 26–31.

Martinson, I. M., Armstrong, G. D., Geis, D., Anglim, M., Gronseth, E. C., MacInnis, M. A., et al. (1978). Home care for children dying of cancer. *Pediatrics, 62,* 106–113.

McGrath, P., Yates, P., Clinton, M., & Hart, G. (1999). "What should I say?" Qualitative findings on dilemmas in palliative care nursing. *The Hospice Journal, 22,* 72–78.

McKinley, D., & Blackford, J. (2001). Nurses' experiences of caring for culturally and linguistically diverse families when their child dies. *International Journal of Nursing Practice, 7,* 251–256.

McKinley, E. D., Garrett, J. M., Evans, A. T., & Danis, M. (1996). Differences in end-of-life decision making among Black and White ambulatory cancer patients. *Journal of General Internal Medicine, 11,* 651–656.

Mills, T. L., & Wilmoth, J. M. (2002). Intergenerational differences and similarities in life-sustaining treatment attitudes and decision factors. *Family Relations, 51,* 46–54.

Mola, G., & Crisci, M. T. (2001). Attitudes towards death and dying in a representative sample of the Italian population. *Palliative Medicine, 15,* 372–378.

Morgan, J. D., & Laungani, P. (Eds.). (2002). *Death and bereavement around the world* (*Vols. 1–5*). Amityville, NY: Baywood.

Mortier, F., Bilsen, J., Vander Stichele, R. H., Bernheim, J., & Deliens, L. (2003). Attitudes, sociodemographic characteristics, and actual end-of-life decisions of physicians in Flanders, Belgium. *Medical Decision Making, 23,* 502–510.

Murphy, S. T., Palmer, J. M., Azen, S., Frank, G., Michel, V., & Blackhall, L. J. (1996). Ethnicity and advance care directives. *Journal of Law, Medicine, & Ethics, 24,* 108–117.

Murray, S. A., Grant, E., Grant, A., & Kendall, M. (2003). Dying from cancer in developed and developing countries: Lessons from two qualitative interview studies of patients and their carers. *British Medical Journal, 326,* 368–372.

Neimeyer, R. A. (Ed.). (2001). *Meaning reconstruction and the experience of loss.* Washington, DC: American Psychological Association.

Ngalula, J., Urassa, M., Mwaluko, G., Isingo, R., & Boerma, J. T. (2002). Health service use and household expenditure during terminal illness due to AIDS in rural Tanzania. *Tropical Medicine and International Health, 7*, 873–877.

Nord, D. (1998). Tramatization in survivors of multiple AIDS-related loss. *Omega, 37*, 215–240.

Nuland, S. B. (1994). *How we die*. New York: Knopf.

Nunez Olarte, J. M., & Guillen, D. G. (2001). Cultural issues and ethical dilemmas in palliative and end-of-life care in Spain. *Cancer Control, 8*, 46–54.

O'Brien, L. A., Grisso, J. A., Maislin, G., LaPann, K., Krotki, K. P., Grecco, P. J., et al. (1995). Nursing home residents' preferences for life-sustaining treatments. *Journal of the American Medical Association, 274*, 1775–1779.

Office of Academic Affiliations. (2002, February). *Hospice and palliative care services in the Department of Veterans Affairs: A report on the TAPC Project Survey*. Retrieved April 4, 2003, from http://www.hospice.va.gov/VA_initiatives/index.htm

O'Gorman, M. L. (2002). Spiritual care at the end of life. *Critical Care Nursing Clinics of North America, 14*, 171–176.

Owen, J. E., Goode, K. T., & Haley, W. E. (2001). End of life care and reactions to death in African-American and White family caregivers of relatives with Alzheimer's Disease. *Omega, 43*, 349–361.

Pacquiao, D. (2001). Addressing cultural incongruities of advance directives. *Bioethics Forum, 17*, 27–31.

Papadatou, D., Martinson, I. M., & Chung, P. M. (2001). Caring for dying children: A comparative study of nurses' experiences in Greece and Hong Kong. *Cancer Nursing, 24*, 402–412.

Papadatou, D., Yfantopoulos, J., & Kosmidis, H. (1996). Death of a child at home or in hospital: Experiences of Greek mothers. *Death Studies, 20*, 215–235.

Parkes, C. M., Laungani, P., & Young, B. (Eds.). (1997). *Death and bereavement across cultures*. London: Routledge.

Perkins, H. S., Cortez, J. D., & Hazuda, H. P. (2004). Advance care planning: Does patient gender make a difference? *American Journal of the Medical Sciences, 327*, 25–32.

Puchalski, C. M. (2002). Spirituality and end-of-life care: A time for listening and caring. *Journal of Palliative Medicine, 5*, 289–294.

Rebagliato, M., Cuttini, M., Broggin, L., Berbik, I., de Vonderweid, U., Hansen, G., et al. (2000). Neonatal end-of-life decision making: Physicians' attitudes and relationship with self-reported practices in 10 European countries. *Journal of the American Medical Association, 284*, 2451–2459.

Rhymes, J. A. (1996). Barriers to effective palliative care of terminal patients: An international perspective. *Clinics in Geriatric Medicine, 12*, 407–416.

Richter, J., Eisemann, M., & Zgonnikova, E. (2001). Doctors' authoritarianism in end-of-life treatment decisions. A comparison between Russia, Sweden and Germany. *Journal of Medical Ethics, 27*, 186–191.

Ruiz, P. (2000). Living and dying with HIV/AIDS: A psychosocial perspective. *American Journal of Psychiatry, 157,* 110–113.

Sambamoorthi, U., Walkup, J., McSpiritt, E., Warner, L., Castle, N., & Crystal, S. (2000). Racial differences in end-of-life care for patients with AIDS. *AIDS and Public Policy Journal, 15,* 136–148.

Saunders, C. (1969). The moment of truth: Care of the dying person. In L. Pearson (Ed.), *Death and dying.* Cleveland, OH: Case Western Reserve University Press.

Seale, C. (1998). *Constructing death: The sociology of dying and bereavement.* Cambridge, England: Cambridge University Press.

Shannon, S. E., & Tatum, P. (2002). Spirituality and end-of-life care. *Missouri Medicine, 99,* 571–576.

Shernoff, M. (1998). Individual practice with gay men. In G. P. Mallon (Ed.), *Foundations of social work with lesbian and gay persons* (pp. 77–103). Binghamton, NY: Haworth Press.

Siegel, B., Tenenbaum, A. J., Jamanka, A., Barnes, L., Hubbard, C., & Zuckerman, B. (2002). Faculty and resident attitudes about spirituality and religion in the provision of pediatric health care. *Ambulatory Pediatrics, 2,* 5–10.

Stein, G. L., & Bonuck, K. A. (2001). Attitudes on end-of-life care and advance care planning in the lesbian and gay community. *Journal of Palliative Medicine, 4,* 173–190.

Steinberg, M. D., & Youngner, S. J. (Eds.). (1998). *End-of-life decisions: A psychosocial perspective.* Washington, DC: American Psychiatric Press.

Steinhauser, K. E., Clipp, E. C., McNeilly, M., Christakis, N. A., McIntyre, L. M., & Tulsky, J. A. (2000). In search of a good death: Observations of patients, families, and providers. *Annals of Internal Medicine, 132,* 825–832.

Stillion, J. M., & Papadatou, D. (2002). Suffer the children: An examination of psychosocial issues in children and adolescents with terminal illness. *American Behavioral Scientist, 46,* 299–315.

Strang, S., Strang, P., & Ternestedt, B.-M. (2002). Spiritual needs as defined by Swedish nursing staff. *Journal of Clinical Nursing, 11,* 48–57.

Stroebe, M. S., & Schut, H. (2001). Models of coping with bereavement: A review. In M. S. Stroebe, R. O. Hanson, W. Stroebe, & H. Schut (Eds.), *Handbook of bereavement research: Consequences, coping, and care* (pp. 375–403). Washington, DC: American Psychological Association.

Sullivan, M. C. (2001). Lost in translation: How Latinos view end-of-life care. *Plastic Surgical Nursing, 21,* 90–91.

Sulmasy, D. P. (2002). A biopsychosocial-spiritual model of the care of patients at the end of life. *The Gerontologist, 42*(Special Issue III), 24–33.

Tanida, N. (2000). The view of religions toward euthanasia and extraordinary treatments in Japan. *Journal of Religion and Health, 39,* 339–354.

Temkin-Greener, H., & Mukamel, D. B. (2002). Predicting place of death in the Program of All-Inclusive Care for the Elderly (PACE): Participant versus program characteristics. *Journal of the American Geriatrics Society, 50,* 125–135.

Toombs, K. (1993). *The meaning of illness: A phenomenological account of the different perspective of physician and patient*. Dordrecht, the Netherlands: Kluwer Academic.

Triandis, H. (1994). *Culture and social behavior*. New York: McGraw-Hill.

Van Ness, P. H., & Larson, D. B. (2002). Religion, senescence, and mental health: The end of life is not the end of hope. *American Journal of Geriatric Psychiatry, 10*, 386–397.

Walsh, K., King, M., Jones, L., Tookman, A., & Blizard, R. (2002). Spiritual beliefs may affect outcome of bereavement: Prospective study. *British Medical Journal, 324*, 1551–1555.

Walter, T. (1999). *On bereavement: The culture of grief*. Buckingham, England: Open University.

Werth, J. L., Jr., Blevins, D., Toussaint, K. L., & Durham, M. R. (2002). The influence of cultural diversity on end-of-life care and decisions. *American Behavioral Scientist, 46*, 204–219.

Worden, W. J. (2001). *Grief counseling and grief therapy: A handbook for the mental health practitioner* (3rd ed.). New York: Springer Publishing Company.

Yick, A. G., & Gupta, R. (2002). Chinese cultural dimensions of death, dying, and bereavement: Focus group findings. *Journal of Cultural Diversity, 9*, 32–42.

Young, E., Bury, M., & Elston, M. A. (1999). "Live and/or let die": Modes of social dying among women and their friends. *Mortality, 4*, 269–289.

3

ETHICAL CONSIDERATIONS IN PROVIDING PSYCHOLOGICAL SERVICES IN END-OF-LIFE CARE

JAMES L. WERTH JR. AND PHILLIP M. KLEESPIES

Psychologists who consider providing services to people who are dying and their loved ones not only must be sure they have the appropriate level of training and experience to work with these groups, they must also have an understanding of the ethical issues that may arise and how to resolve them. End-of-life situations can lead to ethical dilemmas for service providers as well as for the dying person and her or his loved ones.

In this chapter, we use the American Psychological Association's (APA; 2002) most recent version of the *Ethical Principles of Psychologists and Code of Conduct* (Ethics Code) as the framework for discussing ethical dilemmas psychologists may face in this area of practice. We then review some of the significant issues near the end of life that may challenge the client and caregivers. Finally, we provide a synopsis of an ethical decision-making model that has been recommended for use with end-of-life dilemmas.

ETHICAL ISSUES FOR PSYCHOLOGISTS WHO WORK WITH DYING INDIVIDUALS AND THEIR LOVED ONES

The APA (2002) Ethics Code begins with a set of aspirational general principles that appear to be based at least in part on the work in bioethics of

Beauchamp and Childress (1979/2001) that were brought into psychology by Kitchener (1984). These meta-principles undergird the Ethical Standards of the APA code and should be at least an implicit part of what psychologists consider as they provide services. Authors writing on end-of-life issues have discussed the varied ways that these principles are interpreted by members of various cultural groups (Ersek, Kagawa-Singer, Barnes, Blackhall, & Koenig, 1998; Hallenbeck & Goldstein, 1999). Our focus in this chapter, however, is less on these general principles than on four aspects of the Ethical Standards that we see as most relevant to the psychologist engaged in end-of-life care and consultation: competence, human relations, privacy and confidentiality, and therapy. In each section we review the relevant standards and apply them to end-of-life situations.

Standard 2: Competence

There are three standards in this section that we discuss in some detail: Boundaries of Competence (2.01), Bases for Scientific and Professional Judgments (2.04), and Personal Problems and Conflicts (2.06). Although the others should not be ignored, these are the most relevant for our discussion.

Boundaries of Competence and Maintaining Competence

It should go without saying that psychologists who wish to provide counseling to people who are dying and their loved ones should have the professional training and experience necessary to provide services that measure up to the standard of care and should work within the boundaries of their competence. No generally accepted guidelines are available regarding the type of training a psychologist needs to work in this area, although one of us has offered a set of recommendations (Werth, 1999d).

One of the points made in this part of the Ethics Code is that if there is evidence that cultural differences are relevant, then the psychologist needs to be prepared for working with various diverse groups (2.01b). The importance of respecting cultural diversity has been promulgated for years (see Sue & Sue, 1999), and the APA recently passed its "Guidelines on Multicultural Education, Training, Research, Practice, and Organizational Change for Psychologists" (2003; see also APA, 1993). Within the end-of-life domain, there are clear differences in experiences, values, and desires among people who vary in any number of demographic characteristics. In fact, the research is too voluminous to recount here, but as we discuss in the section on decisions faced by the dying person and her or his caregivers, in general there are differences based on age, gender, and ethnicity, among other variables, in terms of trust in the medical system, desire to have life-sustaining treatment withheld or withdrawn, completion of advance care directives, and access to and use of pain medication, among other issues (see Blevins & Papadatou, chap. 2; Braun, Pietsch, & Blanchette, 2000; Irish, Lundquist, & Nelsen, 1993;

Spiro, Curnen, & Wandel, 1996; Taylor & Box, 1999; Werth, Blevins, Toussaint, & Durham, 2002).

Another point in this standard is that in "emerging areas" where guidelines for preparatory training do not exist, psychologists take steps to develop competence (2.01e). The APA's Ad Hoc Committee on End-of-Life Issues is currently (in 2003–2004) engaged in research regarding the degree to which psychologists have received, or are engaged in, end-of-life training, research, and care. The committee members are also attempting to secure funding to develop a national, standardized continuing professional education (CPE) program. Until those data are available, however, psychologists will have to rely on consulting with colleagues, working with professionals in other disciplines (see Standard 3, discussed later in this chapter), and attending CPE courses offered through state psychological associations or at national conferences such as the APA's or American Association of Suicidology's annual conventions. This would also be the way to maintain competence, which is another part of this ethical standard (2.03).

Bases for Scientific and Professional Judgments

The text of this standard is short: "Psychologists' work is based upon established scientific and professional knowledge of the discipline" (p. 1064). We want to focus on professional competence in two specific areas related to end-of-life service provision: assessment and diagnosis. Because of our special training, psychologists may be asked to conduct assessments of people who are near the end of life, and thus it is important to be aware of the issues associated with assessing ill individuals as well as having an idea of some of the useful instruments (for a more thorough discussion of assessment, see Kaut, chap. 5; Gibson, Breitbart, Tomarken, Kosinski, & Nelson, chap. 6; and Rosenfeld, Abbey, & Pessin, chap. 7).

Psychological assessments have their place in some end-of-life situations; however, the physical status of the dying person may significantly affect the appropriateness of using instruments and therefore the choice of measures or whether to use them at all. For example, people who are very ill may have great difficulty reading a test instrument. Likewise, given the often rapid daily shifts in clinical status and the deficits in memory that many dying people experience, tests that ask for global ratings of how the person felt in the past 1 to 2 weeks might not give an accurate picture. This means the psychologist must be aware of the various instruments available to measure different areas and the degree to which they are valid and recommended for use with dying individuals. The best resource for reviewing a variety of measures (although there are relatively few psychological instruments included) is the *Toolkit for Measures of End-of-Life Care* (available at http://www.chcr.brown.edu/pcoc/toolkit.htm). The psychologist should also review both theoretical and empirical articles specifically examining various psychological conditions, such as clinical depression, to see what these authors recommend (e.g., Breitbart et al., 2000; Farrenkopf & Bryan, 1999; Rosenblatt & Block, 2001; Rosenfeld, 2000; Werth, 1999a; Werth, Benjamin, & Farrenkopf, 2000; in this volume, see also the chapters by Gibson et al. [chap. 6] and Rosenfeld et al. [chap. 7]). Furthermore, the psychologist must be familiar with assessing for capacity (see Grisso & Appelbaum, 1998; Kleespies, 2004; Werth, 1996).

Concerns about appropriate use of assessment instruments with dying individuals relates to the psychologist's ability to competently detect, differentiate, and diagnose psychological conditions in dying individuals. For example, there can be difficulties determining whether a dying person has major depression because of the inadequacy of assessment instruments, problems with diagnostic criteria overlapping symptoms of the terminal condition, and misunderstandings of the degree to which dying individuals are clinically depressed (Block, 2000; Chochinov, Wilson, Enns, & Lander, 1994, 1997; Rosenfeld, 2000; Werth, 1999a; see also chaps. 6 and 7 in this volume). Furthermore, it can be difficult to differentiate among depression, guilt, delirium, and dementia (Block, 2000; Farrell & Ganzini, 1995). Because appropriate diagnosis and treatment affects the dying person's quality of life and may affect her or his length of life and ability to make her or his own decisions, diagnosis and treatment is a crucial aspect of end-of-life care. Inexperienced clinicians should therefore liberally consult with more seasoned colleagues.

Personal Problems and Conflicts

The final aspect of this standard on which we focus is the potential for a psychologist's own issues to interfere with service provision. There are a few ways that this can be a concern for psychologists providing care in end-of-life situations. First, research has indicated that graduate students were more uncomfortable when working with clients who present with death-related issues than with other types of presenting problems (Kirchberg & Neimeyer, 1991). The degree to which this "death anxiety" (see Neimeyer & Van Brunt, 1995) can be extended to professional psychologists is not clear, but the same societal injunctions that affect graduate students are likely to influence professionals. Thus, the general discomfort with, even denial of (Becker, 1973), dying and death that permeates the U.S. culture could interfere with providing appropriate services (Field & Cassel, 1997), as could ageism (Genevay & Katz, 1990) and ableism (Gill, 2000).

In addition, a psychologist's own personal experiences related to dying and death may influence her or his ability to provide appropriate care to clients near the end-of-life and their families. Katz and Genevay (2002) discussed several ways that the professional's own emotional responses, what some may consider "countertransference," can interfere with optimal care, including unresolved grief work, threats to professional omnipotence, threats to professional omniscience, overidentification, and intimacy needs. If a psychologist experiences a personal loss, she or he may need to take some time before working further with dying clients to reduce the possibility of impairment (Katz & Genevay, 2002; Katz & Johnson, in press).

Summary

Psychologists considering working in the end-of-life arena must ensure that they have and maintain the proper training and experience, which includes awareness of cultural issues, before working with clients who are dying and their loved ones. They must be able to assess appropriately and diagnose psychological conditions that may be present and affecting the quality of life of the dying person. Finally, they must be aware of their own issues associated with dying and death and remove themselves from service provision when their own experiences may unduly interfere with care.

Standard 3: Human Relations

As with Standard 2, in this section we focus specifically on three standards: Multiple Relationships (3.05), Third-Party Requests for Services (3.07), and Cooperation With Other Professionals (3.09).

Multiple Relationships

The most recent revision of the Ethics Code is more clear in stating that not all multiple relationships are unacceptable. Only those in which there is a reasonable expectation that the psychologist's objectivity, competence, or effectiveness will be impaired, or where there is a risk of exploitation or harm are considered unethical (S. Behnke, personal communication, September 2004; see also Fisher, 2003; Knapp & VandeCreek, 2003). This is an important point to emphasize because it is likely that the psychologist providing services to people who are dying could be asked to, or may inadvertently or purposefully, enter into any number of multiple relationships.

In some ways this is similar to issues discussed among providers of HIV-related services who have talked about "bending the frame" of traditional counseling because the typical rules do not work with this clientele (e.g., Eversole, Kitchener, & Burris, 2001; Winiarski, 1991; see, generally, Anderson & Barret, 2001; in this volume, see also chap. 9 by Connor et al.). For example, the psychologist may find herself or himself visiting the client's home or the client's room in a hospital or nursing home or hospice. She or he may be asked or may volunteer to do something around the client's home or help the client with a chore or bodily requirement. Because a spur of the moment decision at times needs to occur (e.g., "Will you help me to the bathroom?"), the therapist needs to have thought ahead of time what boundaries she or he will place on the relationship. In other situations, there will be time for careful consideration and consultation. For example, if the client asks the therapist to serve as her or his durable power of attorney for health care, the therapist can ask to think about the effects of that on their relationship (see, e.g., Eversole et al., 2001). The psychologist, however, needs to try to be ready for requests that demand an immediate answer so that she or he will not offend the client when the initial question is asked.

Clients will differ in the degree to which they request or feel comfortable receiving assistance from their therapist, and different psychologists are likely to draw the lines in different places regarding what they are or are not willing to do. We cannot hope to provide the psychologist with a set of cut-and-dried do's and don'ts in such situations. Rather, it seems important that the clinician go through a decision-making process. Later in the chapter, we outline an ethical decision-making model (Barret, Kitchener, & Burris, 2001a) for use in end-of-life situations (e.g., Barret, Kitchener, & Burris, 2001b; Eversole et al., 2001; Werth, 2002; Werth & Rogers, 2005).

Third-Party Requests for Services

Because dying individuals often reside in institutions (e.g., hospitals, nursing homes) and are cared for by others (e.g., physicians, nurses, loved ones), another person is likely to ask the psychologist to be involved in the care of the client. In such instances, the psychologist must clarify to the dying person the role she or he is taking and how any information received will be used (see also chap. 5 by Kaut and chap. 6 by Gibson et al.). This is especially true if any material may be used in a decision regarding the person's ability to make her or his own decisions (see Appendix F of Working Group on Assisted Suicide and End-of-Life Decisions, 2000).

Because control is often a significant issue near the end of life (see, e.g., Kastenbaum, 1978), the psychologist must minimize the possibility that she or he is doing anything that inappropriately takes away control from the dying person, or the individual's loved ones. If the psychologist has been a part of the person's health care team from early on, this reduces the chances of misunderstanding or lack of cooperation (by anyone). In any event, the bottom line is that the psychologist must be careful not to assume that people understand how and why she or he became involved in this person's care.

Cooperation With Other Professionals

Many authors have asserted that interdisciplinary care is the best way to provide end-of-life services (e.g., Connor, Egan, Kwilosz, Larson, & Reese, 2002). Although discussion of multi- or interdisciplinary care in the medical literature often leaves out psychologists (instead only referring to psychiatrists and social workers), it is clear that psychologists have much to offer their professional colleagues (Working Group on Assisted Suicide and End-of-Life Decisions, 2000; see also Connor et al., chap. 9).

Even though it should be obvious that it is in the dying person's best interest, as well as the best interest of the psychologist and other professionals, to work as a team, if the psychologist is not a part of the health care group (e.g., hospital, hospice, nursing home), there is the possibility that her or his input may not be welcome. In such instances, the ethical responsibility of the psychologist is to use her or his skills to find the best way to become involved to help the person receive the best care possible. Communication is the key in such instances (Hickman, 2002).

Summary

Psychologists need to be prepared to be asked to step outside the traditional therapeutic situation when working with dying individuals. Consideration of boundaries and roles before being put in a difficult situation and consulting with others as soon as possible is crucial when these dilemmas arise. In addition, the psychologist must be clear with dying individuals why they are involved in the situation and how any information received may affect them. Finally, the therapist must be willing and able to cooperate with other professionals to facilitate quality care near the end of life.

Standard 4: Privacy and Confidentiality

In this section, we discuss other issues related to the Standards of Maintaining Confidentiality (4.01), Discussing the Limits of Confidentiality (4.02), and Disclosures (4.05).

Maintaining Confidentiality

One of the most fundamental aspects of psychotherapy is confidentiality. The focus on this tenet has been heightened as a result of the scrutiny on records as a result of the Health Insurance Portability and Accountability Act (HIPAA) Privacy Rule (45 CFR Parts 160–164; see Fisher, 2003). It may therefore seem unnecessary to include discussion of this point in the chapter. Because of the situations in which psychologists working with dying individuals are likely to find themselves, however, one cannot emphasize the importance of confidentiality too often or too strongly. On the other hand, it may be that confidentiality can get in the way of sharing important information, and therefore, the psychologist must also have confidentiality in mind so that she or he can get mutual releases (i.e., a release that allows the psychologist to talk to others and others to talk to the psychologist) signed and therefore share communication with the ill individual's other personal and professional care providers.

Discussing the Limits of Confidentiality

Psychologists are accustomed to discussing the limits of confidentiality (e.g., when the therapist is concerned about the possibility of child abuse; see also 4.05 Disclosures). Certain situations, however, are likely to occur with dying individuals that only rarely arise with other clients. Psychologists may not have thought to discuss these issues with clients before a potential problem arises. Two such issues are the limits of confidentiality if the person becomes incompetent and the limits of confidentiality once the person has died.

If the dying person loses the ability to make health care decisions, then the individual who is her or his health care proxy has access to the dying person's medical and mental health records to the same extent that the dying person would. In the same way, the executor or executrix of the person's estate will have access to the recorded and written records of the work between the client and psychologist (Werth, Burke, & Bardash, 2002).

For some people, the fact that the individual holding power of attorney or the executor or executrix of the person's estate will have access to the person's medical and psychological records may be unimportant; for others, however, there may be concerns that the contents of the sessions may be hurtful in one way or another. In such situations, it is important to discuss who has access to the records after incompetency or death and, perhaps, for the ill person to name the psychologist as the person who holds the rights to the records.

Disclosures

As noted earlier, it may be in the dying person's best interest for the psychologist to get releases signed and to discuss to whom disclosures can be made before and after the person's death. The traditional limits on confidentiality are well known and usually well understood. Yet there is the potential that 4.05(b)(3) may be confusing for the psychologist. This item specifically states that "(b) Psychologists disclose confidential information without the consent of the individual only as mandated by law, or where permitted by law for a valid purpose such as to . . . (3) *protect* the client/patient, psychologist, or others from harm" (APA, 2002, p. 1066, emphasis added). This statement is most often considered to apply when the person is suicidal or homicidal, but recently it has been argued that when the potential is for harm to self, the label of the behavior (i.e., "suicide") is not as important as the potential outcome of the behavior (e.g., high likelihood of serious injury or death within a limited time frame). Cases of advanced anorexia (Werth, Wright, Archambault, & Bardash, 2003) or cases in which end-of-life decisions may hasten death might potentially be included within this broader focus (Werth, 2002; Werth & Rogers, 2005).

In the next major section, we discuss potential ethical issues faced by dying individuals, their loved ones, and their professional caregivers and highlight decisions that may affect the manner and timing of death. With regard to the ethical considerations the psychologist faces, the issue is whether the decision being contemplated is one that might fall under 4.05(b)(3). If so, then the psychologist *may* break confidentiality in an effort to "protect" the dying person (i.e., the language is "permissive rather than mandatory"; Fisher, 2003, p. 98). Extending this analysis from the specific ethical standard to the general standard of care in situations involving the "duty to protect," there is the possibility that the psychologist would not only need to consider break-ing confidentiality but also intervening in some other way to try to prevent harm from occurring. The intricacies of this analysis and the implications are too extensive to include here (see Werth & Rogers, 2005); however, the bottom line is that the psychologist must have thoroughly considered whether the decision being discussed is one that would warrant intervention through disclosure or some other approach.

Summary

Confidentiality is nearly always a significant issue in therapy, and end-of-life counseling is no different. Psychologists need to be aware of the issues associated with maintaining, and not maintaining, confidentiality, as well as discussing some of the unique limits of confidentiality. In addition, service providers must consider when, if ever, they are going to break confidentiality or act in other ways to protect a client who is dying.

The reader will note that we did not discuss whether it is necessary to break confidentiality when a client is considering assisted suicide. Because this topic, as well as the more general debate about whether someone can make a well-reasoned decision to die, is tangential to our focus, we refer interested readers to other sources that discuss these issues in detail (e.g., Barret et al., 2001b; Rosenfeld, 2004; Werth, 1999b, 2002).

Standard 10: Therapy

This section is related to all the preceding material. Here we focus on issues of Informed Consent to Therapy (10.01) and Therapy Involving Couples or Families (10.02).

Informed Consent to Therapy

A thorough informed consent process can prevent or eliminate many potential problems (Kitchener, 2000). Informed consent is crucial not only in therapy, but in assessment, consulting, or other service situations (see also Standards 3.10 and 9.03). The general issues of informed consent are, like the typical considerations associated with confidentiality, well known and well accepted. Thus, the more intriguing aspect of this standard is part (b): discussing situations in which generally accepted guidelines for treatment do not yet exist.

The empirically supported treatment (or evidence-based practice) move-ment (see, e.g., Chambless et al., 1998; Wampold, Lichtenberg, & Waehler, 2002) has become an important, although somewhat controversial, part of the therapy world. Although therapists have been working with dying people for decades, little research (although there are many anecdotes) is available to guide the practitioner. Thus, the informed consent should include a dis-cussion of various approaches to helping the client with the issues she or he is facing as well as a disclosure about the extent of empirical evidence supporting the effectiveness of each approach. Different types of therapies *may* be useful, including cognitive–behavioral and existential, depending on the client and issues (see, e.g., Chochinov & Breitbart, 2000). Couples or family therapy (Nadeau, 1998; Rosen, 1998) can also be helpful as can some forms of group therapy (Greenstein & Breitbart, 2000). Of course, medication is an option and may be useful by itself or as an adjunct to counseling.

Therapy Involving Couples or Families

Communication is a significant issue near the end of life (Haley et al., 2002; Hickman, 2002), especially talking about end-of-life issues—with the dying people not feeling comfortable talking to loved ones about their impending death and vice versa (e.g., Rosen, 1998). The psychologist can play an important role in helping dying persons and their loved ones talk about difficult issues, deal with unfinished business, and talk about the survivors' future without the person. In addition, helping the family–friendship system with grief and anticipatory grief (e.g., Rando, 2000) can be an important role.

The difficulty in such situations arises from the possibility that the psychologist may be privy to information that one or more individuals do not want shared with one or more others. Although this is not unusual in couples or family therapy, the implications in end-of-life situations are heightened by the fact that there is often little time to tread cautiously or lightly. If a secret that was supposed to be kept gets out, the ill person's dying process can become agonizing or the mourning process of the loved one can move from the possibility of developing meaning to developing complicated grief (Neimeyer, Davies, & Prigerson, 2002). It is therefore crucial that the therapist be clear about boundaries regarding secrets in the informed consent process and then sticks to the limits as agreed at the outset.

Summary

Therapy with dying individuals and their loved ones can be extremely rewarding and stressful at the same time. Psychologists can minimize the potential of precipitating or exacerbating problems before and after clients have died by being clear in the informed consent process. They must inform clients of the limits of the state of the field related to care near the end of life and the limits (if they believe there are any) of their ability to maintain secrets shared individually.

General Summary

Although dying and death are not specifically addressed in the newest version of the APA (2002) Ethical Principles of Psychologists and Code of

Conduct, several standards are directly applicable to working with clients who are dying and their loved ones. Space limitations do not permit an extended discussion of each standard, but we have provided references for more information. We now turn to issues for the recipients of psychologists' services.

ETHICAL ISSUES FACED BY DYING PERSONS, LOVED ONES, AND PROFESSIONAL CARE PROVIDERS

The focus of this chapter thus far primarily has been on the ethical issues faced by psychologists as service providers. It would be incomplete, however, if we did not address some of the dilemmas that may be experienced by the dying person, her or his loved ones, and her or his professional care providers (e.g., physicians, nurses, respiratory therapists, dialysis technicians). To work effectively with the client who is dying, the psychologist needs to know the parameters of the difficult ethical decisions that may need to be faced by the individual and those involved in her or his care. In this section, we offer a synopsis of these ethical issues. The reader who is interested in a more comprehensive treatment is referred to sources such as Battin (1994), Beauchamp and Childress (1979/2001), Kleespies (2004), and Rosenfeld (2004).

The section is divided into two parts: (a) issues associated with decisions not to prolong life any longer and (b) issues associated with decisions to attempt to prolong life. We acknowledge that, in reality, these two areas are intertwined.

In addition, we must also emphasize that cultural factors play a significant role in all of the areas to be discussed in this section. In fact, cultural beliefs may be at the root of the dilemma or may help to resolve a situation. Because of this cultural overlay, we will not mention this issue in each of the areas discussed unless the literature is remarkable in some way.

Decisions That Do Not Prolong Life or May Hasten Death

This section will describe three sets of decisions that may affect the manner and timing of death: Refusal of life-sustaining treatment, interventions that may secondarily hasten death, and assisted death.

Refusal of Life-Sustaining Treatment

There is no question that in every state in the United States, competent people (or their surrogates if they are no longer competent) have the legally protected right to withhold or withdraw life-sustaining treatment. It is also unquestionable that physicians, nurses, and other health care providers are ethically and legally able to follow the wishes of a person (or her or his legal designee) to refuse life-sustaining treatment, even if this refusal will likely lead to death (Meisel, 1995; Meisel, Snyder, & Quill, 2000). In fact, it has been estimated that a majority of deaths are preceded by a decision to somehow limit the care that the person receives (*In re L.W.*, 1992). Thus, one of the major decisions facing people who are dying and their loved ones, as well as their health care providers, is whether and when to refuse to start or to continue life-sustaining treatment.

Withholding and withdrawing life-sustaining treatments have long been equated from an ethical perspective. Yet there is evidence that suggests that physicians find withdrawing treatment (once it has been initiated) less preferable to simply withholding it at the outset (Committee on Bioethics, 1994; Singer, 1992; Snyder & Swartz, 1993). One hypothesis about why this might be the case is that it may be easier psychologically for the physician to allow someone to die rather than to take the more active step of stopping treatment and having a resultant death occur (McCamish & Crocker, 1993). A potential risk of preferentially withholding rather than withdrawing treatment, however, is that patients may be influenced not to try a treatment that they might find acceptable. If physicians and patients (or their surrogates) are willing to have treatment withdrawn, it can allow for a trial of treatment when its effectiveness is uncertain. We also note that even though these procedures are legal in all U.S. jurisdictions, states differ in the procedures associated with withholding and withdrawing treatment, so providers must be aware of their states' laws and regulations.

Although the right to refuse life-sustaining treatment is generally accepted in the United States, the psychologist should not assume that all relevant issues are resolved (Kleespies & Mori, 1998). As Kleespies (2004) has indicated, there are a number of critical issues that are still under debate. Thus, for example, there is no consensus on a medical definition of *terminal* (if a time frame is included in the definition). There is also no formal agreement on the criteria for mental competence to make health care decisions. Finally, there is no consensus on how those most vulnerable patients, the incompetent terminally ill who have no family or friends to act as surrogates, can best be represented in end-of-life decisions.

A terminal illness has been defined as an illness for which there is a predictably fatal outcome and for which there is no known cure. Often, this definition is set within a time frame and is limited to cases in which death is expected within 6 months or a year. Medicine, however, is not an exact science, and it is difficult to predict accurately when a patient will die (Mishara, 1999; Thibault, 1997). In one study, for example, only 20% of the physicians who referred patients to a hospice program were accurate in their predictions (with accuracy being defined as between .67 and 1.33 times the actual length of survival; Christakis & Lamont, 2000). Most of the participating physicians (63%) gave predictions that were overly optimistic. Given such findings, it can be argued that it would be less misleading if the definition of terminal illness were not locked into such a time frame. Many treatment providers, however, are heavily influenced by requirements such as those of Medicare that life expectancy be 6 months or less if the patient is to obtain coverage for hospice services.

With regard to determining the capacity to refuse treatment, Grisso and Appelbaum (1998) noted that the following four criteria were most often cited in legal proceedings: (a) the ability to express a choice, (b) the ability to understand information relevant to the illness and proposed treatment, (c) the ability to appreciate the significance of the information disclosed for one's own illness and possible treatment, and (d) the ability to reason with the relevant information and engage in a logical process of weighing treatment options. Not all jurisdictions, however, use all four criteria. Some use various combinations of two or three of these standards. Of course, whether an evaluator uses two, three, or four criteria can make a difference in the threshold for competence or incompetence. A higher threshold may mean that more people are denied the opportunity to make their own decisions, and a lower threshold may mean that fewer vulnerable individuals are protected from their own impaired decision-making abilities. It obviously behooves the psychologist to be aware of which criteria are typically used in the jurisdiction in which she or he practices.

Family members have been recognized in the judicial process as appropriate surrogate decision makers for the incapacitated patient if no health care proxy or guardian has previously been appointed. More problematic, however, are situations in which the patient is terminally ill, lacks capacity to make health care decisions, and has no family or friends to serve as surrogates. In many states, the courts have not taken it on themselves to create a pool of individuals who are readily available to act as guardians for these individuals. The institutional or hospital ethics advisory committee (EAC) has sometimes been asked to fill this void. Yet as Kleespies, Hughes, and Gallacher (2000) have noted, EACs typically consist of hospital staff who, although not part of the patient's treatment team, may identify more with the team than with the patient and who may find it hard not to be influenced by the needs, mores, and values of the institution for which they work. In an era of managed care and efforts at cost containment, this is not a small concern. Given the lack of good alternatives, bioethicists such as Beauchamp and Childress (1979/2001) are of the opinion that the benefits of a good EAC review may outweigh the risks. At the least, it can foster open discussion and debate.

Interventions That May Secondarily Hasten Death

The principle of double effect is often raised in ethical discussions of interventions that may secondarily hasten death. As noted by Kleespies (2004), this ethical principle is taken as justification for performing an act that has a foreseen negative effect (e.g., death) as long as one does not intend the negative effect and only intends a positive effect (e.g., relief from otherwise intractable pain). Battin (1994) has described the four conditions of the principle of the double effect as follows:

> (1) the action must not be intrinsically wrong; (2) the agent must intend only the good effect, not the bad one; (3) the bad effect must not be the means of achieving the good effect; and (4) the good effect must be "proportional" to the bad one, that is, outweigh it. (p. 17)

With the terminally ill client who is suffering, the principle of double effect provides justification for the physician who, for example, prescribes increasing doses of analgesics and sedatives with the intention of easing pain, although a secondary effect might be the slowing of respirations and ending life more quickly. The physician's intent is said to be the relief of suffering, not to kill the patient or assist in the patient's suicide.

The use of double effect reasoning has been disputed in two ways. First, Fohr (1998) has maintained that there is little evidence that the appropriate titration of opioid analgesics hastens death. The implication, then, is that, at least in the case of opioid analgesics, one may not need to think in terms of a double effect. Second, Quill (1993) and Quill, Dresser, and Brock (1997) have questioned whether a physician can always maintain such a clear distinction between intentions as is called for in this principle. Human intentionality is often complex, ambiguous, or even contradictory. Battin (1994) claimed that it is implausible to think that intelligent individuals would not be conscious of both the primary and secondary effects of their decisions, especially if one of those effects is of the magnitude of death. It could, therefore, not be said that they did not in some way intend death to occur.

Some empirical evidence does support the position of Quill and his colleagues and Battin. For example, in a small study on the use of sedatives and analgesics during the withholding and withdrawing of life-sustaining treatment, Wilson, Smedira, Fink, McDowell, and Luce (1992) found that physicians and nurses administered such medications with the intention of hastening death in nearly 40% of the critically ill cases in their sample, but it was never the only reason for doing so. The physicians and nurses concurrently cited relief of pain, anxiety, or air hunger as reasons for using this type and dosage of medication. Proponents of the double effect argument, however, have maintained that it is possible to draw a distinction between "intended results and unintended but accepted consequences" (Annas, 1996, p. 685; see also Sulmasy & Pellegrino, 1999), and, as described later in the chapter, the U.S. Supreme Court also seems to have adopted this position. Given the arguments on both sides of this issue, the dispute over whether the double effect rationale is necessary or sufficient can hardly be said to be settled.

In two cases dealing with the question of a constitutional right to physician-assisted suicide (*Vacco v. Quill*, 1997; *Washington v. Glucksberg*, 1997), the U.S. Supreme Court ruled that there is no constitutional right to physician-assisted suicide but allowed that individual states could make the practice legal or illegal within their own jurisdictions. In the process of articulating the Court's decision, Justices O'Connor and Souter wrote concurrences that approved the use of a practice known as palliative terminal sedation; double effect reasoning was fundamental to their thinking about this issue.

Palliative terminal sedation refers to the use of high doses of sedatives and analgesics to render a consenting patient unconscious as a way of relieving extremes of intractable pain and suffering (Quill & Byock, 2000). The main indications for its use have been to relieve severe physical suffering when all reasonable alternatives have failed. A case example might be that of a person with unbearable head pain secondary to irreversible swelling of the brain. It has also been used to produce unconsciousness before terminal extubation from a ventilator so that the individual does not experience agonal respirations or air hunger. In effect, the person is sedated until there are no signs of pain and discomfort, and, with the person's or surrogate's prior consent, life-sustaining treatments are withheld or withdrawn until death occurs.

There has been considerable discussion about the moral complexity of terminal sedation. Orentlicher (1997) has referred to it as "essentially euthanasia" (p. 1239); whereas Krakauer and colleagues (2000) have argued that there is a difference between terminal sedation and euthanasia, and the difference hinges on the fact that in terminal sedation the physician is titrating the medication to comfort rather than giving a lethal infusion. To say that, in some sense, the physician does not intend the patient's death, however, strains the boundaries of the principle of the double effect.

Yet another practice has gained some acceptance and in which death is hastened: terminal dehydration (also referred to as voluntarily cessation of eating and drinking). In this process, a terminally ill person who is competent and otherwise able to take nourishment makes a voluntary decision to refuse food and fluids. The individual is allowed to die a gradual death by dehydration (Miller & Meier, 1998; Quill & Byock, 2000; Quill, Lo, & Brock, 1997). Ethically and legally, this type of death has been considered an extension of the well-established right to refuse artificial nutrition and hydration under similar circumstances. Such a death is not said to be painful (Ganzini et al., 2003). Often terminally ill people lose their appetites and greatly reduce their food and fluid intake. Any discomfort from the process itself, or from the underlying disease, can usually be managed with standard palliative measures.

This manner of death has been accepted by many hospice and palliative care physicians (Quill et al., 1997). Yet it seems morally complicated in the sense that it blurs the boundary between the refusal of life-sustaining treatment and suicide. The person is, in essence, ending her or his life by intentional inaction.

As Miller and Meier (1998) have pointed out, this sort of death may be relatively painless, but it is not necessarily swift. Depending on the person's physical condition, dying can take anywhere from several days to 3 or 4 weeks. During this time, the dying person can become confused or delirious. In such a compromised state, questions can arise about whether her or his decision remains voluntary. In addition, we do not have some basic information about terminal dehydration—for example, how frequently is it chosen, how often people are successful in carrying it out, and what are the emotional costs and benefits for the individual and her or his family. In short, little is known about this manner of death except by anecdotal account.

Assisted Death

The issue of assisted death is very controversial and potentially distracting from more frequently encountered end-of-life issues. Because there are more comprehensive resources available on this topic (e.g., Kleespies, 2004; Rosenfeld, 2004; Working Group on Assisted Suicide and End-of-Life Decisions, 2000; for the APA's resolution on "assisted suicide," go to http://www.apa.org/pi/eol/activities.html#4), we will not spend a great deal of time on it in this chapter. It is a fact, however, that, although it is only legal in the state of Oregon (Oregon Death With Dignity Act, 1995), assisted death occurs on a regular basis throughout the United States (Emanuel et al., 2000: Meier et al., 1998; Quill, Meier, Block, & Billings, 1998).

Given the advances in our ability to control physical pain, one might ask what, if not pain, gives rise to requests for assistance in dying? Relative to this question, Lavery, Boyle, Dickens, Maclean, and Singer (2001) conducted a small study in which they interviewed persons with HIV disease who considered pursuing assisted suicide or voluntary euthanasia. Two main factors seemed to be associated with such considerations: (a) fear of disintegration and (b) loss of community. Fear of disintegration seemed to refer to the progressive loss of function associated with advancing disease, whereas loss of community seemed to refer to the progressive decline of desire and opportunity to initiate and maintain close personal relationships.

Although the findings of Lavery and colleagues' study can only be regarded as suggestive, they are consistent with observations of terminally ill persons who requested assisted death in Oregon (e.g., Hedberg, Hopkins, & Southwick, 2002; Sullivan, Hedberg, & Hopkins, 2001), in Washington (Back, Wallace, Starks, & Pearlman, 1996), and in the Netherlands (van der Maas, van Delden, Pijnenborg, & Looman, 1991), which indicate that there is a strong psychological or emotional component that is part of the suffering that drives patients to request aid in dying. Thus, when Coombs Lee and Werth (2000) reviewed the experiences of individuals who chose assisted suicide under the Oregon Death with Dignity Act (1995), they found that the majority of the individuals reported that their choices were driven by concern over loss of general control and loss of control over bodily functions.

The essential ethical arguments for and against assisted suicide have been outlined by Battin (1995) and the APA Working Group on Assisted Suicide and End-of-Life Decisions (2000). Those in favor have argued primarily on the basis of the principles of autonomy and mercy or compassion. Autonomy means that the individual has the right to determine, to the extent that it does not interfere with other moral obligations, the course of her or his own life. Dying is a part of the life trajectory and the person also has the right to determine the course and conditions of her or his own death. One objection to this point is that a truly autonomous choice is rarely possible with a dying person because those who are near death are likely to be depressed and otherwise emotionally overwrought. A complicating factor, however, has been that depression, and even other major mental illnesses, have not been found necessarily to preclude competent decision making (Werth et al., 2000; see also chaps. 5 and 6 in this volume; for evidence of this point, see Grisso & Appelbaum, 1998).

The basis of the concern about mercy or compassion is that no one should have to endure pointless and unwanted suffering when she or he is dying. If the physician cannot relieve the patient's suffering by other means and the patient wishes to die to bring her or his agony to an end, the physician should assist the individual in ending her or his life in the most comfortable way. In contrast, as Battin (1995) has noted, opponents of assisted suicide have primarily argued (a) that killing is intrinsically wrong, (b) that assisted suicide puts us on the slippery slope in that it could be abused and vulnerable people could be coerced into accepting it, and (c) that the physician's role as beneficent healer would be compromised if she or he were to engage in bringing about death.

Those who have put forth the first of these points hold that the taking of human life is morally unacceptable; those who disagree note that the taking of life in war and in cases of capital punishment is accepted. If that is so, should it not also be acceptable when it is the choice of a competent, dying person? Those who have been concerned with the slippery slope or potential for abuse issue have argued that cost pressures, insensitivity, and the tendency to follow the easiest course will put physicians and health care institutions at risk of promoting assisted death when it may not be justified. In contrast, Orentlicher (2000; see also Werth, 2000) has pointed out that all of the slippery slope arguments for prohibiting assisted suicide are arguments that apply equally well to the withdrawal or withholding of life-sustaining treatment (where there is also significant potential for abuse). Furthermore, medical ethicists (e.g., Beauchamp & Childress, 1979/2001) seem to believe that the medical community has been able to develop and maintain adequate safeguards in allowing competent patients to refuse life-sustaining treatment. Would this not suggest that assisted suicide could also be regulated to protect against abuses? Finally, with regard to the physician's role, the argument has been that permitting physicians to be involved in assisting in death is a violation of the principles of beneficence and nonmaleficence and will undermine patients' trust in them as healers. Proponents of physician-assisted death (e.g., Jamison, 1997), however, have countered by pointing out that, again, a physician's actions in withdrawing or withholding life-sustaining treatment could also be viewed as violating beneficence and the "do no harm" dictum. In addition, they have argued that many patients might trust their physicians more if they believed that they would not be abandoned to suffer without relief.

The ethical arguments for and against assisted death have often seemed closely matched, and clearly the debate is ongoing. Because physician-assisted death has been legalized in Oregon, the accumulating data about how it is used and about any potential abuses may shed light on this complicated issue, although because much of the debate is based on personal values and moral philosophy, the issue may not be amenable to logical resolution. In any event, although psychologists' roles in helping individuals with these decisions is controversial, there is little debate that providing care for loved ones after the death is an appropriate role for psychologists when requested (Werth, 1999c).

Decisions to Attempt to Prolong Life

Many people who have a terminal illness, or their loved ones, wish to prolong life for as long as possible. They may believe that life, under any conditions, has an intrinsic value, or they may, for various reasons, be unprepared to accept that death is approaching. These individuals, at times, encounter conflict with the health care system when their treatment providers believe that continued efforts at sustaining life should be discontinued.

Futility

Before assisted death entered the limelight, the most controversial end-of-life issue had to do with "futility of treatment." This term refers to the opinion, usually on the part of the treating physician or treatment team, that the individual's medical condition is such that further efforts at acute or curative care will be of no benefit and should be withheld or withdrawn. The debate over futility of treatment has been intensified in modern times by the expectation of some in the medical community that a reduction in allegedly futile treatments near the end of life might help to reduce the nation's escalating health care expenditures, an argument for which there is little hard evidence (Emanuel & Emanuel, 1994; Field & Cassel, 1997).

It is unfortunate efforts to define futility of treatment have not been particularly successful. Definitions have ranged from treatment that will probably only produce an insignificant outcome to treatment that is likely to be more burdensome than beneficial to treatment that has proved useless in the last 100 similar cases (see Beauchamp & Childress, 1979/2001; Kleespies, 2004). No consensus has been reached on any of these definitions, in part because in most medical situations near the end of life, nothing is absolute. Instead, there are probable or likely outcomes that can have different degrees of relevance to the various parties involved. Thus, the dying person, her or his surrogate, the treatment staff, and the hospital administration may all have different definitions and thresholds for what, if anything, is considered "futile" treatment (Truog, Brett, & Frader, 1992).

From the perspective of the patient or consumer, this situation raises serious concerns about whether decisions about futility of treatment will be influenced unduly by the physician's values and biases as opposed to the patient's values and wishes. In fact, there have been several well-known court cases (e.g., the case of Helga Wanglie; Miles, 1991) in which such concerns were at issue and were eventually decided in favor of the person and her or his family. Moreover, it recently has been argued that because of strong evidence about the negative bias of health care providers in evaluations of the quality of life of persons with disabilities (see, e.g., Gill, 2000), the prospect of decision-making based solely on notions of futility is particularly dangerous for disabled people (Werth, in press).

Ethically, the dispute over futility has been between those who invoke the principle of autonomy or self-determination and those who argue for the integrity of the practice of medicine and distributive justice (Finucane & Harper, 1996; Truog, 2000). As noted earlier, when so-called futility cases have gone to court, the courts have almost unanimously ruled on the side of the patient's or surrogate's autonomous choice. Such legal opinions have, in their turn, left health care professionals feeling disenfranchised and as though they have no moral weight in the decision-making process. The demands of medical treatment, however, require the participation of the medical staff and place obligations on them. Do they not have a right to have a significant voice in treatment decisions?

Given that both parties in the futility debate (i.e., the medical staff and the patients) have, at times, felt that they were at risk of being left out of the decision-making process, it has been recommended that definition-based approaches to futility be abandoned in favor of a case-by-case, fair process approach. The approach was formulated by a task force of the Houston Bioethics Network, a consortium of ethics committees from hospitals in the Houston area (Halevy & Brody, 1996). The Houston Policy acknowledges that no policy on futility can be value free and entirely objective. It offers a series of steps for resolving futility dilemmas on an individual case basis. The process gives voice to each of the involved parties (i.e., patient, surrogate, and treatment providers) and requires a thorough institutional review of each case. The physician is not permitted to make unilateral decisions that treatment is futile.

Under the policy, the physician who is of the opinion that treatment is futile must first discuss with the patient or surrogate the nature of the illness or injury, the prognosis, the reasons for considering treatment futile, and the available options, including palliative and hospice care. She or he must clarify that, if the intervention is not provided, the patient will not be abandoned and will be given comfort care and support. The physician is also to present the options of transferring care to another physician or health care institution and of obtaining a second, independent opinion.

If agreement cannot be reached and the patient or surrogate does not wish to arrange transfer, the physician must obtain a second medical opinion and present the case to an institutional review committee (e.g., an ethics advisory committee). The patient or surrogate must be permitted to be present at the case review and encouraged to express her or his views. If the review committee agrees that the treatment is medically inappropriate, the treatment, under this policy, could be discontinued despite the objections of the patient or surrogate. If, however, the review committee does not concur with the physician's opinion about futility, then orders to limit or end interventions would not be accepted as valid.

Although there is considerable support for this type of an approach to futility questions, there is as yet no universal agreement that it is an acceptable way to proceed, and its legal status remains untested. Two states, however, Texas and California, have passed statutes (California Probate Code, 2000; Texas Health and Safety Code, 1999) that allow physicians to write DNR (do not resuscitate) orders over a patient's or surrogate's objections if they follow such a fair process approach.

Allocation of Scarce Health Care Resources

Many people in our society wish to prolong their lives by gaining access to scarce and expensive life-sustaining treatments, those which are not in sufficient supply for all who are in need. Rationing is a method of attempting to allocate such limited resources, and justice demands that it be done in a fair and equitable way. The problem, however, is that no consensus has been established for how such decisions should be made. In fact, deep, value-based divisions may prevent agreement on the relevant criteria.

The need to limit the provision of particular life-sustaining treatments to some people, while excluding others, is exemplified in the field of organ transplantation, which we use here as the primary focus for discussion of allocating scarce resources. As medical technology has improved, the proportion of appropriate transplant candidates has increased, but there has been a persistent shortage of donated organs. This situation led Schmidt (1998) to state that decisions about the allocation of organs are always life-and-death decisions because there will always be someone on the waiting list who is passed over this time and will not make it to the next time. Decisions about who gets an organ transplant can be divided into three stages (Schmidt, 1998). First, the person must be referred for evaluation to a transplant program. Second, she or he must be admitted to the waiting list for such a program. Finally, the person must be selected from the waiting list.

The fact is that much of the selection takes place in the referral stage and the admission to waiting list stage. Yet there has been little information gathered on why some people are referred and others are not, or on why some individuals are accepted to the waiting list and others are not. In one study of racial differences in access to kidney transplants, however, Ayanian, Cleary, Weissman, and Epstein (1999) found that African American patients were less likely than Caucasian patients to want a kidney transplant but, among patients who were very certain that they wanted a transplant, African Americans were substantially less likely to have been referred, to have been placed on a waiting list, or to have received a transplant. The investigators in this study controlled for coexisting illnesses and various other possible confounding factors.

Acceptance to a waiting list for a transplant generally reflects judgments of medical suitability and the prospect of a successful transplant. People tend to be excluded if they have complicating medical conditions such as diabetes or an incurable infection. On a behavioral level, those who are judged as likely to have difficulty with postoperative treatment compliance are often excluded. There are strong negative side effects from the antirejection drugs given after a transplant and a strict postoperative treatment regimen must be followed or the transplanted organ may be lost. If an individual cannot tolerate the side effects and is likely to break the treatment regimen impulsively, some have argued that it is irresponsible to give this person a transplanted organ, especially because there are others who are likely to make better use of it. Others have argued, however, that these judgments are fraught with difficulty because no reliable predictors have been found for postoperative behavior. According to Schmidt (1998), most transplant surgeons will admit that they make subjective judgments in this regard and that they sometimes misjudge a case.

For those who have been put on a waiting list, various principles have been proposed for the allocation of organs. They could be allocated according to who has the greatest medical need, who can pay, who is making the greatest societal contributions, and so forth. In the United States, Beauchamp and Childress (1979/2001) argued that distributive justice requires that such decisions be made on the basis of medical utility (i.e., on the basis of the patient's medical needs and her or his prospects for successful treatment). In general, the Council on Ethical and Judicial Affairs of the American Medical Association has agreed with this position and has specified five factors that may be taken into account in allocation decisions (Clarke et al., 1995): (a) the likelihood of benefit to the patient, (b) the impact of treatment in improving the quality of the patient's life, (c) the duration of benefit, (d) the urgency of the patient's condition, and, in some instances, (e) the amount of resources required for successful treatment. These factors are intended to maximize the number of lives saved, the number of years of life saved, and the quality of life of those saved, while also taking into account the costs involved.

Although the use of these five factors can provide useful guidance, there can be difficulties with each of them and they must be applied with great caution. With the first factor (likelihood of benefit), problems can occur because predictions of outcome in medicine are imprecise. The council (Clarke et al., 1995) therefore recommended that only substantial differences in the likelihood of benefit be considered relevant. Thus, it would be more justifiable to prefer a patient with an 80% chance of graft survival over someone with a 10% chance than it would be to prefer someone with a 60% chance over someone with a 40% chance.

With the second factor, quality of life is a uniquely personal perception (see Kleespies, 2004). The council, however, focused more on improvements in functional status, something that is not necessarily synonymous with how someone assesses improvements in her or his overall quality of life. In terms of the third factor (duration of benefit), it should be noted that it is not always appropriate to give scarce resources to those with the longest expected life span. Such an approach could lead to age-based discrimination, and it is difficult to predict life span on an individual level. The fourth factor (urgency of need) was seen by the council as most applicable in situations of intermittent rather than persistent scarcity. Thus, giving priority to the most urgent cases is justifiable when it comes to intensive care unit (ICU) beds because beds in an ICU turn over rapidly and less urgent cases gain access rapidly. With transplants, however, applying an urgency criterion alone might result primarily in saving those lives that were of extremely poor quality and might have a short duration of life.

Finally, the fifth factor (amount of resources) can become important if resources are limited and the ability of candidates to benefit from those resources is equal, but some patients require fewer resources. Thus, if one had a heart and a liver to transplant and there were three transplant candidates, one of whom needed a liver, one of whom needed a heart, and one of whom needed a heart and a liver, other things being equal, it would save more lives to give priority to the patients who needed only a heart transplant and only a liver transplant. The council cautioned, however, that this criterion should be applied only when it is relatively certain that conserving resources will save more lives.

There are certain potential criteria that the council deemed ethically unacceptable. Although health care in the United States is generally allocated on the basis of the ability to pay, such an ability is not an ethically acceptable criterion when it comes to the need for scarce and life-saving resources. In addition, a person's social worth or contribution to society usually should not be a consideration in allocation decisions. In a pluralistic society, it is difficult to arrive at a definition of social worth. A social worth criterion can also lead to age-based rationing because some might argue that the elderly are no longer making positive contributions to the social good. Such an approach, however, fails to take into account the variation in productivity among older age groups. Finally, factors such as substance abuse, poverty and homelessness, transportation problems, and antisocial or aggressive personality traits should not become criteria for automatically excluding patients from treatment. Rather, the decision makers should consider the possibility of whether rehabilitation or additional support might improve the person's potential to benefit from treatment. The council has cautioned against invoking moral judgments about a patient's behavioral contributions to her or his illness as a basis for allocation decisions.

Summary

A variety of decisions near the end of life involve ethical considerations, and these can lead to dilemmas or disagreements among the dying person, loved ones, and health care professionals. Psychologists who are directly involved with an ill individual, the person's family, or both, as well as psychologists brought in as consultants, must be aware of the various influences on people's considerations and decision making. Although in these situations, the ethical issues are more on the shoulders of the other participants, the psychologist can serve as an important resource and mediator. We also need to emphasize that psychologists are not prevented from being involved in discussions about any of these end-of-life decisions, and therefore they can focus their energy on helping others instead of being concerned about their own ethical responsibilities or limits.

RESOLUTION OF ETHICAL DILEMMAS

We have now at least briefly reviewed several ways that psychologists, or those to whom they are providing services, may be confronted with ethical dilemmas. The nature of a dilemma is such that there is more than one possible response that appears, at least at first, to be plausible, possible, and acceptable (Kitchener, 2000). In such situations, the psychologist could come up with a seat-of-the-pants response that seems to make sense at the time or, if time allows, she or he could consult with at least one other professional. It makes more sense (ethically as well as professionally and legally and in terms of risk management) for the provider to use a comprehensive decision-making model in which the steps are documented and consultation is integrated into the process. There are several such models in the literature (e.g., Cottone & Claus, 2000; Hansen & Goldberg, 1999).

The model that we highlight here was developed and illustrated in the context of service provision for persons with HIV disease (see Anderson & Barret, 2001), and it serves as the basis for an ethical decision-making training sponsored by the APA Office on AIDS. Of specific relevance here is that the model has been applied in cases involving end-of-life situations (e.g.,

Barret et al., 2001b; Eversole et al., 2001) and in other places has been advocated for when end-of-life ethical dilemmas arise (e.g., Werth, 2002). Here we merely highlight the nine steps in the model (Barret et al., 2001a):

1. Pause and identify your personal responses to the case.
2. Review the facts of the case.
3. Conceptualize an initial plan based on clinical issues.
4. Consult agency policies and professional ethical codes to see if your plan is congruent with them.
5. Analyze your plan in terms of the five ethical meta-principles (autonomy, beneficence, nonmaleficence, fidelity, and justice).
6. Identify legal issues.
7. Refine your plan so that it
   - is most congruent with your personal values,
   - advances clinical issues as much as possible,
   - permits you to operate within agency policies and professional ethics codes,
   - minimizes harm to the client and relevant others,
   - maximizes all other ethical principles to the extent possible, and
   - allows you to operate within the law.
8. Choose a course of action and share it with your client.
9. Implement the course of action, then monitor and document the outcomes.

We must emphasize that consultation and documentation (and documentation of the consultation) are important aspects throughout the model.

Barret, Kitchener, and Burris (2001b) used this model to analyze a case involving a client who was considering suicide, and Eversole, Kitchener, and Burris (2001) used the framework to examine boundary issues with a dying client. Werth (2002) suggested that this model held promise for situations in which a psychologist was involved in a case that included end-of-life issues.

CONCLUSION

For a therapist to practice up to the standard of care in any clinical area, she or he must have sufficient knowledge and experience (or supervision, or both). The other chapters in this book provide some of that information with regard to the end-of-life arena. The practitioner must also be aware of the ethical and legal considerations that may or may not constrain her or his work. We have provided an overview of ways that the recent standards in the APA (2002) Ethics Code may be relevant in end-of-life situations and outlined some of the types of end-of-life decisions that dying clients, their loved ones, and their health care providers may need to make that have ethical implications. We hope the interested reader will also review some of the sources we cited for additional information and perspectives.

REFERENCES

American Psychological Association. (1993). Guidelines for providers of psychological services to ethnic, linguistic and culturally diverse populations. *American Psychologist, 48*, 45–48.

American Psychological Association. (2002). Ethical principles of psychologists and code of conduct. *American Psychologist, 57*, 1060–1073.

American Psychological Association. (2003). Guidelines on multicultural education, training, research, practice, and organizational change for psychologists. *American Psychologist, 58*, 377–402.

Anderson, J. R., & Barret, B. (2001). *Ethics in HIV-related psychotherapy: Clinical decision making in complex cases.* Washington, DC: American Psychological Association.

Annas, G. (1996). The promised end: Constitutional aspects of physician-assisted suicide. *New England Journal of Medicine, 335*, 683–687.

Ayanian, J., Cleary, P., Weissman, J., & Epstein, A. (1999). The effect of patients' preferences on racial differences in access to renal transplantation. *New England Journal of Medicine, 341*, 1661–1669.

Back, A. L., Wallace, J. I., Starks, H. E., & Pearlman, R. A. (1996). Physician-assisted suicide and euthanasia in Washington state: Patient requests and physician responses. *Journal of the American Medical Association, 275*, 919–925.

Barret, B., Kitchener, K. S., & Burris, S. (2001a). A decision model for ethical dilemmas in HIV-related psychotherapy and its application in the case of Jerry. In J. R. Anderson & B. Barret (Eds.), *Ethics in HIV-related psychotherapy: Clinical decision making in complex cases* (pp. 133–154). Washington, DC: American Psychological Association.

Barret, B., Kitchener, K. S., & Burris, S. (2001b). Suicide and confidentiality with the client with advanced AIDS: The case of Phil. In J. R. Anderson & B. Barret (Eds.), *Ethics in HIV-related psychotherapy: Clinical decision making in complex cases* (pp. 299–314). Washington, DC: American Psychological Association.

Battin, M. P. (1994). *The least worst death: Essays in bioethics on the end of life.* New York: Oxford University Press.

Battin, M. P. (1995). *Ethical issues in suicide.* Englewood Cliffs, NJ: Prentice Hall.

Beauchamp, T., & Childress, J. (2001). *The principles of biomedical ethics* (5th ed.). New York: Oxford University Press. (Original work published 1979)

Becker, E. (1973). *The denial of death.* New York: Free Press.

Block, S. D. (2000). Assessing and managing depression in the terminally ill patient. *Annals of Internal Medicine, 132*, 209–218.

Braun, K. L., Pietsch, J. H., & Blanchette, P. L. (2000). *Cultural issues in end-of-life decision-making.* Thousand Oaks, CA: Sage.

Breitbart, W., Rosenfeld, B., Pessin, H., Kaim, M., Funesti-Esch, J., Galietta, M., et al. (2000). Depression, hopelessness, and desire for hastened death in terminally ill patients with cancer. *Journal of the American Medical Association, 284,* 2907–2911.

California Probate Code, Section 4736 (West 2000).

Chambless, D. L., Baker, M. J., Baucom, D. H., Beutler, L. E., Calhoun, K. S., Daiuto, A., et al. (1998). Update on empirically validated therapies, II. *The Clinical Psychologist, 51,* 3–16.

Chochinov, H. M., & Breitbart, W. (2000). *Handbook of psychiatry in palliative medicine.* New York: Oxford University Press.

Chochinov, H. M., Wilson, K. G., Enns, M., & Lander, S. (1994). Prevalence of depression in the terminally ill: Effects of diagnostic criteria and symptom threshold judgments. *American Journal of Psychiatry, 151,* 537–540.

Chochinov, H. M., Wilson, K. G., Enns, M., & Lander, S. (1997). "Are you depressed?" Screening for depression in the terminally ill. *American Journal of Psychiatry, 154,* 674–676.

Christakis, N. A., & Lamont, E. B. (2000). Extent and determinants of error in doctors' prognoses in terminally ill patients: Prospective cohort study. *British Medical Journal, 320,* 469–473.

Clarke, O., Glasson, J., Epps, C., Jr., Plows, C., Ruff, V., August, A., et al. (1995). Ethical considerations in the allocation of organs and other scarce medical resources among patients. *Archives of Internal Medicine, 155,* 29–40.

Committee on Bioethics, American Academy of Pediatrics. (1994). Guidelines on forgoing life-sustaining treatment. *Pediatrics, 93,* 532–536.

Connor, S. R., Egan, K. A., Kwilosz, D. M., Larson, D. G., & Reese, D. J. (2002). Interdisciplinary approaches to assisting with end-of-life care and decision making. *American Behavioral Scientist, 46,* 340–356.

Coombs Lee, B., & Werth, J. L., Jr. (2000). Observations on the first year of Oregon's Death With Dignity Act. *Psychology, Public Policy, and Law, 6,* 268–290.

Cottone, R. R., & Claus, R. E. (2000). Ethical decision-making models: A review of the literature. *Journal of Counseling and Development, 78,* 275–283.

Emanuel, E. J., & Emanuel, L. L. (1994). The economics of dying: The illusion of cost savings at the end of life. *New England Journal of Medicine, 330,* 540–544.

Emanuel, E. J., Fairclough, D. L., Clarridge, B. C., Blum, D., Bruera, E., Penley, W. C., et al. (2000). Attitudes and practices of U.S. oncologists regarding euthanasia and physician-assisted suicide. *Annals of Internal Medicine, 133,* 527–532.

Ersek, M., Kagawa-Singer, M., Barnes, D., Blackhall, L. J., & Koenig, B. A. (1998). Multicultural considerations in the use of advance directives. *Oncology Nursing Forum, 25,* 1683–1690.

Eversole, T., Kitchener, K. S., & Burris, S. (2001). Multiple roles with a dying client: The case of Pat. In J. R. Anderson & B. Barret (Eds.), *Ethics in HIV-related psychotherapy: Clinical decision making in complex cases* (pp. 277–297). Washington, DC: American Psychological Association.

Farrell, K. R., & Ganzini, L. (1995). Misdiagnosing delirium as depression in medically ill elderly patients. *Archives of Internal Medicine, 155,* 2459–2464.

Farrenkopf, T., & Bryan, J. (1999). Psychological consultation under Oregon's 1994 Death With Dignity Act: Ethics and procedures. *Professional Psychology: Research and Practice, 30,* 245–249.

Field, M. J., & Cassel, C. K. (Eds.). (1997). *Approaching death: Improving care at the end of life.* Washington, DC: National Academy Press.

Finucane, T., & Harper, M. (1996). Ethical decision-making near the end of life. *Clinics in Geriatric Medicine, 12,* 369–377.

Fisher, C. B. (2003). *Decoding the ethics code: A practical guide for psychologists.* Thousand Oaks, CA: Sage.

Fohr, S. A. (1998). The double effect of pain medication: Separating myth from reality. *Journal of Palliative Medicine, 1,* 315–328.

Ganzini, L., Goy, E. R., Miller, L. L., Harvath, T. A., Jackson, A., & Delorit, M. A. (2003). Nurses' experiences with hospice patients who refuse food and fluids to hasten death. *New England Journal of Medicine, 349,* 359–365.

Genevay, B., & Katz, R. S. (Eds.). (1990). *Countertransference and older clients.* Thousand Oaks, CA: Sage.

Gill, C. J. (2000). Health professionals, disability, and assisted suicide: An examination of relevant empirical evidence and Reply to Batavia. *Psychology, Public Policy, and Law, 6,* 526–545.

Greenstein, M., & Breitbart, W. (2000). Cancer and the experience of meaning: A group psychotherapy program for people with cancer. *American Journal of Psychotherapy, 54,* 486–500.

Grisso, T., & Appelbaum, P. S. (1998). *Assessing competence to consent to treatment: A guide for physicians and other health professionals.* New York: Oxford University Press.

Halevy, A., & Brody, B. (1996). A multi-institution collaborative policy on medical futility. *Journal of the American Medical Association, 276,* 571–574.

Haley, W. E., Allen, R. S., Reynolds, S., Chen, H., Burton, A., & Gallagher-Thompson, D. (2002). Family issues in end-of-life decision making and end-of-life care. *American Behavioral Scientist, 46,* 284–298.

Hallenbeck, J., & Goldstein, M. K. (1999). Decisions at the end of life: Cultural considerations beyond medical ethics. *Generations, 23,* 24–29.

Hansen, N. D., & Goldberg, S. G. (1999). Navigating the nuances: A matrix of considerations for ethical-legal dilemmas. *Professional Psychology: Research and Practice, 30,* 495–503.

Hedberg, K., Hopkins, D., & Southwick, K. (2002). Legalized physician-assisted suicide in Oregon, 2001. *New England Journal of Medicine, 346,* 450–452.

Hickman, S. E. (2002). Improving communication near the end of life. *American Behavioral Scientist, 46,* 252–267.

In re L.W., 482.N.W.2d 60 (Wis. 1992).

Irish, D. P., Lundquist, K. F., & Nelsen, V. J. (Eds.). (1993). *Ethnic variations in dying, death, and grief.* Washington, DC: Taylor & Francis.

Jamison, S. (1997). *Assisted suicide: A decision-making guide for health professionals.* San Francisco: Jossey-Bass.

Kastenbaum, R. (1978). In control. In C. A. Garfield (Ed.), *Psychosocial care of the dying patient* (pp. 227–240). New York: McGraw-Hill.

Katz, R. S., & Genevay, B. (2002). Our patients, our families, ourselves: The impact of the professional's emotional responses on end-of-life care. *American Behavioral Scientist, 46,* 327–339.

Katz, R. S., & Johnson, T. (Eds.). (in press). *When the helping professional weeps: Emotional and countertransference responses in end-of-life care.* New York: Brunner-Routledge.

Kirchberg, T. M., & Neimeyer, R. A. (1991). Reactions of beginning counselors to situations involving death and dying. *Death Studies, 15,* 603–610.

Kitchener, K. S. (1984). Intuition, critical evaluation and ethical principles: The foundation for ethical decisions in counseling psychology. *The Counseling Psychologist, 12*(3), 43–55.

Kitchener, K. S. (2000). *Foundations of ethical practice, research, and teaching in psychology.* Mahwah, NJ: Erlbaum.

Kleespies, P. M. (2004). *Life and death decisions: Psychological and ethical considerations in end-of-life care.* Washington, DC: American Psychological Association.

Kleespies, P. M., Hughes, D., & Gallacher, F. (2000). Suicide in the medically ill and terminally ill: Psychological and ethical considerations. *Journal of Clinical Psychology, 56,* 1153–1171.

Kleespies, P. M., & Mori, D. L. (1998). Life-and-death decisions: Refusing life-sustaining treatment. In P. M. Kleespies (Ed.), *Emergencies in mental health practice: Evaluation and management* (pp. 145–173). New York: Guilford Press.

Knapp, S., & VandeCreek, L. (2003). An overview of the major changes in the 2002 APA ethics code. *Professional Psychology: Research and Practice, 34,* 301–308.

Krakauer, E. L., Penson, R., Truog, R., King, L., Chabner, B., & Lynch, T. (2000). Sedation for intractable distress of a dying patient: Acute palliative care and the principle of double effect. *The Oncologist, 5,* 53–62.

Lavery, J. V., Boyle, J., Dickens, B. M., Maclean, H., & Singer, P. A. (2001). Origins of the desire for euthanasia and assisted suicide in people with HIV-1 or AIDS: A qualitative study. *Lancet, 358,* 362–367.

McCamish, M., & Crocker, N. (1993). Enteral and parenteral nutrition support of terminally ill patients: Practical and ethical perspectives. *Hospice Journal, 9,* 107–129.

Meier, D. E., Emmons, C. A., Wallenstein, S., Quill, T. E., Morrison, R. S., & Cassel, C. K. (1998). A national survey of physician-assisted suicide and euthanasia in the United States. *New England Journal of Medicine, 338,* 1193–1201.

Meisel, A. (1995). *The right to die* (2nd ed.). New York: Wiley.

Meisel, A., Snyder, L., & Quill, T. (2000). Seven legal barriers to end-of-life care. *Journal of the American Medical Association, 284*, 2495–2501.

Miles, S. (1991). Informed demand for "nonbeneficial" medical treatment. *New England Journal of Medicine, 325*, 512–515.

Miller, F. G., & Meier, D. E. (1998). Voluntary death: A comparison of terminal dehydration and physician-assisted suicide. *Annals of Internal Medicine, 128*, 559–562.

Mishara, B. L. (1999). Synthesis of research and evidence on factors affecting the desire of terminally ill or seriously chronically ill persons to hasten death. *Omega, 39*, 1–70.

Nadeau, J. W. (1998). *Families making sense of death.* Thousand Oaks, CA: Sage.

Neimeyer, R. A., Prigerson, H. G., & Davies, B. (2002). Mourning and meaning. *American Behavioral Scientist, 46*, 235–251.

Neimeyer, R. A., & Van Brunt, D. (1995). Death anxiety. In H. Wass & R. A. Neimeyer (Eds.), *Dying: Facing the facts* (3rd ed., pp. 49–88). Philadelphia: Taylor & Francis.

Oregon Death With Dignity Act. (1995). Or. Rev. Stat. §§127.800–127.995.

Orentlicher, D. (1997). The Supreme Court and physician-assisted suicide— rejecting assisted suicide but embracing euthanasia. *New England Journal of Medicine, 337*, 1236–1239.

Orentlicher, D. (2000). The implementation of Oregon's Death With Dignity Act: Reassuring, but more data are needed. *Psychology, Public Policy, and Law, 6*, 489–502.

Quill, T. E. (1993). The ambiguity of clinical intentions. *New England Journal of Medicine, 329*, 1039–1040.

Quill, T. E., & Byock, I. R. (2000). Responding to intractable terminal suffering: The role of terminal sedation and voluntary refusal of food and fluids. *Annals of Internal Medicine, 132*, 408–414.

Quill, T. E., Dresser, R., & Brock, D. (1997). The rule of double effect: A critique of its role in end-of-life decision-making. *New England Journal of Medicine, 337*, 1768–1771.

Quill, T. E., Lo, B., & Brock, D. W. (1997). Palliative options of last resort: A comparison of voluntarily stopping eating and drinking, terminal sedation, physician-assisted suicide, and voluntary active euthanasia. *Journal of the American Medical Association, 278*, 2099–2104.

Quill, T. E., Meier, D. E., Block, S. D., & Billings, J. A. (1998). The debate over physician-assisted suicide: Empirical data and convergent views. *Annals of Internal Medicine, 128*, 552–558.

Rando, T. A. (Ed.). (2000). *Clinical dimensions of anticipatory mourning.* Champaign, IL: Research Press.

Rosen, E. J. (1998). *Families facing death* (rev. ed.). San Francisco: Jossey-Bass.

Rosenblatt, L., & Block, S. D. (2001). Depression, decision making, and the cessation of life-sustaining treatment. *Western Journal of Medicine, 175*, 320–325.

Rosenfeld, B. (2000). Assisted suicide, depression, and the right to die. *Psychology, Public Policy, and Law, 6*, 467–488.

Rosenfeld, B. (2004). *Assisted suicide and the right to die: The interface of social science, public policy, and medical ethics*. Washington, DC: American Psychological Association.

Schmidt, V. (1998). Selection of recipients for donor organs in transplant medicine. *Journal of Medicine and Philosophy, 23*, 50–74.

Singer, P. A. (1992). Nephrologists' experience with and attitudes toward decisions to forego dialysis. *Journal of the American Society of Nephrology, 7*, 1235–1240.

Snyder, J., & Swartz, M. (1993). Deciding to terminate treatment: A practical guide for physicians. *Journal of Critical Care, 8*, 177–185.

Spiro, H. M., Curnen, M. G. M., & Wandel, L. P. (1996). *Facing death*. New Haven, CT: Yale University Press.

Sue, D. W., & Sue, D. (1999). *Counseling the culturally different* (3rd ed.). New York: Wiley.

Sullivan, A., Hedberg, K., & Hopkins, D. (2001). Legalized physician-assisted suicide in Oregon, 1998–2000. *New England Journal of Medicine, 344*, 605–607.

Sulmasy, D. P., & Pellegrino, E. D. (1999). The rule of double effect: Clearing up the double talk. *Archives of Internal Medicine, 159*, 545–550.

Taylor, A., & Box, M. (1999). *Multicultural palliative care guidelines*. Sydney, Australia: Palliative Care Australia. Retrieved March 10, 2004, from http://www.pallcare.asn.au/mc/mccontents.html

Texas Health and Safety Code, Section 166 (1999).

Thibault, G. (1997). Prognosis and clinical predictive models for critically ill patients. In M. Field & C. Cassel (Eds.), *Approaching death: Improving care at the end of life* (pp. 358–362). Washington, DC: National Academy Press.

Truog, R. (2000). Futility in pediatrics: From case to policy. *Journal of Clinical Ethics, 11*, 136–141.

Truog, R., Brett, A., & Frader, J. (1992). The problem with futility. *New England Journal of Medicine, 326*, 1560–1564.

Vacco v. Quill, 117 S.Ct. 2293 (1997).

van der Maas, P., van Delden, J., Pijnenborg, L., & Looman, C. (1991). Euthanasia and other medical decisions concerning the end of life. *Lancet, 338*, 669–674.

Wampold, B. E., Lichtenberg, J. W., & Waehler, C. A. (2002). Principles of empirically supported interventions in counseling psychology. *The Counseling Psychologist, 30*, 197–217.

Washington v. Glucksberg, 117 S.Ct. 2258 (1997).

Werth, J. L., Jr. (1996). *Rational suicide? Implications for mental health professionals*. Washington, DC: Taylor & Francis.

Werth, J. L., Jr. (1999a). Clinical depression and desire for death among persons with terminal illnesses. *Social Pathology, 5*, 22–36.

Werth, J. L., Jr. (1999b). Mental health professionals and assisted death: Perceived ethical obligations and proposed guidelines for practice. *Ethics and Behavior, 9*, 159–183.

Werth, J. L., Jr. (1999c). The role of the mental health professional in helping significant others of persons who are assisted in death. *Death Studies, 23,* 239–255.

Werth, J. L., Jr. (1999d). When is a mental health professional competent to assess a person's decision to hasten death? *Ethics and Behavior, 9,* 141–157.

Werth, J. L., Jr. (2000). How do the mental health issues differ in the withholding/withdrawing of treatment versus assisted death? *Omega, 41,* 259–278.

Werth, J. L., Jr. (2002). Legal and ethical considerations for mental health professionals related to end-of-life care and decision-making. *American Behavioral Scientist, 46,* 373–388.

Werth, J. L., Jr. (in press). Concerns about decisions related to withholding/withdrawing life-sustaining treatment and futility for persons with disabilities. *Journal of Disability Policy Studies.*

Werth, J. L., Jr., Benjamin, G. A. H., & Farrenkopf, T. (2000). Requests for physician assisted death: Guidelines for assessing mental capacity and impaired judgment. *Psychology, Public Policy, and Law, 6,* 348–372.

Werth, J. L., Jr., Blevins, D., Toussaint, K. L. , & Durham, M. R. (2002). The influence of cultural diversity in end-of-life care and decisions. *American Behavioral Scientist, 46,* 204–219.

Werth, J. L., Jr., Burke, C., & Bardash, R. J. (2002). Confidentiality in end-of-life and after-death situations. *Ethics and Behavior, 12,* 205–222.

Werth, J. L., Jr., & Rogers, J. R. (2005). Assessing for impaired judgment as a means of meeting the "duty to protect" when a client is a potential harm-to-self: Implications for clients making end-of-life decisions. *Mortality, 10,* 7–21.

Werth, J. L., Jr., Wright, K. S., Archambault, R. J., & Bardash, R. J. (2003). When does the "duty to protect" apply with a client who has anorexia nervosa? *The Counseling Psychologist, 31,* 427–450.

Wilson, W. C., Smedira, N. G., Fink, C., McDowell, J. A., & Luce, J. M. (1992). Ordering and administration of sedatives and analgesics during the withholding and withdrawal of life support from critically ill patients. *Journal of the American Medical Association, 267,* 949–953.

Winiarski, M. G. (1991). *AIDS-related psychotherapy.* New York: Pergamon.

Working Group on Assisted Suicide and End-of-Life Decisions. (2000). *Report to the Board of Directors.* Washington, DC: American Psychological Association. Retrieved January 25, 2004, from http://www.apa.org/pi/aseolf.html

4

SELF-DETERMINATION, SUBSTITUTED JUDGMENT, AND THE PSYCHOLOGY OF ADVANCE MEDICAL DECISION MAKING

PETER H. DITTO

The human struggle to perfect the art of medicine has been dominated throughout virtually its entire history by a singular goal: to keep people alive as long as possible, using any means available. Life was always a victory. Death was always a defeat.

THE PROBLEM

During the last few decades, however, rapid advances in medical technology have complicated this exclusive focus on extending the quantity of human life. Physicians now have the ability to maintain lives of very low

I gratefully acknowledge the contributions of the ADVANCE Project research team to the ideas expressed in this chapter. Financial support for many of the studies discussed in the chapter was provided by grants from the Agency for Healthcare Research and Quality (HS08180), the Applied Psychology Center at Kent State University, and the Summa Health System Foundation.

quality (e.g., states characterized by little or no cognitive function, or severe and chronic pain), with minimal hope for recovery. These technological advances have brought to the fore an important ethical and practical problem. Can physicians' noble struggle to sustain human life be abandoned in some instances to allow people to die rather than continue living in conditions that many view as "fates worse than death" (Ditto, Druley, Moore, Danks, & Smucker, 1996)?

The answer to this question, of course, involves a complicated web of ethical and legal issues, one of which is a distinction between actively terminating life (e.g., euthanasia or physician-assisted suicide), and more passive measures such as simply not using certain "heroic" treatments that can sustain life in low quality of states (e.g., cardiopulmonary resuscitation or artificial feeding and fluids). This is an important distinction because whereas actively terminating the life of seriously ill individuals has been ethically and legally controversial (President's Commission for the Study of Ethical Problems in Medicine and Biomedical and Behavioral Research [President's Commission], 1983), the latter issue has been much less so. There is consensus in ethical debate and legal decision supporting individual's rights to refuse medical treatment, particularly medical treatments that serve only to prolong life in low-quality states (*Cruzan v. Director, Missouri Department of Health*, 1990; President's Commission, 1983).

At an ethical level then, allowing people to make their own choices about whether to use or forgo life-sustaining medical treatment has presented little problem. Many people say that they do not want treatment to prolong their life when faced with debilitating and incurable illness, and we accept people's right to refuse such treatment. The problem that remains, however, is a practical one. Decisions about whether to use or forgo life-sustaining treatment are typically made only when an individual is very ill and often quite near the end of life. By this time, many patients have already lost the capacity to make (or at least express) choices for themselves (Bradley, Walker, Blecher, & Wettle, 1997). In other words, at exactly the point at which individuals are faced with crucial life-or-death decisions, decisions that are consensually accepted as theirs to make, many people are too sick to make them.

THE SOLUTION

In 1969, attorney Luis Kutner suggested a solution to this problem that he dubbed "the living will." Within a few years, physician William Modell (1974) and philosopher Sissela Bok (1976) made similar proposals. The solution they offered was elegant in its simplicity. If individuals are often too sick to make decisions for themselves near the end of life, they should simply record their preferences for the use of life-sustaining medical treatment *before* they get sick in what has since come to be called an *advance medical directive*, or *advance directive* for short.

As the name implies, an advance directive can be defined as any statement given in advance of decisional incapacity directing the provision of life-sustaining treatment in incapacitated states. Advance directives come in two basic forms. *Proxy advance directives* simply designate a proxy or surrogate decision maker to make decisions for the patient when the person is no longer able (e.g., a durable power of attorney for health care). Such directives convey the legal right to make treatment decisions for an incapacitated patient but do not necessarily contain any explicit guidance regarding what those decisions should be.

The second type of directive, and the one that will be the primary focus of this chapter, is called an *instructional advance directive*. The prototypical example of an instructional directive is Kutner's (1969) living will, in which individuals record some kind of instructions regarding the types of medical care they would like to receive should they become so sick that they can no longer make decisions for themselves. Instructional advance directives vary in their formality, from legal documents prepared with the help of an attorney, to notations made in medical charts (a well-known example being a DNR, or do-not-resuscitate order), to verbal statements made to loved ones or physicians. They also vary in their specificity, from general statements such as "no heroic measures," to statements regarding the general values or goals a patient would like to guide their medical care (e.g., Doukas & McCollough, 1991), to careful delineations of specific medical treatments to be used or withheld in specific medical conditions (e.g., Emanuel, 1991). Regardless of their particular form, all instructional directives share the essential characteristic of making plans for the use of life-sustaining medical treatment in advance of decisional incapacity, and this simple strategy for allowing individuals to maintain control over their medical treatment at the end of life seemed to many people to be just what the doctor ordered.

Indeed, advance directives seemed such a simple solution to a difficult problem, so imminently commonsensical, that it took little more than a decade for advance directives to be institutionalized in American medicine despite the inherent challenge they pose to the generally paternalistic inclinations of the U.S. medical establishment. Advance directives are advocated by virtually every relevant organization including the American Medical Association (Orentlicher, 1990) and the American Association of Retired Persons (1988). Legislation supporting advance directives (instructional, proxy, or both) has been passed in all 50 states and the District of Columbia, and these state laws are reinforced at the federal level by the Patient Self-Determination Act (1990), which stipulates that all hospitals receiving Medicaid or Medicare reimbursement must ascertain whether patients have or wish to have advance directives. Advance directives also enjoy strong support among the general public (Emanuel, Barry, Stoeckle, Ettelson, & Emanuel, 1991).

THE PROBLEM WITH THE SOLUTION

It is remarkable that this institutionalization of advance directives in U.S. law and medical practice has developed in the almost total absence of empirical evidence demonstrating their effectiveness. Over the last decade, a substantial body of policy and law has been fashioned to encourage the use of advance directives with little attention paid to empirical research examining whether they achieve the medical outcomes they are intended to achieve, and even more fundamentally, without any clear agreement in the field regarding *what* outcomes they are intended to achieve.

By way of illustration, compare the development of advance directive policy to how policy might develop around the use of a traditional medical procedure, such as a drug therapy. It is hard to imagine major organizations and legislative bodies endorsing the use of a particular medication in the absence of data to suggest that it accomplished the medical outcome it was intended to accomplish, and without even a clear sense of what outcome it was intended to accomplish. Yet with a behavioral procedure such as the use of advance directives, it all seemed so commonsensical that policy simply leapt forward ahead of science.

The goal of this chapter then is to help science begin to play catch up. In particular, I argue for the crucial role of psychological science in the development of empirically informed policies regarding the use of advance directives. As is so aptly demonstrated in this volume, end-of-life decision making is an inherently psychological affair, and policy and law advocating advance directives rest on a number of psychological assumptions of questionable validity. I begin the chapter by presenting a conceptual analysis of advance directives and making explicit two key psychological assumptions underlying their effective use in end-of-life decision making. I then examine the validity of these assumptions in light of both direct empirical examination as well as a wealth of relevant research and theory from social and cognitive psychology. Although my conclusion is that the psychological foundation of advance directives is a shaky one, I end the chapter by examining the value of a psychological analysis for guiding future research and policy development and hope to demonstrate that by bringing the full force of state-of-the-art psychological science to bear on the problem, the noble goals embodied by the advance directive movement are more likely to be realized.

ADVANCE DIRECTIVES AS ACTS OF COMMUNICATION

Policy and law advocating advance directives flows directly from a belief in the ethical priority of *self-determination* in medical decision making (*Cruzan v. Director, Missouri Department of Health*, 1990; Dresser, 2003; President's Commission, 1983). The fundamental right of individuals to control decisions about the important outcomes in their lives, especially regarding their own bodily integrity, is well founded in U.S. law and embodied by the traditional American values of personal liberty and the right to privacy. Not only are these rights generally acknowledged as giving competent patients the freedom to refuse any form of medical treatment (even if that treatment is necessary to sustain their life), but ethicists and legal scholars are equally well agreed that the right to self-determination is not diminished when a formally competent individual becomes decisionally incapacitated because of illness or injury (Dresser, 2003).

Yet how can individuals who are currently incompetent make decisions for themselves when they, by definition, lack the ability to do so? The key is a process that has come to be referred to as *substituted judgment* (Baergen, 1995; President's Commission, 1983). Substituted judgment is the process of making decisions for another person that the person would make for himself or herself if able. In that way, the interpersonal judgment can be substituted for the personal one, and the incapacitated individual can maintain, through the vehicle of a surrogate decision maker (e.g., a loved one or physician), the ability to express choices even though he or she currently lacks decision making capacity.

The substituted judgment standard is consensually accepted as a more desirable method of making decisions for incapacitated patients than, for example, making decisions on the basis of the surrogate's contemporaneous beliefs about what is in the patient's best interest (Buchanan & Brock, 1990; President's Commission, 1983). The logic of this order flows precisely from the ethical priority accorded to patient self-determination. Rather than representing the surrogate's beliefs about what is best for the patient, the substituted judgment standard directs surrogate decision makers to remove their own wishes from the decision-making process and strive only to represent the patient's preferences regarding the use of life-sustaining medical treatment.

The same logic that makes the substituted judgment standard the preferred method of surrogate decision making, however, is what makes it such a difficult standard to meet. If substituted judgment is to achieve its goal of maintaining the incapacitated individual's control over treatment decisions, it is not enough that the surrogate decision maker try, in good faith, to represent the patient's wishes. Substituted judgment can only maintain patient autonomy if the surrogate is successful in accurately representing the choices the incapacitated person would make for himself or herself if able. As such, reliance on substituted judgment in end-of-life decision making assumes that the surrogate decision maker has an intimate understanding of the patient's preferences regarding the use of life-sustaining medical treatment and can use that understanding to mimic the patient's choices in any medical eventuality that might arise.

How, though, are surrogates supposed to gain the understanding necessary to accurately recreate patients' treatment decisions? This is where advance directives enter the picture. Advance directives (in particular, instructional advance directives) are intended as the medium through which the surrogate comes to understand the patient's preferences for the use of life-sustaining medical treatment. That is, although advance directives are typically viewed as legal documents or medical procedures, they are most fundamentally *acts of communication* (Ditto et al., 2001). The central goal of an advance directive is to communicate the wishes of the (currently) incapacitated patient to surrogate decision makers faced with the difficult task of making the medical decisions for the patient that the patient would have made for himself or herself if able. It is only if this communication process is negotiated successfully that advance directives can achieve their intended goal of maintaining the decisional autonomy of incapacitated patients.[1]

Two Assumptions

Making explicit the essential links between patient self-determination, substituted judgment, and the communicative function of advance directives serves to highlight the complicated set of psychological processes involved in effective end-of-life medical decision making. Specifically, policy and law advocating instructional advance directives as a means of honoring incapacitated patients' wishes about the use of life-sustaining medical treatment rests on two key psychological assumptions.

The first and most general assumption is that instructional advance directives improve the ability of surrogate decision makers to predict accurately incapacitated patients' preferences for life-sustaining medical treatment. I call this the *communication assumption* because accurate substituted judgment is the essential evidence that an instructional advance directive has served the communicative function that is its raison d'être. Surrogates cannot honor a patient's wishes if they do not understand them. When instructional advance directives are advocated as a way of honoring patient's wishes, the underlying assumption is that the directive will communicate the patient's wishes to the surrogate in a way that will allow the surrogate to make the same decisions for the patient that the patient would make for himself or herself.

---

[1]In their influential analysis of the ethical basis of surrogate decision making, Buchanan and Brock (1990) distinguished between three standards for making decisions for others: the best interest standard, the substituted judgment standard, and the advance directive standard. Separation of the latter two, however, implies that somehow an advance directive can speak *directly* for the patient, without interpretation. I believe that it makes more conceptual (and certainly more psychological) sense to fold the advance directive standard into the substituted judgment standard, as I do in this analysis. Any advance directive, no matter how specific and detailed, must be interpreted by others (whether it be the incapacitated patients' loved ones or a physician) before action based on that information can be initiated. Thus, it makes more psychological sense, I would argue, to view advance directives as informing substituted judgment, rather than conceiving of the advance directive standard as separate from (and in Buchanan and Brock's analysis, preferable to) the substituted judgment standard.

This communication assumption, however, itself rests on an even more fundamental assumption about the ability of individuals to predict their *own* preferences for future medical treatment. Substituted judgment is a process of *interpersonal* prediction in which a surrogate decision maker attempts to use whatever information he or she is able to gather from the currently incapacitated patient's past life as an autonomous agent, potentially including the patient's instructional advance directive, to predict how that patient would want to be treated in the current state of serious illness. It is important to note, however, that any preferences the patient might have stated prior to the current debilitating illness (including any preferences stated in an instructional advance directive) are themselves merely predictions. That is, treatment preferences stated in a living will are best construed as *intrapersonal* predictions that relatively healthy individuals make about how they believe they would want to be treated if they were to become seriously ill. Like any other predictions, predictions made in a living will can be right or wrong, and this possibility introduces an additional complication into decisions guided by advance directives. Preferences stated in an advance directive can only further the cause of improving surrogate substituted judgment if the patient is able to anticipate her or his own unique personal reactions to future disease states and predict accurately whether she or he would want to receive or forgo various life-sustaining treatments if she or he were to experience such states.

Said in another way, a second key assumption underlying the use of instructional advance directives is that preferences for life-sustaining medical treatment remain stable over time and across changes in the individual's physical, psychological, and social condition. This *stability assumption* is what puts the "advance" in advance directives. If treatment preferences change substantially over time or with changes in an individual's life condition, then wishes stated months or years before an incapacitating illness may misrepresent the patient's current treatment wishes and consequently misinform a surrogate attempting to use those prior preferences as input into their substituted judgments.[2]

TESTING THE COMMUNICATION AND STABILITY ASSUMPTIONS

Policy and laws advocating advance directives assume that advance directives effectively communicate patients' life-sustaining treatment wishes

---

[2]Emanuel (1994) has argued that advance directives should not be taken as representing the individual's current wishes for treatment because incompetent individuals are, by definition "wishless." Even if one accepts this argument, the issue of stability is still important because one would want decisions to reflect the most recent version of an individual's prior wishes. That is, Emanuel's argument changes the issue only slightly to concern not whether an advance directive completed at some point in the past reflects an incapacitated individual's "current" wishes for treatment, but whether it represents the wishes he or she would have stated immediately prior to incapacitation.

and that patients' wishes remain stable over time; however, each of these assumptions has now received direct examination in the burgeoning literature on end-of-life decision making and each is representative of broader issues that have received considerable empirical and theoretical attention by social, cognitive, and health psychologists. In the sections that follow, I take up each of these assumptions in turn and briefly review the research bearing on them. Because these assumptions apply primarily to instructional rather than proxy advance directives, the following discussion focuses primarily on living wills.

The Accuracy of Substituted Judgment

Many studies have examined the ability of potential surrogate decision makers to predict accurately patients' wishes regarding the use of life-sustaining medical treatment (e.g., Uhlmann, Pearlman, & Cain, 1988). Of course, the ideal method of examining this question is impossible. Incapacitated patients cannot be awakened and queried about whether their surrogates' beliefs about their treatment wishes are consistent with their actual wishes. Instead, studies have examined the accuracy of surrogate-substituted judgment by having surrogates predict the wishes of fully competent "patients" in what can best be described as a kind of end-of-life *Newlywed Game*. That is, just as in the old television game show in which couples tried to predict how their partners would respond to a given question, a host of studies have been conducted in which an individual records his or her treatment preferences for various end-of-life scenarios, and a surrogate decision maker (e.g., a loved one or physician) is asked to try to predict those preferences. These studies have used a number of end-of-life scenarios (e.g., irreversible coma, end-stage cancer, debilitating stroke) and examined predictions for a number of life-sustaining treatments (e.g., cardiopulmonary resuscitation, artificial feeding and fluids, blood transfusion), but the results have been remarkably consistent. Studies have repeatedly shown that whether it be physicians or nurses predicting one of their patient's wishes or individuals predicting the wishes of a family member, surrogates can seldom predict a patient's life-sustaining treatment wishes at levels of accuracy that exceed those expected from chance guessing (Baergen, 1995; Uhlmann et al., 1988).

This research has often been taken as support for the necessity of living wills on the basis of the assumption that allowing a surrogate to read a patient's advance directive would improve the accuracy of the surrogate's predictions (Baergen, 1995). This, of course, is an empirical question and as such is the acid test of the efficacy of instructional advance directives. If the communication assumption is correct, then surrogates exposed to a patient-completed instructional directive should be significantly more accurate in their ability to predict that patient's life-sustaining treatment wishes than surrogates who make their predictions without the benefit of exposure to the directive.

This issue was addressed by Ditto et al. (2001) in a randomized controlled trial examining surrogate accuracy after four advance directive interventions. Participants in the study were 401 older adults (outpatients at a network of family practices who were selected solely on the basis of their being older than 65 years) and each of these patients' self-designated surrogate decision makers (defined for the patients as "the individual you would want to make medical decisions for you if were no longer able"). Patients in the intervention conditions were randomly assigned to complete one of two types of instructional directives. To capture the range of possible advance directive strategies, some participants completed a traditional "disease and treatment" living will (Emanuel, 1991) in which patients indicated their desire to receive or forgo a list of several life-sustaining treatments in a number of end-of-life medical scenarios, and other participants completed a value-based or "function and outcome" living will (derived from a cognitive model of health-state evaluations posited by Ditto et al., 1996) in which patients generated a list of the activities that were so important to their quality of life that they would not want to continue living if they could not engage in them. In addition, some patients completed these directives alone, and the directives were then given to their self-designated surrogate decision makers (almost all of whom were either spouses or children of the patient), but other patients actually completed the directives together with their surrogate and were encouraged to discuss the reasoning behind their choices with their surrogates as they went along. The key outcome measure was the surrogates' ability to predict patients' preferences for four life-sustaining treatments in nine end-of-life scenarios. Accuracy in the intervention conditions was compared with the accuracy of a control group of patient–surrogate pairs in which the surrogates made their predictions without the benefit of exposure to a patient-completed advance directive (characteristic of past research on the accuracy of substituted judgment).

The results of the study could not have been more clear and consistent. Surrogates provided with either type of directive were no more accurate in their predictions of patients' desires for life-sustaining treatment than were surrogates making predictions without the benefit of a directive. This was true for every scenario and treatment examined and was consistent across a number of analyses examining the interventions' effectiveness within various patient and surrogate subgroups. Most striking, however, was the ineffectiveness of the discussion intervention in improving the accuracy of substituted judgment. The ineffectiveness of an advance directive document alone to improve surrogate decisions might have been expected, based on past writings skeptical of the usefulness of written directives in the absence of a broader process of advance care planning (Emanuel, Danis, Pearlman, & Singer, 1995). More surprising was the finding that allowing surrogates to discuss an advance directive with the patient immediately before the predictive task similarly produced no improvement in the accuracy of surrogates' substituted judgment relative to the control (no advance directive) condition.

The results of the Ditto et al. (2001) study represent a significant challenge to the first key assumption underlying the effective use of instructional advance directives by suggesting that living wills are not necessarily effective in communicating one's treatment wishes to others. Although these results should certainly not be taken to suggest that no method of advance directive documentation or discussion can improve the accuracy of surrogate-substituted judgment, the fact that surrogate judgment showed significant inaccuracy even under the relatively ideal situations created in this study (e.g., possession of a thorough living will supplemented by a structured patient–surrogate discussion) suggests that improving the ability of surrogate decision makers to honor their loved one's end-of-life treatment wishes is considerably more daunting a task than has been previously assumed.

Indeed, the ineffectiveness of advance directives to improve surrogate judgment found in the Ditto et al. (2001) study suggests that there are likely additional psychological barriers that may undermine the effectiveness of advance directives in surrogate decision making. A quick perusal of the psychological literature produces a number of likely suspects. Cognitive psychologists, for example, have found that people often have considerable difficulty perceiving similarities between two story problems and are unable to use the solution provided in the first problem to solve a second, similar problem (Gick & Holyoak, 1980). The use of living wills in surrogate decision making is similarly an exercise in information transfer, and given the unfamiliarity and complexity of the issues surrounding end-of-life medical decisions, one might expect transfer to be especially difficult in this domain.

More generally, a long tradition of research in social psychology has documented a host of errors and biases that characterize interpersonal judgments (Nisbett & Ross, 1980), and these biases are particularly likely to reveal themselves under conditions of uncertainty such as those surrounding end-of-life medical decisions. For example, adhering to the substituted judgment standard requires surrogates to concern themselves only with discerning those treatments that the patient wants, regardless of surrogates' own personal preferences or any beliefs surrogates might hold about what will best promote the patient's well-being (Baergen, 1995). Social psychological research, however, has long reported the difficulty people have in separating their own traits, attitudes, and wishes from their perceptions of others (e.g., Holmes, 1968). Specifically, one of the most replicated findings in the social perception literature is that people overestimate the extent to which their own opinions and behavioral choices are shared by others (e.g., Mullen & Hu, 1988). That is, people "project" their own characteristics onto others as they assume that the majority of people are likely to behave and believe as they do.

My research group examined this tendency in the context of end-of-life decisions by having surrogates predict patients' treatment preferences in a variety of medical scenarios and recording surrogates' own preferences in those same scenarios as well (Fagerlin, Ditto, Danks, Houts, & Smucker, 2001). In two studies using different populations of patient–surrogate pairs, surrogates were found to show a disproportionate tendency to make errors of projection (i.e., mispredict that the patient had the same treatment preference that they themselves did in a given scenario). In fact, surrogates' predictions of the patients' preferences were consistently found to be more similar to their own preferences than to those of the patients. Evidence of projection bias has been found in physicians' predictions of their patients' wishes as well (Schneiderman, Kaplan, Pearlman, & Teetzel, 1993). These results highlight the difficulty that surrogate decision makers are likely to have in separating their own personal preferences from those of the patients whose wishes they are attempting to honor. They also provide just one example of how the basic social psychological literature on judgmental bias can be fruitfully applied to the problem of identifying potential sources of error in surrogate medical decision making.

The Durability of Life-Sustaining Treatment Wishes

Implicit in the preceding discussion of surrogate inaccuracy is that to the extent that surrogates' predictions deviate from patients' actual preferences, it is the surrogate who is at "fault." In any case of misprediction, the predictor would seem the obvious place to start the search for sources of error; in this case, however, it is worth considering that at least part of the problem may be more fundamental.

Stated another way, surrogates can only be expected to predict patients' preferences for end-of-life treatment as well as patients can predict their own. The very task of having surrogates attempt to predict patients' life-sustaining treatment preferences assumes that patients have genuine, authentic preferences that remain stable over time and across decision context. To the extent that a patient's preferences change over time or are significantly affected by transitory aspects of the decision context such as the patient's physical condition or emotional state, the surrogate's task becomes considerably more difficult as he or she is faced with the problem of trying to hit the proverbial "moving target." Thus, questions about the stability of life-sustaining treatment preferences over time are crucial to placing the problem of surrogate inaccuracy in its appropriate context. In fact, the stability issue is really the psychological lynchpin of the entire enterprise of encouraging the use of advance directives in end-of-life medical decision making. If individuals cannot generate preferences for life-sustaining treatment that remain stable over time and across changes in health and decision context, then the appropriateness of policies encouraging healthy individuals to decide how they would like to be treated in future states of incapacitating illness must be questioned.

A number of studies have examined the extent to which preferences for life-sustaining treatment remain stable over time (e.g., Danis, Garrett, Harris, & Patrick, 1994; Ditto et al., 2003). Like studies of surrogate predictive accuracy, participants are asked to record their preferences for various life-sustaining treatments in hypothetical medical scenarios. After a designated time interval (from a few months to 2 years), participants are asked to record their preferences again, and the concordance of these wishes between measurements is examined.

In a recent review of these studies (Jacobson, Ditto, Coppola, Danks, & Smucker, 2005), my research group conducted a meta-analysis that included 11 such studies (a few more were identified but could not be included in analyses because they did not report the necessary data) and found that the average stability of life-sustaining treatment preferences across all judgments and all studies was 71% (the range of overall stability levels across studies was 57% to 89%). Drawing simple conclusions from this figure is complicated by the fact that our analyses also identified a number of factors moderating levels of stability such as the nature of the treatment decision (preferences to refuse treatment tended to be more stable than preferences to receive treatment), the severity of the medical scenario (preferences were more stable for scenarios describing the most and least serious medical conditions than for more moderate scenarios), and certain characteristics of the participants (e.g., individuals who had completed advance directives had more stable preferences than individuals who had not). The important point for the current purposes, however, is the general one that life-sustaining treatment preferences show substantial instability over time, with typically about one third of preferences stated at any given point being expected to change within time periods as short as 2 years.

Of course, change in treatment preferences over time is not inherently problematic. A person may change his or her preferences for considered reasons on the basis of new information or personal experience (e.g., a friend's or relative's experience with life-sustaining treatment). Although such a person would be expected to be cognizant of the change in preferences and, consequently, to review and update his or her living will accordingly, preference change is more of a problem if an individual's preferences change without any awareness of the change. Importantly, my research group has found evidence that life-sustaining treatment preferences often change without awareness (Gready et al., 2000). The study followed a sample of older adults over 2 years and measured both actual change in life-sustaining treatment preferences and participants' perception of whether their preferences had changed. For every judgment examined, the majority of participants whose preferences had actually changed over the 2 years were unaware of this change; that is, they mistakenly believed that the preferences they stated during the second interview were identical to those stated during their first interview.

Although this finding may seem surprising at first blush, it is actually quite consistent with numerous studies in the psychological literature demonstrating a tendency for people to overestimate the stability of their attitudes and beliefs over time (e.g., Markus, 1986). In fact, a long tradition of social psychological research suggests that attitudes and preferences are often constructed "online" rather than accessed from a stable set of values and considered priorities (Slovic, 1995). Individuals are unlikely to be sensitive to changes in constructed preferences because there is no memory of past preferences that can be accessed to compare with one's current opinion. This should be particularly true with regard to topics such as life-sustaining medical treatment about which individuals have little concrete information or direct experience.

To the extent that a preference is constructed at the time it is expressed, it is also likely to be dependent on the context in which it is made. This context-dependency also seems to be characteristic of life-sustaining treatment preferences. For example, like other types of medical (McNeil, Pauker, Sox, & Tversky, 1982) and nonmedical judgments (Tversky & Kahneman, 1981), life-sustaining treatment preferences have been found to be dramatically affected by small changes in the way the eliciting questions are framed (Forrow, Taylor, & Arnold, 1992). More important, experience with illness has also been shown to change preferences for life-sustaining treatment (Danis et al., 1994; Ditto, Jacobson, Smucker, Danks, & Fagerlin, 2004). In the clearest demonstration of this phenomenon, Ditto, Jacobson, et al. used a prospective design to examine the life-sustaining treatment preferences of participants who were hospitalized for at least 48 hours during the course of a 2-year study. Upon their release from the hospital, participants' preferences were assessed and could then be compared with those stated at annual interviews conducted before and several months after the hospitalization. This comparison revealed that participants' desires for life-sustaining treatment showed a significant "hospitalization dip." Specifically, participants reported less desire to receive life-sustaining treatment immediately after hospitalization than they had prior to hospitalization. If we were to consider just these two data points, one might suspect that confrontation with the discomforts of hospitalization caused an enduring change in participants' attitudes about the value of extending life through aggressive medical treatment. Instead, patients' change in preferences was found to be fleeting, with desire for life-sustaining treatment returning to near pre-hospitalization levels at the annual interview conducted at least 3 months after hospitalization. The fact that preferences solicited in the immediate aftermath of hospitalization did not remain stable, but returned to pre-hospitalization levels in the months after the event, suggests that life-sustaining treatment preferences are dependent in an important way on the current context in which they are made.

Research showing that life-sustaining treatment preferences change over time and are dependent on decision context coincides nicely with a growing body of social psychological studies documenting more general difficulties people seem to have predicting their future preferences, behavior, and emotions (e.g., Loewenstein & Schkade, 1999). This new field of "affective forecasting" has provided evidence for a number of systematic biases in people's predictions of how they are likely to react to future events. For example, people often hold inaccurate theories about what makes them happy or sad (Loewenstein & Schkade, 1999); underestimate the impact that subtle, everyday events have on their overall well-being (Schkade & Kahneman, 1998); and fail to appreciate their own ability to adapt to negative life events (Gilbert, Pinel, Wilson, Blumberg, & Wheatley, 1998). As such, this body of work raises significant doubts about the wisdom of asking people to make predictions regarding how they are likely to behave or choose in future situations, particularly to the extent that that future situation is dramatically different from the individual's current life situation. This, of course, is exactly the psychological act that one is asked to perform in an instructional advance directive.

IS THE LIVING WILL DEAD?

To summarize the material presented so far, policy and law advocating the use of instructional advance directives is based on the assumptions that living wills improve the ability of surrogates to understand (and therefore honor) patients' end-of-life wishes and that patients are able to state wishes in their living wills that will reflect accurately the decisions they will want made for them if they become too ill to make decisions for themselves. Empirical research directly examining each of these assumptions, however, raises significant doubts about their validity. Surrogates have considerable difficulty predicting patients' wishes for life-sustaining treatment even when they have seen and discussed an instructional directive completed by the patient. Life-sustaining treatment preferences show substantial instability even over relatively short periods of time and are dependent on the state of the individual at the time the preferences are solicited. A review of the general psychological literature also raises fundamental doubts about the ability of individuals to meet the psychological demands underlying the effective use of advance directives. A long tradition of research on biases in interpersonal perception suggests that surrogate accuracy may be undermined by difficulties transferring information from living wills to actual end-of-life decisions and by persistent biases in social judgment. A more recent but increasingly substantial body of research on affective forecasting raises similar questions about the ability of individuals to predict their own future wishes and suggests that individuals' attempts to make advance decisions are also likely to be prone to bias and error.

There is a story often recounted about Lyndon Johnson, who when he took over the presidency after John F. Kennedy's assassination was left with a group of advisors heavily populated with Ivy League academic types. After allowing these advisors to spout their statistics and voice their abstract theoretical concerns, President Johnson liked to respond with a parsimonious but insightful question, "Therefore, what?" Johnson wanted to know how all the elegant research and theory might be translated into an effective and feasible course of action. It is this challenge that I take up in the final sections as I sketch and evaluate a few possible answers to President Johnson's query as it relates to research on instructional advance directives.

Abolish Advance Directives?

The first and most draconian conclusion one might draw from the research reviewed thus far is that the psychological obstacles facing the effective use of instructional advance directives are insurmountable, and so the policy of encouraging their use should be abandoned. I believe such a drastic conclusion, however, is premature for a number of reasons.

First, it ignores the possibility that the same theory and research that has identified important problems with end-of-life decision making can be used to point the way toward possible solutions to those problems. I take up this issue more fully in the next section.

Second, despite their problems as communicators of individual's end-of-life wishes, there is evidence that the process of completing and discussing advance directives provides psychological benefits for patients and their loved ones. The Ditto et al. (2001) study, for example, found that the discussion interventions produced in both patients and surrogates a sense of mutual understanding and comfort with end-of-life decision making. In another study, the presence of an advance directive reduced stress and increased positive emotion among family members who had recently decided to withdraw the life support of a loved one (Tilden, Tolle, Nelson, & Fields, 2001).

Finally, although instructional directives may not improve decisions made by family members, there is evidence that they are more effective in improving the accuracy of decision makers with little or no past relationship with the patient. In a satellite project of the Ditto et al. (2001) study, Coppola, Ditto, Danks, and Smucker (2001) examined whether living wills improved the predictive accuracy of the patients' primary care physicians and a group of hospital-based (e.g., emergency room) physicians who had had no prior contact with the patient. As with family surrogates, neither directive improved the accuracy of primary care physicians. The predictions of hospital-based physicians, which generally showed lower accuracy than those of both family surrogates and primary care physicians, improved significantly when these physicians read the disease-and-treatment-based directive. These data suggest that although living wills hold little value for decision makers well acquainted with the patient, they may be more helpful when decisions fall to individuals, such as estranged family members or emergency room physicians, who have little prior relationship with the patient.

Build a Better Living Will

These data suggest that there is hope—a pulse—for living wills. As such, it may be possible to resuscitate them and construct a better living will by building on the accumulating body of relevant theory and research in the medical and psychological literatures. It is important to recognize that the Ditto et al. (2001) study is perhaps most valuable in laying out an approach for evaluating the effectiveness of instructional advance directives. The trial itself examined only two of the many varieties of existing advance directives. Similarly, the discussion intervention, although intensive, was a brief, single-session affair with neither an underlying theoretical focus nor an explicit educational component. It is certainly possible that more effective methods of improving the accuracy of surrogate decision making can be developed. It is crucial in this regard, however, that these methods be constructed on the basis of state-of-the-art research in communication and social cognition rather than the mixture of common sense and political consensus that has guided the development of many current advance directive documents (e.g., living will forms developed by state legislatures).

Moreover, new approaches must move beyond the idea of simple documents to develop a more comprehensive process of advance care planning (Emanuel et al., 1995). One element of this is situating the completion of any living will document within an ongoing series of discussions that includes both family members and medical professionals. Also important, however, is developing ways to help people document life-sustaining treatment preferences that are likely to be more durable over time and across changes in health status. For example, psychological research has begun to identify some conditions under which people are better or worse at predicting future emotional reactions (Wilson, Kraft, & Dunn, 1989), and this research might form the basis for techniques to improve the quality of people's predictions of their future treatment preferences. Technological advancements, such as the use of interactive video (or even virtual reality) simulations might also have potential to help individuals imagine possible end-of-life scenarios in more vivid and realistic ways. Finally, as research continues to document the trajectory of changes in life-sustaining treatment preferences over time, it can be used to develop sensible policies for how to interpret instructional advance directives once completed. For example, along with the current legal requirement that patient's advance directive status be checked upon hospital admission (Patient Self-Determination Act, 1990), a simple provision could be added requiring that the date of any documented directive be checked and that "expired" directives (e.g., directives completed too long ago or when the individual was in a dramatically different state of health) be discussed and recompleted.

Self-Determination Revisited

There is certainly potential to develop empirically based policies to improve the ability of incapacitated patients to maintain control over their own treatment decisions. Before we proceed too far down this path, however, it is worth considering whether this goal is as important to everyday people as it clearly has been to the ethicists and policymakers who have been the driving force in the advance directive movement.

For example, despite years of enthusiastic advocacy by major health care organizations and the widespread passage of state and federal law encouraging their use, relatively few Americans complete advance directives. Although approximately 80% of American adults report having an estate will (Emanuel et al., 1991), fewer than 25% are estimated to have an advance directive (Eiser & Weiss, 2001). Completion rates are even lower for many ethnic groups (Morrison, Zayas, Mulvihill, Baskin, & Meier, 1998), and even individuals with chronic illnesses show rates of advance directive completion that are generally only slightly greater than rates observed in nonpatient populations (Holley, Stackiewicz, Dacko, & Rault, 1997).

Similarly, a number of recent studies have found that people facing real decisions about end-of-life treatment seem less concerned with the ability to predict specific treatment decisions than they are with gaining a general sense of control over the dying process and reducing the burden on surrogate decision makers (Ditto et al., 2001). Many patients are quite satisfied leaving end-of-life medical decisions to their families (Holley et al., 1997) and feel comfortable letting surrogates override their living wills if the surrogate thinks it is in their best interest (Sehgal et al., 1992). Because some individuals are aware that they cannot have all the facts regarding their illness when they are completing their living will, they prefer that someone who has the information to make the decision would reflect their best interest at the time the decision must be made (Terry et al., 1999).

All of this suggests a quite different picture of end-of-life decision making than that portrayed in the opening sections of this chapter. Policy and law advocating advance directives have always been motivated by the perceived desire of incapacitated patients to maintain control over their own medical decisions (hence the name, Patient Self-Determination Act). Rather than yearning to micromanage their own deaths; however, research increasingly suggests that many people are more interested in delegating control over end-of-life decisions to those they trust. Such people may be unconcerned about whether their surrogates can predict with precision their responses to hypothetical end-of-life scenarios, and in fact may be quite aware that they have trouble predicting their own wishes in such situations as well.

Recognizing that the desire for specific control over end-of-life decisions is not a universal goal requires that we broaden our view of how to evaluate the effectiveness of advance directives. Additional research is needed to examine individual and cultural variations in what people perceive as the desired outcomes of advance care planning and how the process can be tailored to meet these expectations. This research is likely to find that proxy directives (e.g., durable powers of attorney for health care) may be a more desirable approach than instructional directives for many people. More generally, we have suggested that people may often be more interested in advance directives documenting how end-of-life decisions should be made and who should make them (what we have termed *process preferences*) than in traditional directives cataloging more specific treatment preferences (Hawkins, Ditto, Danks, & Smucker, 2005). Such process directives might strike an ideal balance between individuals' desire to exert some general level of control over the care they receive near the end of life and their desire to delegate the specific decisions made to individuals they trust to have their best interests at heart and all the relevant facts in hand when the time to make the final decision arrives.

CODA

The institutionalization of advance directives in American medicine stands in stark contrast to a growing body of research questioning the psychological assumptions on which advance directives are based. Because research has raised significant doubts about the ability of instructional directives to fulfill their promise of helping to honor the wishes of dying patients, blanket endorsements such as those offered by the American Medical Association (Orentlicher, 1990) and others are clearly premature.

It is equally clear, however, that more research is sorely needed before specific alternative policies for guiding end-of-life decision making can be proposed. The discussion of practical recommendations in this chapter raises more questions than it answers. Thoughtful policy development will require a concerted research effort, and state-of-the-art psychological research must be a crucial component of this effort. The issues involved in end-of-life decision making are inherently psychological, and yet psychology as a field has been slow in focusing its attention on the issue. This volume, I hope, will represent a turning point in this regard and stimulate more psychologists, including basic researchers in social and cognitive psychology, to begin to explore the psychological processes involved in end-of-life decision making.

REFERENCES

American Association of Retired Persons. (1988). *Tomorrow's choices: Preparing now for future legal financial and health care decisions.* Washington, DC: Author.

Baergen, R. (1995). Revising the substituted judgment standard. *Journal of Clinical Ethics, 6,* 30–38.

Bok, S. (1976). Personal directions for care at the end of life. *New England Journal of Medicine, 295,* 367–369.

Bradley, E., Walker, L., Blecher, B. B., & Wettle, T. (1997). Assessing capacity to participate in discussions of advance directives in nursing homes: Findings from a study of the Patient Self Determination Act. *Journal of the American Geriatrics Society, 45,* 79–83.

Buchanan, A. E., & Brock, D. W. (1990). *Deciding for others: The ethics of surrogate decision making.* Cambridge, England: Cambridge University Press.

Coppola, K. M., Ditto, P. H., Danks, J. H., & Smucker, W. D. (2001). Accuracy of primary care and hospital-based physicians' predictions of elderly outpatients' treatment preferences with and without advance directives. *Archives of Internal Medicine, 161,* 431–440.

Cruzan v. Director, Missouri Department of Health, 497 U.S. 261 (1990).

Danis, M., Garrett, J., Harris, R., & Patrick, D. L. (1994). Stability of choices about life-sustaining treatments. *Annals of Internal Medicine, 120,* 567–573.

Ditto, P. H., Danks, J. H., Smucker, W. D., Bookwala, J., Coppola, K. M., Dresser, R., et al. (2001). Advance directives as acts of communication: A randomized controlled trial. *Archives of Internal Medicine, 161,* 421–430.

Ditto, P. H., Druley, J. A., Moore, K. A., Danks, J. H., & Smucker, W. D. (1996). Fates worse than death: The role of valued life activities in health-state evaluations. *Health Psychology, 15,* 332–343.

Ditto, P. H., Jacobson, J. A., Smucker, W. D., Danks, J. H., & Fagerlin, A. (2005). *Context changes choices: A prospective study of the effects of hospitalization on life-sustaining treatment preferences.* Unpublished manuscript.

Ditto, P. H., Smucker, W. D., Danks, J. H., Jacobson, J. A., Houts, R. M., Fagerlin, A., et al. (2003). The stability of older adults' preferences for life-sustaining medical treatment. *Health Psychology, 22,* 605–615.

Doukas, D. J., & McCullough, L. B. (1991). The values history: The evaluation of the patient's values and advance directives. *Journal of Family Practice, 32,* 145–153.

Dresser, R. (2003). Precommitment: A misguided strategy for securing death with dignity. *Texas Law Review, 81,* 1823–1847.

Eiser, A. R., & Weiss, M. D. (2001). The underachieving advance directive: Recommendations for increasing advance directive completion. *American Journal of Bioethics, 1,* W10.

Emanuel, L. L. (1991). The health care directive: Learning how to draft advance care documents. *Journal of the American Geriatrics Society, 39,* 1221–1228.

Emanuel, L. L. (1994). Appropriate and inappropriate use of advance directives. *Journal of Clinical Ethics, 5,* 357–359.

Emanuel, L. L., Barry, M. J., Stoeckle, J. D., Ettelson, L. M., & Emanuel, E. J. (1991). Advance directives for medical care—a case for greater use. *New England Journal of Medicine, 324,* 889–895.

Emanuel, L. L., Danis, M., Pearlman, R. A., & Singer, P. A. (1995). Advance care planning as a process: Structuring the discussions in practice. *Journal of the American Geriatrics Society*, *43*, 440–446.

Fagerlin, A., Ditto, P. H., Danks, J. H., Houts, R. M., & Smucker, W. D. (2001). Projection in surrogate decisions about life-sustaining medical treatments. *Health Psychology*, *20*, 166–175.

Forrow, L., Taylor, W. C., & Arnold, R. M. (1992). Absolutely relative: How research results are summarized can affect treatment decisions. *American Journal of Medicine*, *92*, 121–124.

Gick, M., & Holyoak, K. (1980). Analogical problem solving. *Cognitive Psychology*, *12*, 306–355.

Gilbert, D. T., Pinel, E. C., Wilson, T. D., Blumberg, S. J., & Wheatley, T. (1998). Immune neglect: A source of durability bias in affective forecasting. *Journal of Personality and Social Psychology*, *75*, 617–638.

Gready, R. M., Ditto, P. H., Danks, J. H., Coppola, K. M., Lockhart, L. K., & Smucker, W. D. (2000). Actual and perceived stability of preferences for life-sustaining treatment. *Journal of Clinical Ethics*, *11*, 334–346.

Hawkins, N. A., Ditto, P. H., Danks, J. H., & Smucker, W. D. (2005). Micromanaging death: Process preferences, values, and goals in end-of-life medical decision making. *The Gerontologist*, *45*, 107–117.

Holley, J. L., Stackiewicz, L., Dacko, C., & Rault, R. (1997). Factors influencing dialysis patients' completion of advance directives. *American Journal of Kidney Diseases*, *30*, 356–360.

Holmes, D. S. (1968). Dimensions of projection. *Psychological Bulletin*, *69*, 248–268.

Jacobson, J. A., Ditto, P. H., Coppola, K. M., Danks, J. H., & Smucker, W. D. (2005). *The stability of life-sustaining treatment preferences over time: A meta-analysis.* Unpublished manuscript.

Kutner, L. (1969). Due process of euthanasia: The living will, a proposal. *Indiana Law Journal*, *44*, 539–554.

Loewenstein, G., & Schkade, D. A. (1999). Wouldn't it be nice? Predicting future feelings. In D. Kahneman, E. Diener, & N. Schwarz (Eds.), *Well-being: The foundations of hedonic psychology* (pp. 85–105). New York: Russell Sage Foundation.

Markus, G. B. (1986). Stability and change in political attitudes: Observed, recalled, and "explained." *Political Behavior*, *8*, 21.

McNeil, B. J., Pauker, S. G., Sox, H. C., Jr., & Tversky, A. (1982). On the elicitation of preferences for alternative therapies. *New England Journal of Medicine, 306*, 1259–1262.

Modell, W. (1974). A "will" to live. *New England Journal of Medicine*, *290*, 907.

Morrison, R. S., Zayas, L. H., Mulvihill, M., Baskin, S. A., & Meier, D. E. (1998). Barriers to completion of health care proxies: An examination of ethnic differences. *Archives of Internal Medicine*, *158*, 2493–2497.

Mullen, B., & Hu, L. (1988). Social projection as a function of cognitive mechanisms: Two meta-analytic integrations. *British Journal of Social Psychology*, *27*, 333–356.

Nisbett, R., & Ross, L. (1980). *Human inference: Strategies and shortcomings of social judgment*. Englewood Cliffs, NJ: Prentice-Hall.

Orentlicher, D. (1990). Advance medical directives. *Journal of the American Medical Association, 263*, 2365–2367.

Patient Self-Determination Act of 1990, Publ. L. No. 101-508, 4206, 4751 of the Omnibus Reconciliation Act of 1990.

President's Commission for the Study of Ethical Problems in Medicine and Biomedical and Behavioral Research. (1983). *Deciding to forego life-sustaining treatment: Ethical, medical, and legal issues in treatment decisions*. Washington, DC: U.S. Government Printing Office.

Schkade, D. A., & Kahneman, D. (1998). Does living in California make people happy? A focusing illusion in judgments of life satisfaction. *Psychological Science, 9*, 340–346.

Schneiderman, L. J., Kaplan, R. M., Pearlman, R. A., & Teetzel, H. (1993). Do physicians' own preferences for life-sustaining treatment influence their perceptions of patients' preferences? *Journal of Clinical Ethics, 4*, 28–33.

Sehgal, A., Galbraith, A., Chesney, M., Schoenfeld, P., Charles, G., & Lo, B. (1992). How strictly do dialysis patients want their advance directives followed? *Journal of the American Medical Association, 267*, 59–63.

Slovic, P. (1995). The construction of preferences. *American Psychologist, 50*, 364–371.

Terry, P. B., Vettese, M. A., Song, J., Forman, J., Haller, K. B., Miller, D. J., et al. (1999). End-of-life decision making: When patients and surrogates disagree. *Journal of Clinical Ethics, 10*, 286–293.

Tilden, V. P., Tolle, S. W., Nelson, C. A., & Fields, J. (2001). Family decision-making to withdraw life-sustaining treatments from hospitalized patients. *Nursing Research, 50*, 105–115.

Tversky, A., & Kahneman, D. (1981). The framing of decisions and the psychology of choice. *Science, 211*, 453–458.

Uhlmann, R. F., Pearlman, R. A., & Cain, K. C. (1988). Physicians' and spouses' predictions of elderly patients' resuscitation preferences. *Journal of Gerontology, 43*, M115–M121.

Wilson, T. D., Kraft, D., & Dunn, D. S. (1989). The disruptive effects of explaining attitudes: The moderating effect of knowledge about the attitude object. *Journal of Experimental Social Psychology, 25*, 379–400.

5

END-OF-LIFE ASSESSMENT WITHIN A HOLISTIC BIO-PSYCHO-SOCIAL-SPIRITUAL FRAMEWORK

KEVIN P. KAUT

There is much about death and dying that has yet to be explained by science.

—Walter (1996, p. 358)

Death is certain, yet drastically underexamined. The notion of death is often intellectualized, but rarely internalized as part of a cognitive and affective perspective on life itself. We are aware of its reality—reminded daily in obituaries and media reports of the recently deceased. Yet the thought of dying and the realization of mortality may be deferred until the time it is closer at hand. Death comes in many forms, including sudden trauma and brief illness, which, unfortunately, may rob individuals of the opportunity to address the most important issues of life prior to one's final exit. Alternatively, disease or chronic health ailments can gradually erode health and strength, thereby prolonging the process of dying (see Emanuel & Emanuel, 1998). Indeed, modern advances in medicine may alter the very nature and progression of end-of-life "trajectories" (e.g., Lynn, 1997) with significant implications for the psychological, social, and emotional experience of the dying person (Emanuel & Emanuel, 1998; Kaut, 2002; Muir & Arnold, 2001; Walter, 1996).

Despite the inevitability of death, it is avoided, essentially removed from public consideration in favor of an emphasis on health, vitality, and longevity (McPhee, Rabow, Pantilat, Markowitz, & Winker, 2000). Nevertheless, death remains a reality, most poignantly evident when individuals are diagnosed with terminal conditions. In these cases the complex social and emotional characteristics of each individual in her or his own life context may be challenged by a medical establishment focused principally on disease and death as enemies to be confronted with biomedical technology (for further discussion, see Kaplan, Foreword; Stillion, chap. 1).

Dying can certainly be viewed from a purely reductionistic perspective, characterized by an emphasis on cellular physiology, biological systems, and pathological processes (e.g., Rothschild, 1997; Steinhauser, Clipp, et al., 2000). It is becoming increasingly clear, however, that discussions of treatment for individuals in the midst of illness and dying must incorporate a broader perspective of the individual, including a consideration of the emotional, social, and spiritual[1] context in which the person lives (Emanuel & Emanuel, 1998; Kaut, 2002; Kearney & Mount, 2000; Steinhauser, Clipp, et al., 2000; Sulmasy, 2002). One perspective initially proposed by Engel (as cited in Nicassio & Smith, 1995) represented an attempt to identify the interconnections among the biological facets of life (e.g., genetics, biological systems) and the broader socioemotional and relational circumstances surrounding the individual (e.g., interpersonal relationships; community and culture). An adaptation of this perspective for end-of-life assessment (see Figure 5.1; Blevins, Kaut, Kopera-Frye, & Werth, 2001) emphasizes the diverse factors (e.g., psychological, biomedical, pharmacological, social, environmental) contributing in some way to an individual's adaptive strengths and weaknesses affecting the process of dying and death. Similar to the perspective of health status offered by Hoffman (2000), the current model focuses on a person's level of adaptive behavior near the end of life and underscores the need to consider intrapersonal characteristics (e.g., cognition, affect, personality), the person's actual biomedical status and treatment milieu, and the broader social and environmental circumstances that can affect adaptation and quality of life while dying.

Recognizing the relationships among biological, psychological, social, and spiritual dimensions may be interesting from an academic perspective, but this is of minimal value if models offer limited directions for clinical practice. In particular, for professionals providing psychological or spiritual end-of-life care (e.g., psychologists, counselors, social workers, clergy), the tendency may be to focus on their isolated position in an overall model (e.g.,

---

[1]Throughout this chapter I use the term "spiritual"; however, I do so in the most general sense so that it can include all potential belief systems that serve as a means of understanding the larger world and one's place in it. Because I cannot hope to include reference to all forms of belief systems, I encourage the reader to substitute whatever terms make sense, including non-Western/non-Judeo-Christian systems, as well as more general perspectives such as "life philosophy," "existential concerns," "meaning-making," and so forth. Similarly, as Blevins and Papadatou (chap. 2) emphasize, culture is inherent in all aspects of a person's life. I therefore have not repeatedly mentioned the cultural aspects of all the issues I discuss, hoping the reader will automatically infer these aspects.

Kellehear, 2000; Mauritzen, 1988; Smith, 1993) rather than perceiving a model as a complete framework through which they can view their role as a comprehensive care provider (Kaut, 2002). Implicit in this latter perspective is the notion that mental health and spiritual care providers benefit from an understanding and integration of multiple levels of human functioning when assessing client needs across the various domains believed to influence adaptive behavior near the end of life (e.g., psychological, social, spiritual).

The model presented in Figure 5.1 provides one framework for conceptualizing an assessment of a patient's end-of-life experience; however, it does not include the preponderance of the belief system patients use to make meaning near the end of life. Thus, Figure 5.2A represents the perspective developed in this chapter, emphasizing the spiritual or existential elements of a person's life. Specifically, the spiritual life context of the dying person is conceptualized as reflecting the physical, cognitive, and social circumstances affecting the process of dying; the model's components is further clarified in subsequent sections. Conceptually similar to Maslow's notion of human needs and motivation (see Marrone, 1999), this perspective suggests that an individual's expression of spirituality within an end-of-life context is influenced by his or her biological status, biomedical treatments, psychological resources, and sociocultural factors. In addition, an individual's spiritual experience and level of spiritual awareness might also reflect elements of existentialism as offered by Frankl (1963, 1969; see also Eliason, Hanley, & Leventis, 2001), thus underscoring the importance of human needs and the search for meaning when preparing for death. Not all persons will approach the end of life in the same way and are unlikely to have the same set of needs and expectations regarding a "good" or "healthy" death as the end of life approaches (e.g., Block, 2001; Emanuel & Emanuel, 1998; Smith & Maher, 1991). Nevertheless, the intent of this chapter is to illustrate the utility of a conceptual framework for gathering information and providing patient care, while underscoring the need for an eclectic perspective, particularly among those who traditionally focus on mental health and spiritual or existential needs of the dying. Cultural characteristics of the individuals involved will affect all aspects of the end-of-life situation, perhaps especially in the spiritual realm.

A MODEL FOR ASSESSMENT NEAR THE END OF LIFE

The presentation of this framework is accompanied by the inclusion of a vignette depicting an individual's end-of-life process. Case studies can effectively relate principles important for end-of-life care (see, e.g., Block, 2001; Kagawa-Singer & Blackhall, 2001; Lynn, 1997), and the vignette segments selected here are intended to reflect briefly the issues, emotions, and needs emerging throughout a dying trajectory. Each vignette segment represents

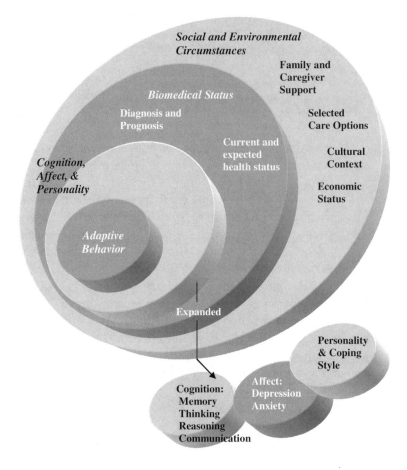

Figure 5.1. Biopsychosocial models of human behavior. Model of adaptive behavior near the end of life, reflecting multiple dimensions contributing to a patient's general level of adaptive functioning.

the experience of a dying person at various points along a unique end-of-life progression and is also depicted by the circles at various points along the timeline presented in Figure 5.2B. Essentially, assessment and intervention near the end of life must be considered within the context of a dying person's life, and context here is best assessed through a bio-psycho-social-spiritual framework—that is, the one portrayed in Figure 5.2A.

Conceptualizing Life in the Context of Dying

The diagnosis was presented to the family by a young physician emerging from surgery; confidently, yet respectfully, he delivered the news. An adenocarcinoma (i.e., a malignant tumor in the glandular tissues), originating in one location and spreading to other organs, had been confirmed. Weeks after the onset of physical symptoms and various medical

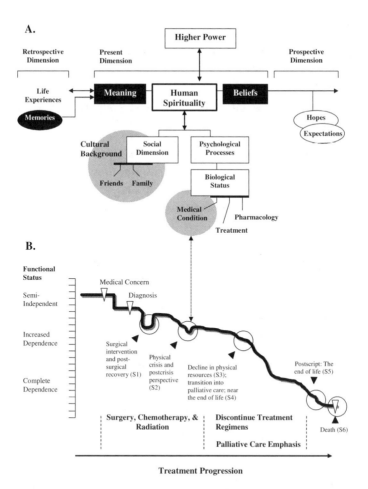

A.

B.

Figure 5.2. Framework for assessment near the end of life assessment near the end of life. (A) Multiple dimensions involved in assessment. Assessment requires a consideration of biological (e.g., medical condition, health status, treatment regimen and pharmacology), psychological (cognitive and affective behavior), and sociocultural (family, relationships) domains. Assessment of the dying patient requires an understanding of how these factors influence quality of life, including spirituality, which can be reflected in a sense of meaning shaped by life experiences and accomplishments, a belief in a higher power or systematic theology, or an alternative belief system (e.g., New Age philosophy). The present dimension is at the center of the vertical perspective (i.e., bottom up—from biological to spiritual), which should be considered in the context of a person's life history through the recollection of important events or memories (i.e., retrospective dimension), and an appreciation of how past and present circumstances shape beliefs about the future (i.e. prospective dimension). (B) An example of end-of-life progression, from diagnosis to death. Trajectories differ among diseases and individuals, and professional caregivers must understand how a particular illness course affects the current levels of functioning in a dying person, as well as how expected changes in function may alter her or his ability to deal with important life and death issues. *Note.* The areas circled on the timeline are in approximate order with the vignette segments (i.e., S1–S6) presented in the text (adapted from Kaut, 2002). From "Religion, Spirituality, and Existentialism Near the End of Life," by K. P. Kaut, 2002. *American Behavioral Scientist, 46*(2), p. 225. Adapted with permission.

tests, the final diagnosis and prognosis were offered. In the weeks ahead were many decisions to make regarding postsurgical treatments and various approaches to curative and palliative care. An end-of-life scenario had developed, and the trajectory of dying was now a reality.

The situation depicted in this first vignette segment represents an early period in a patient's end of life trajectory (see Figure 5.2B, S1), reflecting the first of various medical interventions attempted in this patient's progression toward death. The context of dying and death may be changing, but the process of dying often remains medicalized, particularly in the modern era of medical advancements, aggressive treatments, and a pursuit of longevity. Even chronic conditions of the 21st century, such as heart disease, respiratory distress, and cancer, are now associated with prolonged periods of illness and survival, quite possibly resulting in extended periods of living in preparation for death (Nicassio & Smith, 1995; Walter, 1996). Following a definitive diagnosis, there are many interventions that can be considered in the medical context of illness and dying, including surgery, chemotherapy, radiation treatments, and pharmacological approaches. Modern medicine has clearly improved chances of survival, the quality of living, and even the quantity of years lived. It has also influenced the very nature of dying, however.

Recent literature devoted to understanding and improving the process of dying underscores the need to prepare for death while seeking appropriate ways to ensure quality of life in the context of dying (e.g., Emanuel & Emanuel, 1998; Patrick, Engelberg, & Curtis, 2001; Singer, Martin, & Kelner, 1999; Steinhauser, Clipp, et al., 2000). Phrases such as "good death" or "healthy death" (Smith & Maher, 1991) suggest that in some way the sting of death can be lessened, and the process of dying can be experienced with a sense of closure and growth (Larson & Tobin, 2000). This notion is found most notably in the early writings of Kubler-Ross (1975), who portrayed the gravity and sadness associated with terminal illness, yet characterized the process as an opportunity for personal growth and development. Given the ability to prolong life while providing better palliative support of the whole person while dying (Kearney & Mount, 2000; Patrick et al., 2001; Walter, 1996), it is anticipated that the notion of extending life will be associated with opportunities for a higher quality of living while preparing to die. To accomplish this, many facets of the dying person's experience must be carefully assessed and specifically addressed. Indeed, extending the length of life without attention to the social and emotional circumstances would be viewed as antithetical to what many might consider a "good death" (see Singer et al., 1999).

The various domains identified in Figure 5.2A (e.g., biological, psychological, social) represent key elements in the consideration of a person's adaptive approach to the end of life. The end-of-life trajectory presented in Figure 5.2B reflects a declining level of physical independence, illustrated throughout various phases of a patient's terminal condition (and depicted in the vignette discussed throughout this chapter). Importantly, adaptive behavior is the outcome of the processes identified in these models (Figure 5.2A and 5.2B), defined as an optimal level of performance across a variety of life-skills domains, including cognition (e.g., awareness, thinking, memory, decision making), communication, and relationship involvement. Essentially, evaluating the emotional and spiritual experience of a dying person (refer to Figure 5.2A) requires a full examination of how she or he lives in the present, how she or he has functioned in the past (retrospective dimension), and a consideration of her or his beliefs, hopes, and expectations for the future (prospective dimension) as the illness progresses.

Conceptualizing the life of a dying person necessitates an "attitude of assessment" rather than a process grounded in traditional principles of client evaluation. This perspective is predicated on the need to observe behavior, collect information, and identify a person's adaptive strengths and weaknesses. Rather than providing a scheme for systematically evaluating a dying person, this framework is intended to guide the practitioner in the process of assembling and organizing information. This requires an understanding of the singular and contextual factors defining a person's experience near the end of life, developed through the process of hearing and accepting a patient's "own story" as reflected in her or his behaviors, relationships, memories, and beliefs (personal communications with chaplains L. Gregson and D. Engle, February 14, 2002).

The Assessment Relationship: Integrating Process and Knowledge

The process of evaluating a client's needs at the end of life entails a consideration of how biomedical, psychosocial, and personal history influence his or her sense of spirituality. As noted in Figure 5.2A the assessment process must ultimately be viewed from a multidimensional perspective, with the goal of helping a client move through the end of life process in a manner that helps him or her embrace his or her own sense of spirituality.

The Biological Dimension

Entering into the life of a dying person requires sensitivity, openness, awareness, and recognition of the many issues that influence behavior and shape the process of dying (see Emanuel & Emanuel, 1998; Lynn, 1997). Importantly, the life of the dying person must be appreciated as having a history and a future—each contributing to the context within which the person experiences the present (Cherny, Coyle, & Foley, 1994; refer also to Figure 5.2A). It is vital to focus on a patient's personal identity rather than viewing her or him as "terminally ill" or a "dying person." It is understandable that physical and biomedical issues may be prominent among the rather diverse concerns expressed by dying patients (see Table 5.1); the nature of their medical pathology may overshadow their identity (e.g., "cancer patient"). Nevertheless, the professional caregiver's attempt to understand "who the

TABLE 5.1
Issues of Importance and Areas of Assessment for
Terminally Ill Patients Near the End of Life

Domain and issue	Suggested references addressing this issue
Physical	
Pain	Cherny et al., 1994; Emanuel & Emanuel, 1998
Anorexia	Emanuel & Emanuel, 1998
Cleanliness	Steinhauser, Christakis, et al., 2000
Fatigue, drowsiness/insomnia	Emanuel & Emanuel, 1998
Vomiting, diarrhea	Singer et al., 1999
Dyspnea, suffocation	Rothschild, 1997
Somatic (bodily) changes	Cherny et al., 1994
Prolongation of dying	Singer et al., 1999
Psychological	
Fear of dying	Block, 2001; Quill, 2000
Sadness, worry, grief	Block, 2001
Depression	Cherny et al., 1994
Existential distress	Cherny et al., 1996
Death anxiety	Chochinov, 2002
Anxiety	Block, 2001; Cherny et al., 1994
Psychological distress	Chochinov, 2002; Cherny et al., 1996
Mental pain/suffering	Shuster, Breitbart, & Chochinov, 1999
Dignity	Chochinov, 2002; Steinhauser, Christakis, et al., 2000
Fear of abandonment	Rothschild, 1997
Social–Familial	
Concern about family	Block, 2001
Fear of being a burden	Emanuel et al., 2000
Sharing time with friends	Steinhauser, Christakis, et al., 2000
Communication	Stewart et al., 1999
Family relationships	Singer et al., 1999
Decision Making and Planning	
Funeral/burial arrangements	Lynn, 1997; Steinhauser, Clipp, et al., 2000
Do-not-resuscitate orders	Fins et al., 1999
Legal and financial issues	Block, 2001; Steinhauser, Christakis, et al., 2000
Health care proxy	Fins et al., 1999
Spiritual	
Existential distress	Cherny et al., 1994
Peace with God	Steinhauser, Christakis, et al., 2000
Unmet spiritual needs	Moadel et al., 1999
Meaning of pain and suffering	Block, 2001
Identify spiritual self/needs	Kaut, 2002

Note. For a discussion of cultural considerations and a set of related references, see Blevins and Papadatou (chap. 2).

person is" may be a first step toward successfully entering into the person's trajectory and is a prerequisite for end-of-life assessment.

The process of end-of-life assessment must also begin with knowledge of the issues that may influence the mental, spiritual, and even physical health of the dying person. An individual confronted with a terminal condition may be thrust into a very different life context as she or he deals with the reality of her or his own mortality. Amid the many issues that may emerge at this time, there may be specific concerns about the nature of the physical condition, chief of which may be the presence of pain and the treatment of physical distress (Emanuel & Emanuel, 1998). Given that persistently unrelieved symptoms and organic problems may result in depressive symptomology (see Cherny et al., 1994), and the current belief that the experience of "total pain" itself may have many components (e.g., socioemotional, spiritual, even financial considerations; see Kearney & Mount, 2000, p. 359), it is imperative that end-of-life caregivers appreciate the vertical (i.e., bottom-up) perspective advocated in the holistic model presented here (Figure 5.2A).

One example of a relevant framework for considering the relationship between physical needs and more advanced social and cognitive issues in life is Maslow's hierarchy of human needs (see Marrone, 1999). It is hoped that the dying person will have time to examine issues of personal, social, and spiritual importance as she or he considers her or his life in the context of dying (Block, 2001; Exley, 1999; Lynn, 1997; Patrick et al., 2001). This requires energy and effort, however—drawing on the physical, cognitive, and emotional resources of the body (refer to Figure 5.2A). The preparedness to engage in valued end-of-life activities, such as spending time with family and friends or communicating with others (see Table 5.1; Steinhauser, Christakis, et al., 2000; Stewart, Teno, Patrick, & Lynn, 1999), can be undermined if the biological needs of the body are not appropriately met. Moreover, the impact of medical treatments and pharmacological regimens may weaken the body or otherwise alter consciousness and temperament. Importantly, the biological status of the person must be clarified and continually monitored to ensure a suitable level of comfort from which the individual may explore other issues as she or he prepares to die.

Of particular relevance here is a perspective offered by Lynn (1997), who noted the importance of understanding the dying person's body, with its associated "limits and possibilities determined by its ailments [suffered] over time" (p. 1635). The notion of "limits and possibilities" is consistent with the principle of adaptive behavior assessment advocated here and emphasizes the need to consider the strengths and weaknesses of the person, while also recognizing her or his own movement through the illness within a given time frame. Essentially, the temporal dimension of illness is relevant (i.e., how the physical condition has changed since diagnosis) and may provide insight into the person's experience, in addition to the cumulative impact an illness may have had on current levels of strength, resolve, and hope for the future.

Indeed, the initial entry point into the life context of a person who is dying will likely involve consideration of various biomedical issues, including the nature of the disease (e.g., cancer, congestive heart failure), current physical condition (e.g., cancer stage, level of physical decline), medicinal and mechanical support, and treatment schedules (e.g., chemotherapy, radiation)—all of which reinforce the physical and reductionistic nature of dying (see Cherny, Coyle, & Foley, 1996; Morrison, Meier, & Cassel, 1996; Rothschild, 1997). Ultimately, the care provider must recognize the impact physical conditions have on the cognitive and affective nature of a person who is dying but must also be able to look past the physical dimension and find the living human being caught within the confines of physical constraints.

Assessment of the biomedical domain requires specific inquiry into patient health status (i.e., diagnosis and prognosis), treatment implications, pharmacological interventions, and treatment side effects. This may be uncommon practice among mental health professionals, because their respective professional literatures on end-life-care rarely discuss the relevance of biomedical knowledge to the actual provision of care. Thus, the delivery of mental health or spiritual services is often described with minimal emphasis on the biological condition—generally approached from a discipline-specific perspective. Accordingly, it is reasonable that counselors will focus almost exclusively on the particular dimension of need expressed by a patient (e.g., death anxiety, depression), especially in cases of limited-term involvement. A broader level of patient knowledge, however, would provide a richer context within which to consider the diverse issues affecting the dying person's current condition and anticipated trajectory. Importantly, without knowledge of a person's illness trajectory or an understanding of treatment effects on cognition and behavior, the provider may miss critical opportunities to address the needs of the dying patient and family.

The Psychological Dimension

> Although the patient's surgery was behind her, she was once again in crisis after an acute episode of angina, but was made comfortable after appropriate medical intervention. An intravenous morphine line had been inserted into a surgically implanted delivery port to eliminate the need for repeated injections in the months ahead. The nursing staff, engaged in the business of cancer care, steadily moved in and out of the room to monitor the patient and satisfy written orders. Under the influence of morphine, the patient was relaxed and relatively pain free. She had embarked upon the road to physical recovery; however, this road would surely challenge the very core of her cognitive and emotional being, as the truly hard issues of life and death lie ahead.

The biomedical approach to treating a terminal illness is naturally focused on the biological pathology underlying the disease. A physical crisis experienced in the midst of various treatment efforts (refer to Figure 5.2B, S2) would likely be approached from a reductionistic perspective, focused principally on the pathology itself. However, amid the complex biomedical interventions that so often characterize an end-of-life scenario (e.g., morphine, surgical ports, monitoring devices, treatment regimens), one will find a patient—a person—with emotional, psychological, relational, and spiritual needs. The hard issues of life are not necessarily biomedical in nature (e.g., treatment selection) but are deeply personal and relational. Medical treatment can provide care for the body, but a care provider must recognize the underlying psychological, social, and spiritual–existential issues that also require attention (see Kearney & Mount, 2000).

Steinhauser, Clipp, and colleagues (2000) noted that the care provider attending to the patient near the end of life may be disadvantaged when initially meeting with the dying person (e.g., when confronting a physical crisis) because he or she has but a cross-sectional perspective of the individual at one point in the illness. As noted earlier, when the caregiver has limited prior knowledge of the patient, the moment of entering into the person's life may provide but a shallow perspective in the midst of physical or emotional distress. A full appreciation of the terminally ill person necessitates a deeper understanding of present circumstances and the historical context of the illness trajectory.

Entering the life of a patient at a point of physical crisis requires an evaluation of dimensions other than the obvious medical scenario, including the patient's cognitive and affective status. The assessment of adaptive functioning should involve a consideration of maladaptive tendencies, such as excessive worry, self-isolation, and an attitude of "giving up" (see Cherny et al., 1994). It is understandable that a principal concern for many patients may be a fear of dying (Block, 2001), coupled with concerns about family members, issues regarding one's level of burden to others (Emanuel, Fairclough, Slutsman, & Emanuel, 2000), and anxiety regarding the very nature of death itself (Cherny et al., 1994; Chochinov, 2002). Distress in the form of mental pain and suffering (Shuster, Breitbart, & Chochinov, 1999) may also interfere with the patient's ability to function optimally in the face of the illness, thus limiting the quality of interactions with family, friends, and others involved in end-of-life care. Therefore, a primary goal of end-of-life assessment should be to identify the types of psychological barriers that undermine introspection, communication, and appropriate decision making.

The process of identifying limitations and resources does not imply a standardized approach to assessment; rather, this may best be viewed as a conversational process involving an attitude of assessment, characterized by an awareness of relevant dimensions of importance and a gradual accumulation of information through discourse with the patient and family. Realistically, there is little need for normative assessment tools or standardized interviews near the end of life (but see McClain, Rosenfeld, & Breitbart, 2003). Even the assessment of cognition relevant to medical decision making capacity may initially be conversational in an effort to identify the thought processes and level of comprehension demonstrated by the patient (Morrison et al., 1996). Essentially, the process of psychological assessment advocated here depends critically on relationship, conversation, and inquiries concerning issues of particular concern or relevance to the dying patient and his or her family (for relevant content domains, see Table 5.1).

Recent perspectives have been offered to facilitate conversation with patients, and are intended to guide clinicians as they gather information relevant to treatment planning and patient care (see Block, 2001; Chochinov, 2002; Kagawa-Singer & Blackhall, 2001; Lo et al., 2002). Ultimately, questions must provide the respondent with an opportunity to share ideas, concerns, and feelings, but to do so in a manner that is naturally blended within the context of conversation. The process necessitates a respect for a supportive exchange grounded within the establishment of a relationship between caregiver and patient. The sensitive and timely delivery of focused questions (see Block, 2001; Chochinov, 2002) can be used to understand better the patient's previous and current coping style, which may represent how she or he deals with significant life events and what, if any, issues are particularly stressful at the present time. The assessment domains presented in Table 5.1 represent a sample of issues to be considered when assessing a dying patient. Questions framed to elicit conversation and answers regarding these issues are important in developing an understanding of the patient and her or his specific level of need.

Conversation and questions are central in the assessment equation, but the health care provider must recognize the critical nature of "relationship" as part of the overall assessment process. To best understand the dying person, one must be willing to participate fully in the experience of the patient. The success of an emotional or spiritual assessment and intervention depends on the provider's ability to establish a presence with the dying person (Kaut, 2002), reflected in the act of being present—physically and emotionally—with the patient. Engaging in conversation and listening to the personal story the patient tells (e.g., life experiences, beliefs, hopes, fears) may permit the assessment of adaptive resources and perspectives on dying and death and may provide important insight into cognitive and linguistic competencies necessary for working through social, emotional, and spiritual concerns. The ability to communicate is essential for addressing nearly every issue deemed relevant to those who are dying, including conversations with family (e.g., Lynn, 1997; Stewart et al., 1999), assessing medical information and treatment decision making (e.g., Lynn, 1997; Morrison et al., 1996), finding meaning in the process of illness and dying (Exley, 1999; Kaut, 2002; Patrick et al., 2001), and discussing spiritual and existential concerns (Anbar, 2001; Kaut, 2002; Koenig, 2002; Smith, 1993; Walter, 1996). Therefore, knowing how a patient's physiological status may influence her or his cognitive and language skills at the present, or in the future, is extremely valuable when planning important conversations, considering cognizance of decisions, and managing details near the end of life.

The Spiritual Dimension

A month since the initial hospitalization and surgery, life with cancer was now a focal point of a family immersed in her terminal condition. Treatment included chemotherapy, radiation, and a rather extensive pharmacological regimen. Improvement had been observed for a short period of time but was now giving way to a noticeable loss in functional independence. Mobility was becoming limited, bodily functions were affected, appetite was decreased, and fatigue was an ever-present challenge. Quality time with family was dictated by her energy level, which often declined as the day progressed. Lapses in memory were noted, occasionally regarding her medication schedule, and in reference to recent events. The emergence of seizures ushered in a new crisis, testing the core of her being, stretching her to confront her condition and impending death, while ushering in a transition into an emphasis on palliative care.

At some point in a dying patient's trajectory, the costs of curative treatment might begin to outweigh the benefits, signifying the need for a consideration of more palliative approaches to end of life care (see Figure 5.2B, S3). Life with a terminal illness may at times seem focused on the illness itself: treating the illness; dealing with alterations in physical and cognitive functioning due to disease progression; managing personal and family schedules affected by the disease; adjusting to diminished energy and life activity. Physical and emotional resources of the patient and family can be challenged, and the emergence of crises (i.e., setbacks or progressive declines) can have an impact on the health, hopes, and perspectives of those engaged in the process of dying. In some cases, it may be here that the emphasis gradually shifts from matters of purely physical importance (e.g., treatments may no longer work; disease is progressing) to "supra-physical" or the psycho-social-spiritual dimensions of a person's life context.

Understanding the complex life context of the dying individual naturally begins with a person-centered perspective, emphasizing the intraindividual characteristics that influence adaptive functioning near the end of life (e.g., mental coping strategies, psychological resources). Adaptive behavior, however, must ultimately be placed within the broader context of social and cultural influences and associated supportive resources. Indeed, where adaptive limitations are present, the provision of care and support is likely to be assumed by members of the immediate family (Emanuel et al., 1999; see also chap. 8 by Allen, Haley, Roff, Schmid, & Bergman). Family members and other significant people contribute significantly to the patient's movement toward the final stage of life—not only in terms of physical support, but also as a source of emotional and spiritual care. In fact, many spiritual or existential belief systems are highly relational in nature, particularly as one relates to a source of power or strength central to a given belief system (see Figure 5.2A). Therefore, the social dimension, consisting of an individual's valued relationships, the nature of interactions with others, and the expressed need for connectedness to important persons in life, may provide a brief glimpse into the very nature of a patient's spirituality and existentialism.

Although difficult to define, spirituality is important in the lives of many people when confronted with death (Cherny et al., 1994; Emanuel & Emanuel, 1998; Kaye & Raghavan, 2002; Shuster et al., 1999; Steinhauser, Christakis, et al., 2000; see also chap. 8 by Allen et al.). Mauritzen (1988) has suggested that spirituality may not necessarily require a purely religious perspective even though it is often identified with an adherence to a particular systematic theology or religious tradition (Paulson, 2001). Rather, a broader concept of spirituality includes existentialism and recognizes differences in theological perspective (e.g., belief in God) and the system of beliefs and practices associated with a given religious tradition. Sensitivity to these differences in spiritual perspectives is an important attitude for the end-of-life care provider when entering the life of the dying person. One cannot always anticipate the spiritual condition or convictions of a person struggling with a terminal condition, and caution in this regard is certainly recommended. Some may be estranged from a particular religious tradition or background, and others may simply have no prior experience with organized religion. In these cases, patients may believe that spiritual issues have limited relevance for them; however, this may be an opportunity for the care provider to facilitate an appreciation of a patient's spiritual self, focusing more on the meaning he or she ascribes to her or his life, beliefs about death, and the value of relationships in her or his living and dying. Ultimately, an assessment of this domain requires a respect for the various associations people may have to the notion of spirituality and a recognition that a Western or Judeo-Christian tradition may not be the framework through which many individuals experience and express spirituality.

The model established here (see Figure 5.2A) underscores the notion that human spirituality, regardless of its specific meaning to the dying person, must be viewed as a multidimensional construct influenced by one's biological condition, psychological and affective status, and quality of relationships shared within one's existing social network and cultural experience (Kaut, 2002; Mauritzen, 1988). Assessment near the end-of-life must recognize the relationship between mind, body, and spirit (Kearney & Mount, 2000), recognizing that a dying person's preparedness to examine spiritual issues may depend on the other two domains.

Merely asking a patient about her or his spiritual beliefs or practices may permit a limited assessment of philosophical perspective, religious tradition, or reliance on a personally defined higher power. The status of one's spiritual condition may best be uncovered, however, through the gradual process of discovering the relevant life history of the person in addition to beliefs held about the future. The horizontal dimension in Figure 5.2A represents this process, characterized in part by an examination of the past (i.e., retrospective dimension) and a consideration of the hopes and expectations for the end of life and even existence beyond death (i.e., prospective dimension).

The importance of finding meaning in life and developing a framework of hope for the future emerges prominently in various perspectives of spirituality near the end of life (Block, 2001; Thomas & Retsas, 1999). Walter (1996), in particular, discussed the notion that everyone develops her or his own "spiritual construct" through which she or he seeks a sense of personal identity and meaning. Those with a particular theological perspective, often involving a belief in God (e.g., Catholicism, Judaism, Protestantism), may have developed this construct through religious tradition expressed through adherence to religious observance, literature, and ritual (Kellehear, 2000). Alternatively, a person may possess an eclectic view of one's spiritual self, constructed out of new age philosophies or a combination of principles associated with various beliefs and practices (Walter, 1993). People may even prefer to conceptualize and talk in terms of "existential" issues and considerations, eschewing the terms religious and spiritual in defining their belief system. Regardless of the construct through which people view their lives and prepare for death, the role of the caregiver is to understand the construct and identify how it relates to the sense of meaning (or lack thereof) and level of adaptation expressed in the dying person's approach to the end of life.

The retrospective dimension referred to in Figure 5.2A underscores the value of exploring the life history of the dying patient, which can be accomplished by allowing her or him to reflect on personal experiences and important memories that may have shaped the development of her or his own sense of meaning and purpose. The writings of Frankl (1963, 1969) are of particular relevance here, inasmuch as they emphasize the existential struggle associated with the search for personal meaning. The meaning we ascribe to our lives may be derived from various sources (e.g., family, work, important causes and values, religion and spirituality), and the care provider for persons near the end of life may be in a unique position to help them recognize or articulate a sense of meaning through a process of remembering the past. Indeed, memories may be of particular spiritual significance (Kaut, 2002) because they provide insight into the events, accomplishments, and relationships that contribute to a sense of identity and life meaning.

Allowing the patient to tell her or his own story may appropriately focus attention on the life of the individual rather than her or his impending death. Importantly, this may de-emphasize the patient's current condition (i.e., present dimension, Figure 5.2A), while emphasizing opportunities to invest in the social, emotional, and spiritual issues of living. This may be a difficult perspective to develop, but is critical when working with patients struggling with the many issues surrounding the end of life (refer to Table

5.1). Holistic patient care should ultimately prepare the patient mentally and emotionally for death (Kearney & Mount, 2000; Patrick et al., 2001; Steinhauser, Clipp, et al., 2000; Walter, 1996). It is understandable that some of this preparatory process may necessarily be devoted to working through the details related to death (e.g., treatment decisions, family planning and decision making, funeral arrangements; see Fins et al., 1999; Lynn, 1997); however, it is essential to promote an environment that allows the patient to confront anxieties associated with the fear of death or the mystery of existence after dying. Such questions certainly have no easy answers, yet it is important not only to allow the patient to raise these questions, but also to be prepared to discuss them with patients (Cherny et al., 1996; Chochinov, 2002). Physical and mental comfort can be enhanced through the reduction of anxiety as patients successfully confront issues producing distress (see Kearney & Mount, 2000). Palliative care certainly extends beyond the pharmacological and technical interventions available to promote comfort.

Identifying issues of concern to the patient may be one of the most important functions provided by the professional caregiver near the end of life. Helping the patient verbalize her or his concerns, or at least discuss them openly, may be critical in helping her or him to engage in the process of living while preparing to die. This process is predicated on the provider's willingness to patiently and respectfully "hear and accept" the dying person (chaplain D. Engel, personal communication, February 14, 2002) while promoting a better understanding of a patient's present and future circumstances. However, understanding the patient's present and future concerns involves more than merely asking a standard list of questions pertaining to family, self, and spirituality. Inquiries must be carefully blended within the context of conversation and self-revelation through which the patient discusses the nature of life, meaning, and beliefs about the future. Here, the "prospective dimension" (see Figure 5.2A) enters as an important area of assessment and intervention, given that it may embody the very hopes, anxieties, fears, and expectations a person has about the prospect of dying and the nature of death itself.

Medical uncertainties and related worries about the physical aspects of dying and death may be of significant concern to the dying person (see Table 5.1). It is important to remain sensitive to these issues while being aware of the patient's need for information regarding the effects of treatment or physical changes expected to occur as a condition progresses (see Larson & Tobin, 2000; Lynn, 1997; Steinhauser, Christakis, et al., 2000). Medical personnel are the principal source of information for medical or prognostic queries, addressing questions about existential, theological, and spiritual matters less definitively than issues of biomedical consequence. In these cases, the mental health specialist on the end-of-life care team (e.g., psychologist, counselor, social worker, chaplain; Lo et al., 2002; Lynn, 1997; Muir & Arnold, 2001; Quill, 2000) is essential to address issues of emotional and spiritual importance (but see Anbar, 2001). Importantly, the person providing support for spiritual concerns, regardless of professional discipline, should possess more than a superficial recognition of spirituality. As has been emphasized in this chapter, merely asking questions about a person's spiritual belief system is insufficient (Block, 2001; Cherny et al., 1994; Chochinov, 2002; Kagawa-Singer & Blackhall, 2001; Lo et al., 2002). What is required is the ability to hear nonjudgmentally the person's spiritual beliefs (or lack thereof), while exploring her or his emotional and spiritual needs in ways that promote opportunities for self-examination, cognitive preparation, and growth when possible (see Smith, 1993).

Essentially, some degree of closure regarding future-related anxieties or distress regarding the uncertainties of dying and death may ultimately permit the patient to allocate more mental and emotional resources to the issues of daily living and present relationships.

PREPARING FOR A "GOOD DEATH": A REASONABLE OBJECTIVE?

Death is inevitable, and while there is no way out, there is a way through. (McPhee et al., 2000, p. 2513)

An Attitude of Assessment Near the End of Life

The spreading cancer, having invaded portions of her brain, now produced uncontrollable motor seizures and additional anxiety. Surrounded by family, she struggled to sit up in her hospital bed after a long night in the emergency room. Kneeling at the foot of her bed, an oncologist compassionately explained the circumstances concerning this latest spread of cancer. Family members stood silenced by the news. The ensuing discussion focused on plans for new radiation treatments, but the goal now was solely on palliation and not cure. A new stage in the patient's life, and path toward death, had clearly been reached. One could only speculate about the resources she relied on for support in these moments. As a person of faith, she would find comfort in a beloved pastor's reading of a selected passage of religious text. An apparent source of strength and hope was revealed in this reading, which would ultimately memorialize her life while dying. (See S4 in Figure 5.2B.)

The synthesis of biological, psychological, and spiritual issues near the end of life is a defining characteristic of what some refer to as a "good death" (Emanuel & Emanuel, 1998). Affirming the whole person is central to this perspective (Steinhauser, Clipp, et al., 2000) and is predicated on the belief that dying should be viewed as a period of comfort (i.e., palliative) care and a period within which there is potential for personal growth (Larson & Tobin, 2000; see also Kubler-Ross, 1975). When pain is appropriately managed and the patient has opportunities to prepare for death (Singer et al., 1999;

Steinhauser, Clipp, et al., 2000), there is a greater probability of successful end-of-life work involving mental, emotional, spiritual, and interpersonal issues.

When confronted with the prospect of a terminal illness or when dealing with an ongoing crisis in a medical condition, there may be a reasonable amount of time—albeit limited in some cases—for thinking about and preparing for death (Muir & Arnold, 2001; Walter, 1996). There are likely to be many issues a patient and family must deal with in the weeks, months, or even years leading up to the time of decreased strength, diminished capacity, and eventual death (refer to Table 5.1). Yet within the biomedical context surrounding the patient, with its emphasis on pathology, medical treatments, and decisions for care (e.g., Rothschild, 1997), it cannot be overstated that there is also the need to attend to the social, emotional, and spiritual nature of the person. This is consistent with the tenets of palliative medicine as advocated by modern hospice services (Bradshaw, 1996; Kearney & Mount, 2000). Furthermore, such a comprehensive method of caring is made more difficult in traditional medical settings where there is a tendency to compartmentalize the provision of care to different members of the health care team. Integrated care through interdisciplinary collaboration underscores the importance of communication and collective planning among medical personnel, social support staff, and clergy—an integration that is most represented in the hospice approach to comfort care and quality of life for the dying patient (e.g., Mauritzen, 1988; for more discussion of hospice, see chap. 9 by Connor, Lycan, & Schumacher).

The effective professional caregiver near the end of life will be sensitive to the many issues that have an impact on the process of dying. Guided by a framework for identifying patient concerns, beliefs, and fears (refer to Table 5.1), an attitude of assessment equips the practitioner with a necessary perspective for entering the life of the dying person and facilitating the exploration of adaptive functioning. The goal of this exploration is to maximize the likelihood of a process resulting in an "appropriate death" for the patient and family (see Smith & Maher, 1991). This does not suggest that the focus on what is referred to as a "good death" is inappropriate, insofar as it reflects the set of circumstances that should be in place to ensure the most optimal conditions for dying (see Emanuel & Emanuel, 1998; Steinhauser, Clipp, et al., 2000). Optimal or appropriate, however, may not be synonymous with "good." Indeed, there is nothing inherently good about death, at least not for those with a life-affirming perspective. Models of "good dying" may actually offend some practitioners, especially those who recognize that emphasizing the idea of a good death may be harmful to a patient and family (see Sachs, 2000).

The idea of a unique end-of-life experience, specific to the patient's own spiritual and existential construct, should be a featured concept in any model of "good" or "appropriate" dying. That which is considered adaptive near the end of life for one person may not be endorsed by another. Individual differences must be understood and respected, and efforts to place death and dying within a preferred scenario may be inappropriate. Chochinov (2002) referred to "dignity-conserving-care" as a framework for assessing various factors relevant to the patient's unique experience of dying (e.g., continuity of self, hopefulness, acceptance, social support; see p. 2255) and noted that this perspective depends on preexisting personality characteristics and resources that influence the way dying and death are approached (see also chap. 2 by Blevins & Papadatou). Patients and families require a level of assessment and intervention based on their unique style of communication, interaction, spiritual adherence, and adaptation to stressors. The end-of-life care provider must be prepared to evaluate these areas in a manner that accepts individual preferences while promoting a level of care and intervention that optimizes the comfort and closure associated with the experience of dying.

The Experience of Dying and the Moment of Death

In the span of a few short months, the disease had exacted a considerable toll on the patient's physical resources. Now, the hospital visits, treatments, and delivery of daily medications to manage the condition were no longer necessary. The disease had gradually weakened the body to the point of continual slumber. Efforts to feed the patient had recently been discontinued. The decision, with the help of hospice support, was to comfort the patient and allow her to die quietly at home. Life was gradually ebbing away, as family members dealt with the business of funeral and burial arrangements. Friends and relatives made their final visits, saying their good-byes and offering support to members of the immediate family. The pastor made one final visit, praying with his dying parishioner and her spouse. Clearly the end of her life was near, and the primary caregivers drew closer together and kept a daily vigil over a dying wife and mother. Death was certain, but waiting for the inevitable was difficult. (See S5 in Figure 5.2B.)

It is questionable whether death can ever be viewed as a beautiful experience. An end-of-life process can be a difficult journey, which can place considerable strain on the dying person, family, and friends. However, the work of Kubler-Ross (1975) and others has suggested that death can mark the final stage of growth (Larson & Tobin, 2000). These efforts are to be applauded for their attempts to better understand the process of dying while underscoring the importance of viewing this stage of life as a time with continued potential for spiritual maturity, relationship development, and individual accomplishment. Where possible, leaving something "behind" for the generations who follow can be viewed as an important component in the establishment of a personal sense of legacy (e.g., see Exley, 1999). Uncovering opportunities for growth or the development of what Exley refers to as "after-death identities" may also be an important function provided by the care provider, especially when patients respond to queries for information concerning the meaning ascribed to life and their hopes for the future (see

Allen et al., chap. 8). From a life span development perspective, dying is certainly an eventual component in every life cycle and may provide opportunities for personal growth. It can also be a time of intense sorrow, depression, anticipatory grief, and overwhelming anxiety—for both the dying patient and family. Despite the various models of good and dignified dying (Block, 2001; Chochinov, 2002; Emanuel & Emanuel, 1998; Singer et al., 1999; Smith & Maher, 1991; Steinhauser, Clipp, et al., 2000), it must be understood that death is likely to remain an issue naturally provoking an attitude of fear and avoidance.

The perspective guiding assessment near the end of life should be to appraise realistically the life context of the dying person, with sensitivity to the preferences and wishes of the individual and family. Some families may value time spent together, with an emphasis on talking, sharing, and relating, whereas other families may prefer less interpersonal conversation and discussion of life events. Differences are likely to be evident across many dimensions of personal and family functioning (e.g., strength of relationships and closeness, openness, intrafamily stress or history of conflict, spiritual emphasis, willingness to provide support, ability to offer assistance and comfort). The professional caregiver must address the individual and familial style influencing the patient near the end of life and identify ways to promote optimal existence and emotional–spiritual comfort while preparing for death. What may be optimal for one person, however, may be viewed as irrelevant or less than optimal for another. Although it is important to use available guides and resources purporting to facilitate good, healthy, or dignified dying, it is imperative that the care provider be prepared for the possibility that these various frameworks may not so easily apply to every life and death context. For many, death will still sting, and families may be left with feelings of emptiness, loss, failure, and emotional pain (see Sachs, 2000).

Family members looking back on the experience of a loved one's death may later recognize the good and beautiful aspects of a comfortable, supportive, and "healthy" death. Nonetheless, the process leading up to the death itself can be emotionally draining, physically taxing, and overwhelming. The business of death is difficult and complicated by many factors, but can be made easier (or at least more tolerable) by a careful attention to the many variables that influence the life of a dying person and that affect the nature of dying and ultimately death itself. Death is the inevitable end-stage event following the erosion of physical reserves over time; therefore, preparing the dying person and family for this eventuality should focus on means to maximize adaptive functioning and promote a realistic affirmation of life's end.

The Proposed Framework in Retrospect: Putting the Pieces Together

Models facilitate an appreciation of the relationships among variables inherent in complex issues. Here, a framework emphasizing a patient's level of adaptive functioning within the context of her or his terminal condition is presented (refer to Table 5.1). Multiple factors are part of an individual's general level of functional independence, and various issues must be addressed to evaluate the strengths and weaknesses of an individual at any one point in time. The many issues of importance to dying persons may generate significant concern in the course of terminal illness (see Steinhauser, Christakis, et al., 2000), thus providing a basis for an assessment rubric near the end of life (see Table 5.1 and Figure 5.2A). Given the relative importance of spirituality within the context of end-of-life care (see Daaleman & VandeCreek, 2000; Kaye & Raghavan, 2002; Kearney & Mount, 2000; Kellehear, 2000; Koenig, 2002; Lo et al., 2002; Smith, 1993), this model offers an overall view of a patient's bio-psycho-social-spiritual existence within a framework that underscores the role of spirituality as crucial to a sense of meaning, strength, and hope at the end of life.

Expressions of concern among terminally ill patients (Table 5.1) represent important themes for assessment near the end of life and should guide the development of questions and the direction of conversation for the care provider engaged in the process of identifying patient needs. Ultimately, the development of a relationship with a dying patient (and the family) is the key to gaining insight into her or his spiritual and emotional condition and should be guided by a set of principles intended to prepare the dying person for a process of dying that is consistent with her or his beliefs, wishes, and spiritual construct. The emphasis of end-of-life mental health care should be to support the dying process, but it should do so with as much focus on life and living as possible. Helping a person adapt well to the physical, emotional, social, and spiritual challenges associated with her or his personal journey toward death is essential and necessitates an attention to opportunities for exploration of one's work, relationships, values, and life meaning.

Near the end of life, when treatment regimens and therapeutic interventions (e.g., radiation, chemotherapy) have given way to palliative care (or become supportive of palliative care goals), and the patient is being supported by the best in comfort medicine, there is yet opportunity to live. Time may truly be of the essence, however, inasmuch as opportunities missed now may never emerge again. At this point in the trajectory toward death, the patient is confronted with the certainty of the end and must be prepared to deal with the realities of life's finality. Here, the professional care provider is in a unique position to remain a presence in the life of the dying person, while facilitating movement toward death.

Although many models, frameworks, and perspectives of care near the end of life are available (one of which is presented here), these are useless without the context of relationship between practitioner and patient. Indeed, it may be the mere presence of another, even if only physical (i.e., sitting at a bedside, quietly present), that best supports the dying patient in death. In the end, it is support of human life that motivates emotional care.

Models and frameworks can provide a starting point, and even serve as a map with which to navigate difficult and unfamiliar terrain. Nevertheless, the true vehicle for support and transition toward death is found in the acceptance and affirmation of a human life—the foundation on which the search for meaning is established and the preparation for death is developed.

POSTSCRIPT

At the end, she was comfortable. There had been no official good-byes, and none were expected. She drifted off into a comatose-like state and simply slept her way toward the final moments of life. Her breathing was not labored, but was variable. There was no evidence of struggle, and she remained relatively still and calm in her hospital bed at home. Family members slept nearby, waiting for the moment when life ebbed away. In the early hours of the morning, she took her final breath, and family gathered by her bedside to say a last good-bye. The final stage of life had been completed, preceded by just a few short months of treatment, continued cancer spread, and palliative care. There was only so much that medicine could offer. In the end, what mattered most was how she lived, her mental preparation for death, and the comfort provided by a devoted husband and family. Days later, at a funeral planned to celebrate her life, she was eulogized in word and song and through the reading of her favorite scripture passage (the 139th Psalm), which affirmed her belief in the omniscience and omnipresence of her God. (See S6 in Figure 5.2B.)

REFERENCES

Anbar, R. D. (2001). The closure and the rings: When a physician disregards a patient's wish. *Pediatric Pulmonology, 31*, 76–79.

Blevins, D., Kaut, K. P., Kopera-Frye, K., & Werth, J. L., Jr. (2001, August). *Adaptive cognitive functioning at the end of life.* Poster session presented at the annual meeting of the American Psychological Association, San Francisco.

Block, S. D. (2001). Psychological considerations, growth, and transcendence at the end of life: The art of the possible. *Journal of the American Medical Association, 285*, 2898–2905.

Bradshaw, A. (1996). The spiritual dimension of hospice: The secularization of an ideal. *Social Science and Medicine, 43*, 409–419.

Cherny, N. I., Coyle, N., & Foley, K. M. (1994). The treatment of suffering when patients request elective death. *Journal of Palliative Care, 10*, 71–79.

Cherny, N. I., Coyle, N., & Foley, K. M. (1996). Guidelines in the care of the dying cancer patient. *Pain and Palliative Care, 10*, 261–286.

Chochinov, H. M. (2002). Dignity-conserving care—A new model for palliative care (helping the patient feel valued). *Journal of the American Medical Association, 287*, 2253–2260.

Daaleman, T. P., & VandeCreek, L. (2000). Placing religion and spirituality in end-of-life care. *Journal of the American Medical Association, 284,* 2514–2517.

Eliason, G. T., Hanley, C., & Leventis, M. (2001). The role of spirituality in counseling: Four theoretical orientations. *Pastoral Psychology, 50,* 77–91.

Emanuel, E. J., & Emanuel, L. L. (1998). The promise of a good death. *Lancet, 351*(Suppl. II), 21–29.

Emanuel, E. J., Fairclough, D. L., Slutsman, J., Alpert, H., Baldwin, D., & Emanuel, L. L. (1999). Assistance from family members, friends, paid care givers, and volunteers in the care of terminally ill patients. *The New England Journal of Medicine, 341,* 956–963.

Emanuel, E. J., Fairclough, D. L., Slutsman, J., & Emanuel, L. L. (2000). Understanding economic and other burdens of terminal illness: The experience of patients and their caregivers. *Annals of Internal Medicine, 132,* 451–459.

Exley, C. (1999). Testaments and memories: Negotiating after-death identities. *Mortality, 4,* 249–267.

Fins, J. J., Miller, F. G., Acres, C. A., Bacchetta, M. D., Huzzard, L. L., & Rapkin, B. D. (1999). End-of-life decision-making in the hospital: Current practice and future prospects. *Journal of Pain and Symptom Management, 17,* 6–15.

Frankl, V. E. (1963). *Man's search for meaning.* New York: Pocket Books.

Frankl, V. E. (1969). *The will to meaning.* New York: Signet.

Hoffman, M. A. (2000). Suicide and hastened death: A biopsychosocial perspective. *The Counseling Psychologist, 28,* 561–572.

Kagawa-Singer, M., & Blackhall, L. J. (2001). Negotiating cross-cultural issues at the end of life: "You got to go where he lives." *Journal of the American Medical Association, 286,* 2993–3001.

Kaut, K. P. (2002). Religion, spirituality, and existentialism near the end of life. *American Behavioral Scientist, 46,* 220–234.

Kaye, J., & Raghavan, K. (2002). Spirituality in disability and illness. *Journal of Religion and Health, 41,* 231–242.

Kearney, M., & Mount, B. (2000). Spiritual care of the dying patient. In H. M. Chochinov & W. Breitbart (Eds.), *Handbook of psychiatry in palliative medicine* (pp. 357–373). Oxford, England: Oxford University Press.

Kellehear, A. (2000). Spirituality and palliative care: A model of needs. *Palliative Medicine, 14,* 149–155.

Koenig, H. G. (2002). A commentary: The role of religion and spirituality at the end of life. *The Gerontologist, 42,* 20–23.

Kubler-Ross, E. (1975). *Death: The final stage of growth.* Englewood Cliffs, NJ: Prentice-Hall.

Larson, D. G., & Tobin, D. R. (2000). End-of-life conversations: Evolving practice and theory. *Journal of the American Medical Association, 284,* 1573–1578.

Lo, B., Ruston, D., Kates, L. W., Arnold, R. M., Cohen, C. B., Faber-Langendoen, K., et al. (2002). Discussing religious and spiritual issues at the end of life: A practical guide for physicians. *Journal of the American Medical Association, 287,* 749–754.

Lynn, J. (1997). An 88-year old woman facing the end of life. *Journal of the American Medical Association, 277,* 1633–1640.

Marrone, R. (1999). Dying, mourning, and spirituality: A psychological perspective. *Death Studies, 23,* 495–519.

Mauritzen, J. (1988). Pastoral care for the dying and bereaved. *Death Studies, 12,* 111–122.

McClain, C. S., Rosenfeld, B., & Breitbart, W. (2003). Effect of spiritual well-being on end-of-life despair in terminally ill cancer patients. *Lancet, 361,* 1603–1607.

McPhee, S. J., Rabow, M. W., Pantilat, S. Z., Markowitz, A. J., & Winker, M. A. (2000). Finding our way—Perspectives on care at the close of life. *Journal of the American Medical Association, 284,* 2512–2513.

Moadel, A., Morgan, C., Fatone, A., Grennan, J., Carter, J., Laruffa, G., et al. (1999). Seeking meaning and hope: Self-reported spiritual and existential needs among an ethnically-diverse cancer patient population. *Psycho-Oncology, 8,* 378–385.

Morrison, R. S., Meier, D. E., & Cassel, C. K. (1996). When too much is too little. *New England Journal of Medicine, 335,* 1755–1759.

Muir, J. C., & Arnold, R. M. (2001). Palliative care and the hospitalist: An opportunity for cross-fertilization. *The American Journal of Medicine, 111(9B),* 10S–14S.

Nicassio, P. M., & Smith, T. W. (Eds.). (1995). *Managing chronic illness: A biopsychosocial perspective.* Washington, DC: American Psychological Association.

Patrick, D. L., Engelberg, R. A., & Curtis, J. R. (2001). Evaluating the quality of dying and death. *Journal of Pain and Symptom Management, 22,* 717–726.

Paulson, D. S. (2001). The hard issues of life. *Pastoral Psychology, 49,* 385–394.

Quill, T. E. (2000). Initiating end-of-life discussions with seriously ill patients. Addressing the "elephant in the room." *Journal of the American Medical Association, 284,* 2502–2507.

Rothschild, S. K. (1997). Medical care of the dying patient. *Medical Update for Psychiatrists, 2(3),* 62–66.

Sachs, G. A. (2000). Sometimes dying still stings. *Journal of the American Medical Association, 284,* 2423.

Shuster, J. L., Breitbart, W., & Chochinov, H. M. (1999). Psychiatric aspects of excellent end-of-life care. *Psychosomatics, 40,* 1–4.

Singer, P. A., Martin, D. K., & Kelner, M. (1999). Quality end-of-life care: Patients' perspectives. *Journal of the American Medical Association, 281,* 163–168.

Smith, D. C. (1993). Exploring the religious-spiritual needs of the dying. *Counseling and Values, 37,* 71–77.

Smith, D. C., & Maher, M. F. (1991). Healthy death. *Counseling and Values, 36,* 42–48.

Steinhauser, K. E., Christakis, N. A., Clipp, E. C., McNeilly, M., McIntyre, L. M., & Tulsky, J. A. (2000). Factors considered important at the end of life by patients, family, physicians, and other care providers. *Journal of the American Medical Association, 284,* 2476–2482.

Steinhauser, K. E., Clipp, E. C., McNeilly, M., Christakis, N. A., McIntyre, L. M., & Tulsky, J. A. (2000). In search of a good death: Observations of patients, families and providers. *Annals of Internal Medicine, 132,* 825–832.

Stewart, A. L., Teno, J. M., Patrick, D. L., & Lynn, J. (1999). The concept of quality of life of dying persons in the context of health care. *Journal of Pain and Symptom Management, 17,* 93–108.

Sulmasy, D. P. (2002). A biopsychosocial-spiritual model for the care of patients at the end of life. *The Gerontologist, 42,* 24–33.

Thomas, J., & Retsas, A. (1999). Transacting self-preservation: A grounded theory of the spiritual dimensions of people with terminal cancer. *International Journal of Nursing Studies, 36,* 191–201.

Walter, T. (1993). Death in the new age. *Religion, 23,* 127–145.

Walter, T. (1996). Developments in spiritual care of the dying. *Religion, 26,* 353–363.

6

MENTAL HEALTH ISSUES NEAR THE END OF LIFE

CHRISTOPHER A. GIBSON, WILLIAM BREITBART, ALEXIS TOMARKEN, ANNE KOSINSKI, AND CHRISTIAN J. NELSON

As humans, we often fear the process that leads to our death more than death itself. This fear is increasingly heightened in technologically advanced cultures as medical technology and the consequent life span of "terminal" individuals progress in tandem. The lives of people who previously would have died relatively rapidly are now often greatly extended (see Stillion, chap. 1). Images of suffering or of dying in isolation are often foremost on the minds of those struggling with terminal illness. Inadequately addressed physical and psychiatric symptoms often interact and have a negative impact on quality of life. Our ability to recognize and treat these symptoms effectively is unfortunately lagging behind our ability to sustain life.

Therefore, the prompt recognition and effective treatment of both psychiatric and physical symptoms becomes critically important to the well-being of our clients with advanced disease. In general, palliative care specialists are expert at managing a broad spectrum of difficult and complex physical symptoms. Managing the psychiatric complications (such as organic mental disorders, depression, suicide, anxiety) and difficult psychosocial issues (such as bereavement, loss, family dysfunction) facing persons with terminal ill-

137

ness and their families, however, can test the limits of even the most skilled practitioner. It is for this reason that a multidisciplinary approach to the management of the client with advanced disease has gained broad acceptance. A psychologist or psychiatrist can play a vital role as a member of such a treatment team. This role includes the assessment and treatment of the psychological complications of terminal illness and the application of psychological and psychiatric techniques to the management of physical symptoms. This chapter is designed to provide such mental health practitioners with a knowledge base specific to the issues and symptoms common in terminal illness and to provide a framework for approaching them effectively.

HOW COMMON ARE PSYCHIATRIC DISORDERS IN TERMINALLY ILL INDIVIDUALS?

People with advanced disease face many stressors during the course of their illnesses. Common stressors include fears of a prolonged and painful death, disability, disfigurement, and dependency on others for care and support. Although such concerns are relatively universal, the level of resultant psychological distress is rather variable and dependent on numerous factors such as personality, coping ability, social support, and medical issues. In addition, the expression of such distress in the form of a psychiatric disorder is also relative. Excellent baseline data on the prevalence of psychiatric disorders in seriously physically ill people is provided by a study conducted by the Psychosocial Collaborative Oncology Group, which evaluated the prevalence of psychiatric disorders in 215 cancer patients (ambulatory or hospitalized, with a wide range of cancer diagnoses and stages of disease) receiving treatment in three major cancer centers (Derogatis et al., 1983). Roughly half (53%) of the patients evaluated were adjusting normally to the stresses of their illnesses with no diagnosable psychiatric disorder. However, 47% presented with a diagnosable psychiatric disorder. Of this 47%, 68% had adjustment disorders with depressed or anxious mood, 13% had major depression, and 8% had an organic mental disorder (delirium).

People with advanced cancer are a particularly vulnerable group for the development of such conditions (Breitbart, 1989b; Chochinov, Wilson, Enns, & Lander, 1994; Massie & Holland, 1987; Twycross & Lack, 1983). The incidence of attendant pain, depression, and delirium all increase with higher levels of physical debilitation and advanced illness (Bukberg, Penman, & Holland, 1984; Foley, 1985; Massie, Holland, & Glass, 1983). Approximately 25% of all individuals with cancer experience severe depressive symptoms, with the prevalence increasing to 77% in those with advanced illness (Bukberg et al., 1984). The prevalence of organic mental disorders (delirium) among people with cancer requiring psychiatric consultation has been found to range from 25% to 40% and as high as 85% during the terminal stages of illness

(Massie et al., 1983). Narcotic analgesics commonly cause confusional states, particularly in the elderly and terminally ill (Breitbart, 1988). People with cancer who have pain are twice as likely to develop a psychiatric complication of cancer than similar persons without pain. Of those who received a psychiatric diagnosis, 39% reported significant pain whereas only 19% of individuals without a psychiatric diagnosis had significant pain (Derogatis et al., 1983). The psychiatric diagnoses of these people with pain were predominantly adjustment disorder with depressed or mixed mood (69%) and major depression (15%).

Persons struggling with AIDS are also prone to develop psychiatric disorders. There have been several reports of psychiatric diagnoses seen in people with AIDS who were hospitalized and thus more seriously ill. Karina et al. (1994) reported that of 357 patients hospitalized with AIDS, 49 (14%) had at least one psychiatric diagnosis. An important finding from this study was that these patients were hospitalized an average of 60 days longer than AIDS patients without such psychiatric illnesses. Differences in purely medical factors did not account for these patients' longer hospitalizations. Perry and Tross (1984) reported on the prevalence of psychiatric disorders seen in medically hospitalized AIDS patients. They found that 65% of patients were diagnosed with an organic mental disorder, and 17% were diagnosed with major depression. The organic mental disorders seen were predominantly AIDS dementia complex (ADC) and delirium, often in combination.

As medical technology and the resultant efficacy of treatment increase, people are increasingly treated in outpatient settings. Their psychosocial concerns and difficulties do not necessarily decrease, however. Tross and Hirsch (1988) reported on the prevalence of psychiatric disorders in an ambulatory sample of 279 persons with AIDS spectrum disorders. The study included asymptomatic gay men, gay men with AIDS-related complex (ARC), and gay men with AIDS. Men with ARC showed the greatest distress and frequency of psychiatric disorder. Three quarters of the men with ARC, half of the persons with AIDS, and two fifths of the asymptomatic gay men were diagnosed as having a psychiatric disorder. The most common psychiatric diagnosis was adjustment disorder, seen in two-thirds of the persons with AIDS and more than half of those with ARC. Depression was present in one quarter of the entire study population. People with AIDS thus have comparable, if not higher, levels of psychiatric distress than persons with cancer. What is striking is that levels of distress are high in asymptomatic gay men and highest in those with ARC. These are presumably the "worried well" for whom waiting for a diagnosis of AIDS is more distressing than finally knowing.

Anxiety in the Person With Advanced Illness

As in the example of people with ARC, physically ill individuals present with a complex mixture of physical and psychological symptoms in the context of an uncertain and frightening reality. Thus, the recognition of anxious symptoms requiring treatment can be quite challenging. Individuals with anxiety complain of tension or restlessness or exhibit jitteriness, autonomic hyperactivity, vigilance, insomnia, distractibility, shortness of breath, numbness, apprehension, worry, or rumination. Often the physical or somatic manifestations of anxiety overshadow the psychological or cognitive ones, and are the symptoms that the person most often presents (Holland, 1989). The clinician must use these symptoms as a cue to inquire about the person's psychological state, which is commonly one of fear, worry, or apprehension. The blanket assumption that a high level of anxiety is an inevitable consequence of the terminal phase of illness is neither helpful nor accurate for diagnostic and treatment purposes. In deciding whether to treat anxiety during the terminal phase of illness, the individual's subjective level of distress is the primary impetus for the initiation of treatment. Other considerations include problematic behavior such as noncompliance because of anxiety, family and staff reactions to the person's distress, and the balancing of the risks and benefits of treatment (Massie, 1989).

Anxiety is a symptom in this population that can have many etiologies. Anxiety may be encountered as a component of an adjustment disorder, panic disorder, generalized anxiety disorder, phobia, or agitated depression. Also, in the terminally ill person with cancer, symptoms of anxiety are most likely to arise from some medical complication of the illness or treatment such as organic anxiety disorder, delirium, or other organic mental disorders (Foley, 1985; Holland, 1989; Massie, 1989). Hypoxia, sepsis, poorly controlled pain, and adverse drug reactions such as akathisia (restlessness) or withdrawal states often present as anxiety. In the dying person, anxiety can represent impending cardiac or respiratory arrest, pulmonary embolism, electrolyte imbalance, or dehydration (Strain, Liebowitz, & Klein, 1981).

Despite the fact that anxiety in terminal illness commonly results from medical complications, psychological factors related to dying and death or existential issues play a role in anxiety, particularly in those who are alert and not confused (Holland, 1989). People frequently fear the isolation and separation of death. Claustrophobic individuals may be afraid of the idea of being confined and buried in a coffin. These issues can be disconcerting to consultants who may find themselves at a loss for words that are consoling to the person. Nonetheless, one should not avoid eliciting these concerns, listening empathically to them, and enlisting pastoral involvement where appropriate. The clinician's basic listening and reflective skills are often all that is required in these situations, although they may be tested to their limits at times.

The specific treatment of anxiety in people who are terminally ill often depends on etiology, presentation, and setting. Nonpharmacological interventions for anxiety and distress include supportive psychotherapy and behavioral interventions that are used alone or in combination. Brief supportive psychotherapy is often useful in dealing with both crisis-related issues as well as existential issues confronted by the terminally ill (Massie, 1989). Psychotherapeutic interventions should include both the client and family, particularly as the person with advanced illness becomes increasingly debilitated and less able to interact. Mental health professionals can assist in seeing that the emotional needs of clients and families are met during the terminal phase of illness. Such needs include continuous, updated information regarding the disease status and treatment options available. This information must be delivered repeatedly and with sensitivity as to what they are currently prepared and able to hear and absorb. Families, especially, require a great deal of reassurance that they and the medical staff have done everything possible for the loved one.

The goals of psychotherapy with the client are to establish a bond that decreases the sense of isolation experienced with terminal illness; to help the client face death with a sense of self worth; to correct misconceptions about the past and present; to integrate the present illness into a continuum of life experiences; and to explore issues of separation, loss, and the unknown that lies ahead (Greenstein & Breitbart, 2000). The therapist should emphasize past strengths and support previously successful ways of coping. This helps the person mobilize inner resources, modify plans for the future, and perhaps even accept the inevitability of death.

It is during the terminal phase of illness that we have the greatest opportunity to effect the process of adaptation to loss (Chochinov & Holland, 1989). Mental health professionals must extend their supportive stance to include both the client and family. Anticipatory bereavement is a common experience that allows dying persons, loved ones, and health care providers the opportunity to prepare mentally for the impending death. Clients and family members should be encouraged to use this period to reconcile differences, extend important final communications and reaffirm feelings and wishes. It is a time is of vital importance that can often set the tone for the subsequent bereavement course.

Relaxation, guided imagery, and hypnosis may help reduce anxiety and thereby increase the person's sense of control. Contrary to many clinicians' assumptions, most people with advanced illness are still appropriate candidates for useful application of behavioral techniques despite physical debilitation. In assessing the utility of such interventions for a person who is terminally ill, the clinician should take into account the mental clarity of the client. Confusional states interfere dramatically with a person's ability to focus attention and thus limit the usefulness of these techniques (Breitbart, 1989b). Occasionally these techniques can be modified so as to include even mildly cognitive impaired individuals. These often involve the therapist taking a more active role by orienting the client, creating a safe and secure environment and evoking a conditioned response to the therapist's voice or presence. A typical behavioral intervention for anxiety in a terminally ill person would include a relaxation exercise combined with some distraction or imagery technique. Typically the individual is first taught to relax with passive breathing accompanied by either passive or active muscle relaxation. Once in such a relaxed state, the client is taught a pleasant, distracting imagery exercise. In a randomized study comparing a relaxation technique with a benzodiazepine in the treatment of anxiety in cancer patients, both treatments were demonstrated to be effective for mild to moderate degrees of anxiety or distress. The drug intervention (alprazolam) was more effective for greater levels of distress or anxiety and had more rapid onset of beneficial effect (Holland et al., 1988).

Relaxation techniques can be prescribed concurrently with anxiolytic medications in highly anxious people with cancer and, as is the case with concurrent use of medications with behavioral techniques for anxiety disorders in nonphysically ill individuals, can be expected to have good efficacy.

Depression in People With Advanced Illness

The incidence of depression in persons with cancer ranges from 10% to 25% and increases with higher levels of disability, advanced illness, and pain (Bukberg et al., 1984; Massie & Holland, 1990; Plumb & Holland, 1977; see also Rosenfeld, Abbey, & Pessin, chap. 7). Certain types of illness are associated with an increased incidence of depression. Individuals with pancreatic cancer for example are more likely to develop depression than people with other types of intraabdominal malignancies (Green & Austin, 1994/1995; Holland et al., 1986). Evaluation of illness-related organic factors, such as corticosteroids (Stiefel, Breitbart, & Holland, 1989), chemotherapeutic agents (Adams, Quesada, & Gutterman, 1984; Denicoff et al., 1987; Holland, Fassanellos, & Ohnuma, 1974; Young, 1982), whole brain radiation (DeAngelis, Delattre, & Posner, 1989), and central nervous system complications (Breitbart, 1989a), which can present as depression should be conducted before the initiation of any treatment.

As the terminally ill person faces death, depressed mood and sadness are often appropriate responses. These emotions can be manifestations of anticipatory grief over the impending loss of one's life, health, loved ones, and personal freedom and autonomy. The diagnosis of a major depressive syndrome in a terminally ill individual often relies more on the psychological or cognitive symptoms of major depression (worthlessness, hopelessness, excessive guilt, and suicidal ideation), rather than the neurovegetative or somatic signs and symptoms of major depression (Endicott, 1984; Massie & Holland, 1987; Plumb & Holland, 1977; see also Rosenfeld et al., chap. 7). Terminal illness itself can produce many of these physical symptoms so characteristic of major depression in the physically healthy. How is the clinician to interpret feelings of hopelessness in the dying person when there is no hope for cure or recovery? Feelings of hopelessness, worthlessness, or suicidal ideation must be explored in detail. Hopelessness that is pervasive and accompanied by a sense of despair or despondency is more likely to represent a symptom of a depressive disorder (Massie & Holland, 1990). Similarly, people often state that they believe they are burdening their families unfairly, causing them great pain and inconvenience. Those beliefs are less likely to represent a symptom of depression than if the person thinks that her or his life has never had any worth or that she or he is being punished for evil things she or he has done.

Depression in individuals with advanced cancer is optimally managed using a combination of psychotherapy, cognitive–behavioral techniques, and antidepressant medications (Massie & Holland, 1990; see also Rosenfeld et al., chap. 7). Psychotherapeutic interventions, either in the form of individual or group counseling, have been shown to reduce psychological distress and depressive symptoms in people with cancer (Massie, Holland, & Straker, 1989; Spiegel & Bloom, 1983; Spiegel, Bloom, & Yalom, 1981). Cognitive–behavioral interventions, such as relaxation and distraction with pleasant imagery, have also been shown to decrease depressive symptoms in clients with mild to moderate levels of depression (Holland et al., 1988). Psychopharmacological interventions are the mainstay of management in the treatment of seriously physically ill people with severe depressive symptoms who meet criteria for a major depressive episode (Massie & Holland, 1990).

Supportive psychotherapy is a useful treatment approach to depression in the terminally ill client. Psychotherapy with the dying person consists of active listening with supportive verbal interventions and the occasional interpretation (Cassem, 1987). Despite the seriousness of the client's plight, it is not necessary for the psychologist or psychiatrist to appear overly solemn or emotionally restrained. Often it is only the psychotherapist, of all the person's caregivers, who is comfortable enough to converse lightheartedly and allow the client to talk about his or her life and experiences, rather than focus solely on impending death. The dying person who wishes to talk or ask questions about death should be allowed to do so freely, with the therapist maintaining an interested, interactive stance. It is not uncommon for the dying individual to benefit from pastoral counseling. If a chaplainry service is available, it should be offered to the client and family.

Although many dying people lose hope of a cure, they are able to maintain hope for better symptom control. For many individuals, hope is contingent on the ability to find continued meaning in their day-to-day existence, yet instilling such meaning can be challenging for the clinician. As a result, we have developed both an individual and group meaning-centered psychotherapy for people with cancer (Gibson & Breitbart, 2003; Greenstein & Breitbart, 2000). We are currently conducting a series of randomized, controlled trials to determine the feasibility and efficacy of these treatments. A preliminary analysis of the efficacy of this intervention revealed stronger effects for enhanced spiritual well-being as well as end-of-life despair (hopelessness and desire for hastened death), whereas depression and anxiety were somewhat less responsive. It is important that an analysis of the data from the 2-month follow-up assessment demonstrated that the benefits of this intervention continued to grow after treatment had concluded. Despite the small number of participants available for analysis, these effects are encouraging. Research into effective interventions for enhancing meaning and spiritual well-being should continue.

Suicide Among Terminally Ill Individuals

Depression is a factor in 50% of all suicides and those experiencing depression are at 25 times greater risk of suicide than the general population (American Psychiatric Association, 2003; Guze & Robins, 1970; Sayar, Acar, & Ak, 2003). The role depression plays in the suicides of terminally ill persons is equally significant. For example, approximately 25% of all people with cancer experience severe depressive symptoms, with about 6% fulfilling *Diagnostic and Statistical Manual of Mental Disorders, Third Edition, Revised (DSM–III–R;* American Psychiatric Association, 1987) criteria for the diagnosis of major depression (Bukberg et al., 1984; Derogatis et al., 1983; Plumb & Holland, 1977). Among those with advanced illness and progressively impaired physical function, symptoms of severe depression rise to 77% (Bukberg et al., 1984). Depression also appears to be important in terms of preferences for life-sustaining medical therapy. Ganzini, Lee, Heintz, Bloom, and Fenn (1994) reported that among elderly depressed patients, an increase in desire for life-sustaining medical therapies followed treatment of depression in those subjects who had been initially more severely depressed, more hopeless, and more likely to overestimate the risks and to underestimate the benefits of treatment. They concluded that although patients with mild to moderate depression are unlikely to alter their decisions regarding life-sustaining medical treatment despite treatment for their depression, severely depressed patients—particularly those who are hopeless—should be encouraged to defer advance treatment directives. In these patients, decisions about life-sustaining therapy should be discouraged until after treatment of their depression.

Terminally ill individuals are at increased risk of suicide relative to the general population. Factors associated with increased risk of suicide in people with advanced disease (Breitbart, 1987, 1990) include suffering, poor prognosis, fatigue and exhaustion, hopelessness, helplessness, substance use, personal and familial history of suicide attempts, and lack of social support. In addition, persons with advanced illness are at highest risk, perhaps because they are most likely to have such complications as pain, depression, and delirium. Psychiatric disorders are frequently present in hospitalized cancer patients who are suicidal. A review of the psychiatric consultation data from Memorial Sloan-Kettering Cancer Center (MSKCC) showed that one third of suicidal cancer patients had a major depression, about 20% experienced delirium, and 50% were diagnosed with an adjustment disorder with both anxious and depressed features at the time of evaluation (Breitbart, 1987, 1990).

Poor prognosis and advanced illness usually go hand in hand. It is thus not surprising that in Sweden, those who were expected to die within a matter of months were the most likely to die by suicide (Bolund, 1985). Of 88 cancer suicides, 14 had an uncertain prognosis, and 45 had a poor prognosis. With advancing disease, the incidence of significant cancer pain increases. Uncontrolled pain in cancer patients is a dramatically important risk factor for suicide. The vast majority of cancer suicides in several studies showed that these patients had severe pain that was often inadequately controlled and poorly tolerated (Bolund, 1985; Farberow, Ganzler, Cuter, & Reynolds, 1971).

Hopelessness is a significantly better predictor of completed suicide than is depression alone (Beck, Kovacs, & Weissman, 1975; Breitbart et al., 2000; Kovacs, Beck, & Weissman, 1975). With the typical cancer suicide being characterized by advanced illness and poor prognosis, hopelessness is commonly experienced. In Scandinavia, the highest incidence of suicide was found in people with cancer who were offered no further treatment and no further contact with the health care system (Bolund, 1985; Louhivuori & Hakama, 1979). Being left to face illness alone creates a sense of isolation and abandonment that is critical to the development of hopelessness.

The prevalence of organic mental disorders among people with cancer requiring psychiatric consultation has been found to range from 25% to 40% (Massie et al., 1983) and as high as 85% during the terminal stages of illness (Massie et al., 1983). Although earlier work suggested that delirium was a protective factor in regard to cancer suicide (Farberow, Shneidman, & Leonard, 1963), clinical experience has found these confusional states to be a major contributing factor in impulsive suicide attempts, especially in the hospital setting.

In our experience, loss of control and a sense of helplessness in the face of cancer are important factors in suicide vulnerability. Control refers to both the helplessness induced by symptoms or deficits due to cancer or its treatments, as well as the excessive need on the part of some people to be in charge of all aspects of living or dying. Farberow et al. (1963) noted that individuals who were accepting and adaptable were much less likely to die by suicide than people with cancer who exhibited a need to be in control of even the most minute details of their care. This need to control may be prominent in some people and cause distress with little provocation. It is not uncommon, however, for cancer-related events to induce a great sense of helplessness even in those who are not typically controlling individuals. Impairments or deficits induced by cancer or cancer treatments include loss of mobility, paraplegia, loss of bowel and bladder function, amputation, aphonia, sensory loss, and inability to eat or swallow. Most distressing to people is the sense that they are losing control of their minds, especially when they are confused or sedated by medications. The risk of suicide is increased in persons with cancer with such physical impairments, especially when accompanied by psychological distress and disturbed interpersonal relationships attributable to these deficit factors.

Another consideration is that cancer is now often a chronic illness. Increased survival is accompanied by increased numbers of hospitalizations, complications, and expenses. Symptom control thus becomes a prolonged process with frequent advances and setbacks. The dying process also can become extremely long and arduous for all concerned. It is not uncommon for both family members and health care providers to withdraw prematurely from the person with cancer under these circumstances, leaving a suicidal person feeling even more isolated and abandoned. The presence of a strong support system for the individual that may act as an external control of suicidal behavior reduces risk of cancer suicide significantly.

Frequency of Suicidal Ideation

Thoughts of suicide probably occur quite frequently, particularly in the setting of advanced cancer, and seem to act as a steam valve for feelings often expressed by people as, "If it gets too bad, I always have a way out." Once they develop a trusting and safe relationship, clients almost universally reveal occasional persistent thoughts of suicide as a means of escaping the threat of being overwhelmed by cancer. Recent published reports, however, suggest that suicidal ideation is relatively infrequent in cancer and is limited to those who are significantly depressed. Chochinov et al. (1995) found that of 200 terminally ill patients in a palliative care facility, 44.5% acknowledged at least a fleeting desire to die; these episodes were brief and did not reflect a sustained or committed desire to die. However, 17 patients (8.5%) reported an unequivocal desire for death to come soon and indicated that they held this desire consistently over time. Among this group, 10 (58.8%) received a diagnosis of depression, compared with a prevalence of 7.7% in patients who did not endorse a genuine, consistent desire for death. Patients with a desire for death were also found to have significantly more pain and less social support than those patients without a desire for death.

At Memorial Hospital, suicide risk evaluation accounted for 8.6% of psychiatric consultations, usually requested by staff in response to a patient verbalizing suicidal wishes (Breitbart, 1987). Among 185 cancer patients with pain studied at Memorial Hospital, suicidal ideation was found in 17% of the study population (Breitbart, 1990). The actual prevalence of suicidal ideation may be considerably higher in that patients often disclose these thoughts only after a stable and ongoing physician–patient relationship has been established.

AIDS and Suicide

There is increased risk of suicide in persons with AIDS (Cote, Biggar, & Dannenberg, 1992; Marzuk et al., 1988). A study of the rate of suicide in

1985 in New York City residents diagnosed with AIDS revealed that the relative risk of suicide in men with AIDS aged 20 to 59 years was 36 times that of men without AIDS in the same age range, and 66 times that of the general population (Marzuk et al., 1988). By comparison, the relative risk of suicide in people with cancer is only twice that of the general population. Suicidal ideation, either lifetime prevalence or current ideation, is also dramatically higher in HIV-infected individuals than in the general population or even in the cancer population (Atkinson et al., 1990; Gutierrez et al., 1990; McKegney & O'Dowd, 1992; Orr, O'Dowd, McKegney, & Natali, 1990). In a study of 91 individuals with AIDS in New York City hospitals, 63.4% of the participants acknowledged some degree of suicidal ideation, and 22% had previous suicide attempts (Gil, Passik, Rosenfeld, & Brietbart, 1998). A study of suicide attempts in the United States (Goodwin, Marusia, & Howen, 2003) found that persons with AIDS were 100 times more likely to have made an attempt compared with the general population. In HIV-seropositive populations of gay men, alcohol or substance abusers, and psychiatric outpatients, prevalence rates of lifetime suicidal thoughts ranged from 50% to 82% (Alfonso et al., 1994; Atkinson et al., 1990; Gutierrez et al., 1990; Orr et al., 1990). It is interesting that HIV-negative individuals in the same populations had similar rates of suicidal ideation, thus suggesting that it is not HIV status per se that accounts for such high rates of suicidal ideation, but rather the psychiatric morbidity found in the at-risk groups. For example, in a more recent study of people who died by suicide in New York City, 133 were found to be HIV seropositive, leading the authors to conclude that HIV-positive individuals were at most 2 times as likely to commit suicide compared with the general population (Marzuk et al., 1997). In addition, approximately 70% had no HIV-related illness at autopsy.

Presenting symptomatology is also an important factor to consider. A review of the psychiatric consultation data at Memorial Sloan Kettering Cancer Center (Breitbart, 1987) revealed that AIDS with Kaposi's sarcoma (KS) was the single most common medical diagnosis among suicidal individuals. People with AIDS and KS who were suicidal frequently had prominent signs of delirium, often superimposed on AIDS dementia. Clinicians must be alert to this increased risk of suicide in clients with AIDS and promote early intervention for such psychiatric complications as delirium, depression, and social isolation.

Management of the Suicidal, Terminally Ill Person

Assessment of suicide risk and appropriate intervention are critical. Early and comprehensive psychiatric involvement with high-risk individuals can often avert suicide in the cancer setting (Dubovsky, 1978). A careful evaluation includes a search for the meaning of suicidal thoughts, as well as an exploration of the seriousness of the risk. The clinician's ability to establish rapport and elicit a client's thoughts is essential as he or she assesses history, degree of intent, and quality of internal and external controls. One must listen sympathetically, not appearing critical or stating that such thoughts are inappropriate. Allowing the client to discuss suicidal thoughts often decreases the risk of suicide. The myth that asking about suicidal thoughts "puts the idea in their head" is one that should be dispelled, especially in cancer (Breitbart, Chochinov, & Passik, 2004; McKegney & Lange, 1971). Clients often reconsider and reject the idea of suicide when the physician acknowledges the legitimacy of their option and the need to retain a sense of control over aspects of their death.

The suicide vulnerability factors described earlier (Breitbart, 1987, 1990) should be used as a guide to evaluation and management. Once the setting has been made secure, assessment of the relevant mental status and adequacy of pain control can begin. Analgesics, neuroleptics, or antidepressant drugs should be used when appropriate to treat agitation, psychosis, major depression, or pain. Underlying causes of delirium or pain should be addressed specifically when possible. Initiation of a crisis-intervention-oriented psychotherapeutic approach, mobilizing as much of the person's support system as possible, is important. A close family member or friend should be involved to support the person, provide information, and assist in treatment planning. Psychiatric hospitalization can sometimes be helpful but is usually not desirable for the terminally ill person. Thus, the medical hospital or home is the setting in which management most often takes place. Although it is appropriate to intervene when medical or psychiatric factors are clearly the driving force in a cancer suicide, in some circumstances usurping control from the individual and family with overly aggressive intervention may be less helpful. This is most evident in those with advanced illness for whom comfort and symptom control are the primary concerns. The goal of the intervention should not be to prevent suicide at all cost, but to prevent suicide that is driven by desperation. Prolonged suffering due to poorly controlled symptoms leads to such desperation, and it is the consultant's role to provide effective management of such problems as an alternative to suicide in the terminally ill individual.

We decided not to discuss the emotionally charged and controversial issue of physician-assisted suicide in this chapter. To do so would have taken us far afield from our focus on the psychosocial aspects of care and into debate about ethics and social policy. For discussion of this issue, see Rosenfeld (2004) and chapter 3 of this book (Werth & Kleespies).

COGNITIVE DISORDERS IN PERSONS WHO ARE TERMINALLY ILL

Cognitive failure is unfortunately all too common in people with advanced illness. The *Diagnostic and Statistical Manual of Mental Disorders,*

Fourth Edition (*DSM–IV*; American Psychiatric Association, 1994) divides cognitive disorders into the following subcategories: (a) delirium, dementia, amnestic, and other cognitive disorders; (b) mental disorders due to a general medical condition (including mood disorder, anxiety disorder, and personality change due to a general medical condition); and (c) substance-related disorders. Although virtually all of these mental syndromes can be seen in the person with advanced cancer, the most common include delirium, dementia, and mood and anxiety disorders resulting from a general medical condition. Lipowski (1987) categorized organic mental disorders into those that were characterized by general cognitive impairment, (i.e., delirium and dementia) and those in which cognitive impairment was selective or limited (i.e., amnesic disorder, organic hallucinosis, organic mood disorder, etc.). With organic mental disorders in which cognitive impairment is selective, limited, or relatively intact, the more prominent symptoms tend to consist of anxiety, mood disturbance, delusions, hallucinations, or personality change. For example, the person with mood disturbance meeting criteria for major depression who is severely hypothyroid or on high-dose corticosteroids is most accurately diagnosed as having a mood disorder due to a general medical condition or substance-induced mood disorder respectively (particularly if organic factors are judged to be the primary etiology related to the mood disturbance).

Delirium and Dementia

Despite little being known about the neuropathogenesis of delirium, its symptoms suggest that it is a dysfunction of multiple regions of the brain (Trzepacz, 1994). Delirium has been characterized as an etiologically non-specific, global, cerebral dysfunction characterized by concurrent disturbances of level of consciousness, attention, thinking, perception, memory, psychomotor behavior, emotion, and the sleep–wake cycle. Disorientation, fluctuation, or waxing and waning of these symptoms, as well as acute or abrupt onset of such disturbances, are other critical features of delirium. Delirium, in contrast with dementia, is conceptualized as a *reversible* process. Reversibility of the process of delirium is often possible even in the individual with advanced illness; it may not be reversible in the last 24 to 48 hours of life, however (Breitbart & Sparrow, 1998). This is most likely because irreversible processes such as multiple organ failure occur during the final hours of life. Delirium at this time is often referred to as terminal restlessness or terminal agitation in the palliative care literature (Breitbart & Sparrow, 1998).

At times, it is difficult to differentiate delirium from dementia because they frequently share such common clinical features as impaired memory, thinking, judgment, and disorientation. Dementia appears in relatively alert individuals with little or no clouding of consciousness. The temporal onset of symptoms in dementia is more subacute or chronically progressive, and one's sleep–wake cycle seems less impaired. Most prominent in dementia are difficulties in short- and long-term memory, impaired judgment and abstract thinking, as well as disturbances (such as aphasia and apraxia) of higher cortical functions. On occasion one will encounter delirium superimposed on an underlying dementia, as in the case of an elderly person or an individual with a paraneoplastic syndrome.

Centeno, Sanz, and Bruera (2004) noted that delirium is the most frequently encountered psychiatric disorder in terminal cancer. These authors found delirium in 26% to 46% of cancer patients admitted to a hospice or hospital. Massie et al. (1983) found delirium in more than 75% of terminally ill cancer patients they studied. Delirium can be due to either the direct effects of cancer on the central nervous system (CNS) or indirect CNS effects of the disease or treatments (medications, electrolyte imbalance, failure of a vital organ or system, infection, vascular complications, and preexisting cognitive impairment or dementia). Early symptoms of delirium can be misdiagnosed as anxiety, anger, depression, or psychosis. In any person showing acute onset of agitation, impaired cognitive function, altered attention span, or a fluctuating level of consciousness, a diagnosis of delirium should be considered (Lipowski, 1987).

Delirium is distressing not only to the patient, but also to caregivers and medical staff. Breitbart, Gibson, and Tremblay (2002) conducted a study examining the experience of delirium in hospitalized cancer patients, their caregivers, and their nurses. Results indicated that the presence of delusions during the delirious episode was the strongest predictor of patient distress. In contrast, severity of illness was the strongest predictor of caregiver distress, whereas delirium severity and the presence of perceptual disturbance were the strongest predictors for nursing staff. This study also demonstrated the impact of delirium on those around the patient in that, of these three groups, caregivers were found to be the most distressed by the experience. This points to the importance of providing support to those around the patient during such episodes (see also chap. 8 by Allen et al. for additional discussion of caregiver issues).

A common error among medical and nursing staff is to conclude that a new psychological symptom is functional without completely ruling out all possible organic etiologies. Given the large numbers of drugs people with cancer require, and the fragile state of their physiologic functioning, even routinely ordered hypnotics are enough to tip people over into a delirium. Narcotic analgesics such as levorphanol, morphine sulfate, and meperidine are common causes of confusional states, particularly in elderly and terminally ill persons (Bruera, Macmillan, Hanson, & MacDonald, 1989). Chemotherapeutic agents known to cause delirium include methotrexate, fluorouracil, vincristine, vinblastine, bleomycin, BCNU, cis-platinum, asparaginase, procarbazine, and the glucocorticosteroids (Adams et al., 1984; Denicoff et al., 1987; Holland et al., 1974; Stiefel et al., 1989; Weddington,

1982; Young, 1982). Except for steroids, most people receiving these agents will not develop prominent CNS effects (Coyle, Breitbart, Weaver, & Portenoy, 1994). The spectrum of mental disturbances related to steroids includes minor mood lability, affective disorders (mania or depression), cognitive impairment (reversible dementia), and delirium (steroid psychosis). The incidence of these disorders range from 3% to 57% in noncancer populations, and they occur most commonly on higher doses (Levy, Abaza, Hawkshaw, & Sataloff, 2001; Perantie & Brown, 2002). Symptoms usually develop within the first 2 weeks on steroids but can occur at any time, on any dose, even during the tapering phase (Stiefel et al., 1989). Prior psychiatric illness or prior mental disturbance on steroids is not a good predictor of susceptibility to, or the nature of, disturbance. These disorders are often rapidly reversible upon reduction or discontinuation (Stiefel et al., 1989).

Management of Delirium in Terminally Ill Individuals

A standard approach for managing delirium in the person with cancer includes a search for underlying causes, correction of those factors and management of the symptoms of delirium. When confronted with a delirium in the terminally ill or dying person with cancer, a differential diagnosis should always be formulated; however, tests should be pursued only when a suspected factor can be identified easily and treated effectively. It is interesting that Bruera, Miller, and McCalion (1990) reported that an etiology was discovered in less than 50% of terminally ill patients with cognitive failure. In addition to seeking out and correcting the underlying cause for delirium, symptomatic and supportive therapies are important (Lipowski, 1987). Fluid and electrolyte balance, nutrition, and vitamins may be helpful. Measures to help reduce anxiety and disorientation (i.e., structure and familiarity) may include a quiet, well-lit room with familiar objects, a visible clock or calendar, and the presence of family. Judicious use of physical restraints, along with one-to-one nursing observation may also be necessary and useful. Often, these supportive techniques alone are not effective, and symptomatic treatment with neuroleptic or sedative medications are necessary. Sedation may be necessary to relieve severe agitation or insomnia (Lipowski, 1987). Haloperidol, a neuroleptic agent that is a potent dopamine blocker, is the drug of choice in the treatment of delirium in the medically ill (Adams, Fernandez, & Anderson, 1986; Fernandez, Holmes, Adams, & Kavanaugh, 1988; Lipowski, 1987; Murray, 1987). In low doses (1–3 mg), it is usually effective in targeting agitation, paranoia, and fear.

The use of neuroleptics in the management of delirium in the dying person remains controversial in some circles (Adams et al., 1986; Breitbart, Bruera, Chochinov, & Lynch, 1995; Fainsinger & Bruera, 1992; Roche, 2003). Some have argued that pharmacological interventions with neuroleptics or benzodiazepines are inappropriate in the dying person. Delirium is viewed as a natural part of the dying process that should not be altered. Another rationale that is often raised is that these individuals are so close to death that aggressive treatment is unnecessary. Parenteral neuroleptics or sedatives may be mistakenly avoided because of exaggerated fears that they might hasten death through hypotension or respiratory depression. Many are unnecessarily pessimistic about the possible results of neuroleptic treatment for delirium. They argue that because the underlying pathophysiologic process often continues unabated (such as hepatic or renal failure), no improvement can be expected in the person's mental status. There is concern that neuroleptics or sedatives may worsen a delirium by making the person more confused or sedated. Clinical experience in managing delirium in dying people with cancer suggests that the use of neuroleptics in the management of agitation, paranoia, hallucinations, and altered sensorium is safe, effective, and quite appropriate. Management of delirium on a case-by-case basis seems wisest. The agitated, delirious dying person should probably be given neuroleptics to help restore calm. For example, Breitbart, Tremblay, and Gibson (2002) found that olanzapine (Zyprexa) was effective in treating delirium in a sample of cancer patients but that response to this medication was significantly better in patients experiencing hyperactive delirium. A "wait and see" approach before using neuroleptics may be most appropriate with individuals who have a lethargic or somnolent presentation of delirium.

Organic Mental Disorders in AIDS

The spectrum of organic mental disorders seen in AIDS is similar to that seen in other terminally ill people (with the exception of HIV dementia) and includes delirium, dementia, organic mood disorder, organic personality disorder, organic hallucinosis, and organic delusional disorders (Perry, 1990). Several factors make organic mental disorders somewhat unique in the person with AIDS. Concomitant substance abuse, as well as neuropsychiatric side effects of antiviral or chemotherapeutic agents, can cause organic mental disorders such as organic mood disorder—manic type (Perry, 1990). Most important is the fact that HIV is neurotropic and thus invades the central nervous system early in infection and can result in dementia due to HIV.

Dementia due to HIV is the most common neurological complication of AIDS (Aronow, Brew, & Price, 1988). The syndrome is characterized by disturbances in motor performance, cognition, and behavior. It is estimated that two-thirds of people with AIDS will develop clinical dementia during the course of their illness (McArthur et al., 2003; Sperber & Shao, 2003). Persons with HIV dementia complex clinically exhibit a triad of cognitive, motor, and behavioral disturbances. Cognitive and intellectual impairment is typically subtle in onset, can progress rapidly or gradually, and is quite variable. The presentation is initially one of memory impairment, mental slowing, and impaired concentration. This can progress to global cognitive impairment with disorientation, confusion, psychosis, and mutism. Motor disturbances can begin with clumsiness, unsteady gait, tremor, and impaired handwriting and lead to ataxia, paraplegia, myoclonus, incontinence, and seizures. Early behavioral symptoms include apathy, withdrawal, depression, and anxiety. Late behavioral changes include paranoia, agitation, confusion, psychosis, hallucinations, and affective disturbances (i.e., mania or depression; Aronow et al., 1988).

The earliest symptoms of HIV dementia are often mistaken for functional psychiatric disturbance such as reactive depression or anxiety. As dementia progresses, the organic nature of psychiatric symptoms becomes more obvious. People often react with disbelief, denial, numbness, anxiety, depression, feelings of hopelessness, and, occasionally, suicidal ideation. Differentiating early HIV dementia from a functional psychiatric disorder can be difficult. Early behavioral changes seen in HIV dementia include irritability, anxiety, and depression. These symptoms are common in major depression, anxiety disorders, and adjustment disorders and are easily misconstrued as an understandable reaction to the diagnosis of a life-threatening illness rather than signs of early encephalopathy (American Psychiatric Association, 1994; Perry, 1990). Formal neuropsychological testing can be helpful to document AIDS dementia complex accurately and distinguish it from depression or adjustment disorder.

The use of pharmacotherapy in persons with AIDS must be prudent and cautious because it is becoming more clear that individuals with neurological complications of AIDS are sensitive to the adverse side effects of psychoactive medications (Fernandez, 2002). Nonpharmacological treatments such as relaxation techniques, hypnosis, and cognitive coping strategies should be used whenever possible to help limit medication use to lower dosages.

PHYSICAL SYMPTOMS

Although the diagnosis and treatment of psychiatric disorders in the person with advanced illness is of importance, pain and other troublesome physical symptoms must also be aggressively treated in efforts aimed at the enhancement of the person's quality of life (Bruera et al., 1990). The deleterious influence of uncontrolled pain on an individual's psychological state is often intuitively understood and recognized. Physical symptoms other than pain can go undetected, however, and cause significant emotional distress. This distress often dissipates when effective management is instituted. Coyle, Adelhardt, Foley, and Portenoy (1990) reported that 70% of terminally ill patients have three or more physical symptoms other than pain. This finding replicates those of earlier papers that elucidated the multiple problems facing terminally ill individuals (Levy & Catalano, 1985). The psychologist or psychiatrist concerned with the assessment and treatment of affective and other syndromes in the terminally ill population must assess these symptoms. The following section briefly reviews psychological interventions that may be useful in the management of some selected distressing symptoms.

Pain

Behavioral interventions are effective in the management of acute procedures related cancer pain and as an adjunct in the management of chronic cancer pain (Fotopoulos, Graham, & Cook, 1979; Spiegel & Bloom, 1983). Hypnosis, biofeedback, and multicomponent cognitive–behavioral interventions have been used to provide comfort and minimize pain in adults, adolescents, and children undergoing bone marrow aspirations, spinal taps, and other painful procedures (Hilgard & LeBaron, 1982; Jay, Elliott, & Varni, 1986; Kellerman, Zeltzer, Ellenberg, & Dash, 1983). In chronic, acute and mild to moderate residual cancer pain, cognitive–behavioral techniques are most effective when they are used as part of a multimodal, multidisciplinary approach (Breitbart, 1989b). Adequate medical assessment and management of cancer pain is essential. Relaxation techniques are used to help the person achieve a less agitated state. Once relaxed, the client with pain can use a variety of imagery techniques including pleasant distracting imagery, transformational imagery, and dissociative imagery (Breitbart, 1989b). Transformational imagery involves the imaginative alteration of either the painful sensation itself, or the context of pain, or both. People can imaginatively change a sensation of pain in their arm, for example, into a feeling of warmth or cold. They can use such imagery as "dipping your arm into a bucket of cold spring water," or "into a vat of warm honey." Such techniques can also be used to alter the context of the pain. Dissociative imagery or dissociated somatization refers to the use of one's imagination to disconnect or dissociate from the pain experience. These techniques can provide much needed respite from pain. Even short periods of relief from pain can break the vicious cycle that entraps many people with cancer.

Anorexia and Weight Loss

Persons with cancer and their families find weight loss demoralizing, perplexing, and distressing. Weight loss and anorexia in terminally ill persons are complex problems that can arise from a number of sources. Although most often a variety of medical factors account for the anorexia and cachexia associated with terminal illness, psychological and psychiatric factors may also play a role in the etiology of anorexia and weight loss. Among the most frequent of such causes are anxiety, depression, and conditioned food aversions (Lesko, 1989).

The treatment of anorexia and weight loss begins with the identification and correction of its reversible causes. For example, when uncontrolled opioid-induced nausea is identified as a key factor in a person's inability to eat, adding an antiemetic may completely control the subsequent anorexia. Once specific causes have been ruled out or corrected, subsequent treatment relies on environmental manipulations (Levy & Catalano, 1985). Frequent administration of favorite foods, nutritional supplements, and fluids can reverse weight loss. Conditioned nausea and vomiting is often responsive to relaxation training and other behavioral techniques (Redd, Andresen, & Minagawa, 1982). Even persons with advanced disease can use these interventions if their sensorium is clear and they are capable of concentrating.

Asthenia

Asthenia is defined as generalized weakness and physical or mental fatigue; as many as two-thirds of people with advanced cancer complain of weakness (Stasi, Abriani, Beccaglia, Terzoli, & Amadori, 2003). It is unfortunate that a treatable cause of asthenia will be identified and corrected in only a minority of cases. The role of psychiatric factors in the presentation of asthenia in the dying person with cancer is small in comparison to that of physical factors. The cause of asthenia more likely arises from some of the following etiologies: malnutrition, infection, profound anemia, metabolic abnormalities, and reactions to medication. Chemotherapeutic agents and radiotherapy are frequently used palliative therapies that can both cause significant weakness.

The psychological and psychiatric treatment of people with asthenia includes client and family education (especially to address the nonpsychological nature of the problem in many cases). Some people who suffer with temporary asthenia from chemotherapy or radiotherapy think that their weakness is a sign of imminent death. An ongoing supportive relationship, which permits the person to express fears and concerns about the meaning of continued weakness and to address distorted ideas that they may have about its prognostic significance, is critically important (Bruera & MacDonald, 1988).

CONCLUSION

As the possibility of cure or prolongation of life becomes remote in the care of the person with advanced cancer or AIDS or other chronic, debilitating, or potentially terminal illnesses, the focus of treatment shifts to symptom control and enhancement of quality of life. Such individuals are uniquely vulnerable to both physical and psychiatric complications. The high prevalence of distressing physical symptoms, such as pain, makes the assessment of psychiatric symptoms difficult. It is critical that physicians and nurses working in the palliative care setting recognize the unique knowledge and skills of psychologists and psychiatrists and the contributions they can make to the care of terminally ill individuals. The role of the psychologist, or other mental health professional, in the care of terminally ill or dying persons is critical to both adequate symptom control and integration of the physical, psychological, and spiritual dimensions of human experience in the last weeks of life. To be most effective in this role, the psychologist must not only have specialized knowledge of the psychiatric complications of terminal illness but also be familiar with the common physical symptoms that plague terminally ill individuals and contribute so dramatically to suffering.

REFERENCES

Adams, F., Fernandez, F., & Anderson, B. S. (1986). Emergency pharmacotherapy of delirium in the critically ill cancer patient. *Psychosomatics, 27,* 33–37.

Adams, F., Quesada, J. R., & Gutterman, J. U. (1984). Neuropsychiatric manifestations of human leukocyte interferon therapy in patients with cancer. *Journal of the American Medical Association, 252,* 938–941.

Alfonso, C. A., Cohen, M. A., Aladjem, A. D., Morrison, F., Powell, D., Winters, R. A., et al. (1994). HIV seropositivity as a major risk factor for suicide in the general hospital. *Psychosomatics, 35,* 368–373.

American Psychiatric Association. (1987). *Diagnostic and statistical manual of mental disorders* (3rd ed., rev.). Washington, DC: Author.

American Psychiatric Association. (1994). *Diagnostic and statistical manual of mental disorders* (4th ed.). Washington, DC: Author.

American Psychiatric Association. (2003). *Practice guideline for the assessment and treatment of patients with suicidal behaviors.* Retrieved January 30, 2004, from http://www.psych.org/psych_pract/treatg/pg/pg_suicidalbehaviors.pdf

Aronow, H. A., Brew, B. J., & Price, R. W. (1988). The management of the neurological complications of HIV infection and AIDS. *AIDS, 2*(Suppl. 1), 151–159.

Atkinson, H., Gutierrez, R., Cotter, L., Grant, I., Pace, P., Brown, S., et al. (1990, June). *Suicide ideation and attempts in HIV illness.* Paper presented at the VI International Conference on AIDS, San Francisco.

Beck, A. T., Kovacs, M., & Weissman, A (1975). Hopelessness and suicidal behavior: An overview. *Journal of the American Medical Association, 234,* 1146–1149.

Bolund, C. (1985). Suicide and cancer II: Medical and care factors in suicide by cancer patients in Sweden, 1973–1976. *Journal of Psychosocial Oncology, 3,* 17–30.

Breitbart, W. (1987). Suicide in cancer patients. *Oncology, 1,* 49–53.

Breitbart, W. (1988). Psychiatric complications of cancer. In M. C. Brain & P. P. Carbone (Eds.), *Current therapy in hematology oncology* (3rd ed., pp. 268–274). Philadelphia: Decker.

Breitbart, W. (1989a). Endocrine-related psychiatric disorders. In J. Holland & J. Rowland (Eds.), *The handbook of psychooncology: The psychological care of the cancer patient* (pp. 356–366). New York: Oxford University Press.

Breitbart, W. (1989b). Psychiatric management of cancer pain. *Cancer, 63,* 2336–2342.

Breitbart, W. (1990). Cancer pain and suicide. In K. M. Foley, J. J. Bonica, V. Ventafridda, & M. Callaway (Eds.), *Advances in pain research and therapy* (Vol. 16, pp. 399–412). New York: Raven Press.

Breitbart, W., Bruera, E., Chochinov, H. M., & Lynch, M. (1995). Neuropsychiatric syndromes and psychological symptoms in patients with advanced cancer. *Journal of Pain & Symptom Management, 10,* 131–141.

Breitbart, W., Chochinov, H., & Passik, S. D. (2004). Psychiatric symptoms in palliative medicine. In D. Doyle, G. Hanks, N. Cherny, & K. Calman (Eds.), *Oxford textbook of palliative medicine* (3rd ed., pp. 746–771). New York: Oxford University Press.

Breitbart, W., Gibson, C., & Tremblay, A. (2002). The delirium experience: Delirium recall and delirium-related distress in hospitalized cancer patients, their spouses/caregivers, and their nurses. *Psychosomatics 43,* 183–194.

Breitbart, W., Rosenfeld, B., Pessin, H., Kaim, M., Funesti-Esch, J., Galietta, M., et al. (2000). Depression, hopelessness, and desire for hastened death in terminally ill patients with cancer. *Journal of the American Medical Association, 284,* 2907–2911.

Breitbart, W., & Sparrow, B. (1998). Management of delirium in the terminally ill. *Progress in Palliative Care, 6,* 107–113.

Breitbart, W., Tremblay, A., & Gibson, C. (2002). An open trial of olanzapine for the treatment of delirium in hospitalized cancer patients. *Psychosomatics 43,* 175–182.

Bruera, E., & MacDonald, R. N. (1988). Asthenia in patients with advanced cancer. *Journal of Pain and Symptom Management, 3,* 9–14.

Bruera, E., Macmillan, K., Hanson, J., & MacDonald, R. N. (1989). The cognitive effects of the administration of narcotics. *Pain, 39,* 13–16.

Bruera, E., Miller, L., & McCalion, S. (1990). Cognitive failure in patients with terminal cancer: A prospective longitudinal study. *Psychosocial Aspects of Cancer, 9,* 308–310.

Bukberg, J., Penman, D., & Holland, J. C. (1984). Depression in hospitalized cancer patients. *Psychosomatic Medicine, 43,* 199–212.

Cassem, N. H. (1987). The dying patient. In T. P. Hackett & N. H. Cassem (Eds.), *Massachusetts General Hospital handbook of general hospital psychiatry* (2nd ed., pp. 332–352). Littleton, MA: PSG.

Centeno, C., Sanz, A., & Bruera, E. (2004). Delirium in advanced cancer patients. *Palliative Medicine, 18,* 184–194.

Chochinov, H. M., & Holland, J. C. (1989). Bereavement. In J. Holland & J. Rowland (Eds.), *The handbook of psychooncology: The psychological care of the cancer patient* (pp. 612–627). New York: Oxford University Press.

Chochinov, H. M., Wilson, K. G., Enns, M., & Lander, S. (1994). Prevalence of depression in the terminally ill: Effects of diagnostic criteria and symptom threshold judgments. *American Journal of Psychiatry, 151*, 537–540.

Chochinov, H. M., Wilson, K. G., Enns, M., Mowchun, N., Lander, S., Levitt, M., et al. (1995). Desire for death in the terminally ill. *American Journal of Psychiatry, 152*, 1185–1191.

Cote, T. R., Biggar, R. J., & Dannenberg, A. L. (1992). Risk of suicide among persons with AIDS—A national assessment. *Journal of the American Medical Association, 268*, 2066–2068.

Coyle, N., Adelhardt, J., Foley, K. M., & Portenoy, R. K. (1990). Character of terminal illness in the advanced cancer patient: Pain and other symptoms during the last four weeks of life. *Journal of Pain and Symptom Management, 5*, 83–93.

Coyle, N., Breitbart, W., Weaver, S., & Portenoy, R. K. (1994). Delirium as a contributing factor to "crescendo" pain: Three case reports. *Journal of Pain and Symptom Management, 9*, 44–47.

DeAngelis, L. M., Delattre, J., & Posner, J. B. (1989). Radiation-induced dementia in patients cured of brain metastases. *Neurology, 39*, 789–796.

Denicoff, K. D., Rubinow, D. R., Papa, M. Z., Simpson, C., Seipp, C. A., Lotze, M. T., et al. (1987). The neuropsychiatric effects of treatment with interleukin-w and lymphokine-activated killer cells. *Annals of Internal Medicine, 107*, 293–300.

Derogatis, L. R., Morrow, G. R., Fetting, J., Penman, D., Piasetsky, S., Schmale, A. M., et al. (1983). The prevalence of psychiatric disorders among cancer patients. *Journal of the American Medical Association, 249*, 751–757.

Dubovsky, S. L. (1978). Averting suicide in terminally ill patients. *Psychosomatics, 19*, 113–115.

Endicott, J. (1984). Measurement of depression patients with cancer. *Cancer, 53*, 2243–2248.

Fainsinger, R., & Bruera, E. (1992). Treatment of delirium in a terminally ill patient. *Journal of Pain and Symptom Management, 7*, 54–56.

Farberow, N. L., Ganzler, S., Cuter, F., & Reynolds, D. (1971). An eight-year survey of hospital suicides. *Life-Threatening Behavior, 1*, 184–202.

Farberow, N. L., Shneidman, E. S., & Leonard, C. V. (1963). *Suicide among general medical and surgical hospital patients with malignant neoplasms.* Washington, DC: U.S. Veterans Administration.

Fernandez, F. (2002). Neuropsychiatric aspects of human immunodeficiency virus (HIV) infection. *Current Psychiatry Reports, 4*, 228–231.

Fernandez, F., Holmes, V. F., Adams, F., & Kavanaugh, J. J. (1988). Treatment of severe refractory agitation with a haloperidol drip. *Journal of Clinical Psychiatry, 49*, 239–241.

Foley, K. M. (1985). The treatment of cancer pain. *New England Journal of Medicine, 313*, 84–95.

Fotopoulos, S. S., Graham, C., & Cook, M. R. (1979). Psychophysiologic control of cancer pain. In J. J. Bonica & V. Ventafridda (Eds.), *Advances in pain research and therapy* (Vol. 2, pp. 231–244). New York: Raven Press.

Ganzini, L., Lee, M. A., Heintz, R. T., Bloom, J. D., & Fenn, D. S. (1994). The effect of depression treatment on elderly patients' preferences for life-sustaining medical therapy. *American Journal of Psychiatry, 151,* 1613–1616.

Gibson, C., & Breitbart, W. (2003). *Individual meaning-centered psychotherapy manual.* Unpublished manuscript.

Gil, F., Passik, S. D., Rosenfeld, B., & Breitbart, W. (1998). Psychological adjustment and suicidal ideation in patients with AIDS. *AIDS Patient Care & STDS, 12,* 927–930.

Goodwin, R. D., Marusia, A., & Howen, C. W. (2003). Suicide attempts in the United States: The role of physical illness. *Social Sciences and Medicine, 56,* 1783–1788.

Green, A., & Austin, C. (1994–1995). Psychopathology of pancreatic cancer. *Psychosomatics, 34,* 208–221.

Greenstein, M., & Breitbart, W. (2000). Cancer and the experience of meaning: A group psychotherapy program for people with cancer. *American Journal of Psychotherapy 54,* 486–500.

Gutierrez, R., Atkinson, H., Velin, R., Patterson, T., Heaton, R., Grant, J., et al. (1990, June). *Coping and neuropsychological correlates of suicidality in HIV.* Paper presented at the VI International Conference on AIDS, San Francisco.

Guze, S., & Robins, E. (1970). Suicide and primary affective disorders. *British Journal of Psychiatry, 117,* 437–438.

Hilgard, E., & LeBaron, S. (1982). Relief of anxiety and pain in children and adolescents with cancer: Quantitative measures and clinical observations. *International Journal of Clinical and Experimental Hypnosis, 30,* 417–442.

Holland, J. C. (1989). Anxiety and cancer: The patient and family. *Journal of Clinical Psychiatry, 50,* 20–25.

Holland, J. C., Fassanellos, S., & Ohnuma, T. (1974). Psychiatric symptoms associated with L-asparaginase administration. *Journal of Psychiatric Research, 10,* 105–113.

Holland, J. C., Korzun, A. H., Tross, S., Silberfarb, P., Perry, M., Comis, R., et al. (1986). Comparative psychological disturbance in pancreatic and gastric cancer. *American Journal of Psychiatry, 143,* 982–986.

Holland, J. C., Morrow, G. R., Schmale, A. M., Derogatis, L. R., Stefanek, S., Berenson, S., et al. (1988). Reduction of anxiety and depression in cancer patients by alprazolam or by a behavioral technique. *Proceedings of the American Society of Clinical Oncology, 6,* 258.

Jay, S., Elliott, C., & Varni, J. (1986). Acute and chronic pain in adults and children with cancer. *Journal of Consulting and Clinical Psychology, 54,* 601–607.

Karina, K., Koutsky, L., Bradshaw, D., Hopkins, S., Katon, W., & Lafferty, W. (1994). Psychiatric comorbidity and length of stay in hospitalized AIDS patients. *American Journal of Psychiatry, 151,* 1475–1478.

Kellerman, J., Zeltzer, L., Ellenberg, L., & Dash, J. (1983). Adolescents with cancer: Hypnosis for the reduction of acute pain and anxiety associated with medical procedures. *Journal of Adolescent Health Care, 4,* 85–90.

Kovacs, M., Beck, A. T., & Weissman, A. (1975). Hopelessness: An indication of suicidal risk. *Suicide, 5,* 98–103.

Lesko, L. (1989). Anorexia. In J. Holland & J. Rowland (Eds.), *The handbook of psychooncology: The psychological care of the cancer patient* (pp. 434–443). New York: Oxford University Press.

Levy, M., & Catalano, R. (1985). Control of common physical symptoms other than pain in patients with terminal disease. *Seminars in Oncology, 12,* 411–430.

Levy, S., Abaza, M. M., Hawkshaw, M. J., & Sataloff, R. T. (2001). Psychiatric manifestations of medications commonly prescribed in otolaryngology. *Ear, Nose, & Throat Journal, 80,* 266–268, 270–271.

Lipowski, Z. J. (1987). Delirium (acute confusional states). *Journal of the American Medical Association, 285,* 1789–1792.

Louhivuori, K. A., & Hakama, J. (1979). Risk of suicide among cancer patients. *American Journal of Epidemiology, 109,* 59–65.

Marzuk, P. M., Tardiff, K., Leon, A. C., Hirsch, C. S., Hartwell, N., Portera, L., et al. (1997). HIV seroprevalence among suicide victims in New York City, 1991–1993. *American Journal of Psychiatry, 154,* 1720–1725.

Marzuk, P. M., Tierney, H., Tardiff, K., Gross, E. M., Morgan, E. B., Hsu, M. A., et al. (1988). Increased risk of suicide in persons with AIDS. *Journal of the American Medical Association, 259,* 1333–1337.

Massie, M. J. (1989). Anxiety, panic and phobias. In J. Holland & J. Rowland (Eds.), *The handbook of psychooncology: The psychological care of the cancer patient* (pp. 300–309). New York: Oxford University Press.

Massie, M. J., & Holland, J. C. (1987). The cancer patient with pain: Psychiatric complications and their management. *Medical Clinics of North America, 71,* 243–258.

Massie, M. J., & Holland, J. C. (1990). Depression and the cancer patient. *Journal of Clinical Psychiatry, 51,* 12–17.

Massie, M. J., Holland, J. C., & Glass, E. (1983). Delirium in terminally ill cancer patients. *American Journal of Psychiatry, 140,* 1048–1050.

Massie, M. J., Holland, J. C., & Straker, N. (1989). Psychotherapeutic interventions. In J. Holland & J. Rowland (Eds.), *The handbook of psychooncology: The psychological care of the cancer patient* (pp. 455–469). New York: Oxford University Press.

McArthur, J. C., Haughey, N., Gartner, S., Conant, K., Pardo, C., Nath, A., et al. (2003). Human immunodeficiency virus–associated dementia: An evolving disease. *Journal of Neurovirology, 9,* 205–221.

McKegney, F. P., & Lange, P. (1971). The decision to no longer live on chronic hemodialysis. *American Journal of Psychiatry, 128,* 47–55.

McKegney, F. P., & O'Dowd, M. A. (1992). Suicidality and HIV status. *American Journal of Psychiatry, 149,* 396–398.

Murray, G. B. (1987). Confusion, delirium, and dementia. In T. P. Hackett & N. H. Cassem (Eds.), *Massachusetts General Hospital handbook of general hospital psychiatry* (2nd ed., pp. 84–115). Littleton, MA: PSG.

Orr, D., O'Dowd, M. A., McKegney, F. P., & Natali, C. (1990, June). *A comparison of self reported suicidal behaviors in different stages of HIV infection.* Paper presented at the VI International AIDS Conference, San Francisco.

Perantie, D. C., & Brown, E. S. (2002). Corticosteroids, immune suppression, and psychosis. *Current Psychiatry Reports, 4,* 171–176.

Perry, S. W. (1990). Organic mental disorders caused by HIV: Update on early diagnosis and treatment. *American Journal of Psychiatry, 147,* 696–712.

Perry, S. W., & Tross, S. (1984). Psychiatric problems of AIDS inpatients at the New York Hospital: A preliminary report. *Public Health Reports, 99,* 200–205.

Plumb, M. M., & Holland, J. C. (1977). Comparative studies of psychological function in patients with advanced cancer. *Psychosomatic Medicine, 39,* 264–276.

Redd, W. H., Andresen, G. V., & Minagawa, R. Y. (1982). Hypnotic control of anticipatory emesis in patients receiving cancer chemotherapy. *Journal of Consulting and Clinical Psychology, 50,* 14–19.

Roche, V. (2003). Etiology and management of delirium. *American Journal of Medical Science, 325,* 20–30.

Rosenfeld, B. (2004). *Assisted suicide and the right to die: The interface of social science, public policy, and medical ethics.* Washington, DC: American Psychological Association.

Sayar, K., Acar, B., & Ak, I. (2003). Alexithymia and suicidal behavior. *Israel Journal of Psychiatry and Relational Sciences, 40,* 165–173.

Sperber, K., & Shao, L. (2003). Neurologic consequences of HIV infection in the era of HAART. *AIDS Patient Care & STDs, 17,* 509–518.

Spiegel, D., & Bloom, J. R. (1983). Group therapy and hypnosis reduce metastatic breast carcinoma pain. *Psychosomatic Medicine, 4,* 333–339.

Spiegel, D., Bloom, J. R., & Yalom, I. D. (1981). Group support for patients with metastatic cancer: A randomized prospective outcome study. *Archives of General Psychiatry, 38,* 527–533.

Stasi, R., Abriani, L., Beccaglia, P., Terzoli, E., & Amadori, S. (2003). Cancer-related fatigue: Evolving concepts in evaluation and treatment. *Cancer, 98,* 1786–1801.

Stiefel, F. C., Breitbart, W., & Holland, J. C. (1989). Corticosteroids in cancer: Neuropsychiatric complications. *Cancer Investigation, 7,* 479–491.

Strain, J. J., Liebowitz, M. R., & Klein, D. F. (1981). Anxiety and panic attacks in the medically ill. *Psychiatric Clinics of North America, 4,* 333–348.

Tross, S., & Hirsch, D. A. (1988). Psychological distress and neuropsychological complications of HIV infection and AIDS. *American Psychologist, 43,* 929–934.

Trzepacz, P. (1994). The neuropathogenesis of delirium. *Psychosomatics, 35,* 374–391.

Twycross, R. G., & Lack, S. A. (1983). *Symptom control in far advanced cancer: Pain relief.* London: Pitman.

Weddington, W. W. (1982). Delirium and depression associated with amphotericin B. *Psychosomatics, 23,* 1076–1078.

Young, D. F. (1982). Neurological complications of cancer chemotherapy. In A. Silverstein (Ed.), *Neurological complications of therapy: Selected topics* (pp. 57–113). New York: Futura.

7

DEPRESSION AND HOPELESSNESS NEAR THE END OF LIFE: ASSESSMENT AND TREATMENT

BARRY ROSENFELD, JENNIFER ABBEY, AND HAYLEY PESSIN

Physically healthy individuals typically expect that most dying persons will experience profound feelings of depression and despair as they approach death. Many healthy people project their own feelings onto the dying person by assuming that in a similar situation they would be despondent. Yet although some feelings of sadness during the last weeks of life are perhaps unavoidable, episodes of severe depression and pervasive feelings of hopelessness are not the norm for dying patients and in some settings are relatively uncommon reactions. Even among terminally ill patients with highly distressing physical symptoms (e.g., pain, fatigue, difficulty performing basic daily activities), the frequency of severe depressive disorders is relatively modest, rarely exceeding 20% to 25% in even the most physically disabled patient populations (Breitbart et al., 2000; see also chap. 6 by Gibson, Breitbart, Tomarken, Kosinski, & Nelson).

Unfortunately, when terminally ill patients do become despondent, many aspects of the dying process can become compromised. Severely depressed patients may avoid making necessary health care decisions or delay making plans for their family and financial affairs. They may refuse visits from friends and family members or avoid engaging in the very conversations that might help ease their remaining days. These behaviors can add substantial complications to the dying process for both the patient and his or her family members. Decisions about necessary medical treatments or estate planning can be delayed until they are simply too late or irrelevant. Family members may also experience more profound grief or depression because of lost opportunities to express their feelings or say good-bye. Ultimately, the presence of untreated depression has dramatic repercussions for many aspects of patient quality of life and, in the context of terminal illness, the quality of one's death.

Although some feelings of sadness and dysphoria are relatively common among terminally ill patients, episodes of severe depression are not. A number of studies have estimated prevalence rates for a Major Depressive Episode[1] among various terminally ill populations. Studies of terminally ill patients with cancer have typically identified rates of severe depression ranging from 10% to 20% although other, less severe forms of depression (e.g., "minor depression"[2] or adjustment disorder with depressed mood) are somewhat more common (Breitbart, Passik, & Rosenfeld, 1999; Chochinov, Wilson, Enns, & Lander, 1994). Rates of depression among patients with AIDS have been slightly, although not markedly, higher, often hovering in the 20% to 25% range (Rosenfeld, 1998).[3] Many researchers who study depression at the end of life incorporate these less severe forms of depression, such as minor depression or adjustment disorder with depressed mood, often inflating their estimates of the frequency of depression by broadening the definition. The clinical importance and overall impact of these milder forms of depression are much less clear than many writers presume, however, particularly as the line between normal and abnormal reactions to the dying process become blurred.

HOPELESSNESS

Whereas research and clinical interest has traditionally focused solely on depression and other forms of psychological distress (e.g., anxiety), the

---

[1]The *Diagnostic and Statistical Manual of Mental Disorders, Fourth Edition, Text Revision* (*DSM–IV–TR*; American Psychiatric Association, 2000) defines a major depressive episode as the presence of either a depressed mood or loss of interest or pleasure in daily activities, along with at least four other symptoms (from a predefined list of nine symptoms) present during the same 2-week period and representing a significant change from previous level of functioning.

[2]Although not defined by the *DSM–IV–TR*, "minor depression" has been used to describe depressive episodes that fail to meet the criteria for a major depressive episode because the number of symptoms does not meet the threshold (five symptoms) defined by the *DSM*.

[3]In fact, rates of depression vary substantially across the spectrum of HIV disease, with relatively high rates observed immediately following the HIV-positive diagnosis and again during periods of severe deterioration (e.g., after the first AIDS-defining illness, during the terminal phase of the illness). During intervening periods (i.e., during periods of relatively good health), people with HIV disease typically return to their baseline level of psychological functioning.

construct of hopelessness has increasingly emerged as an important and distinct phenomenon that is particularly salient near the end of life. Indeed, a growing body of research suggests that hopelessness may have an even more substantial impact on quality of life (and death) than severe depressive disorders.

Long-considered simply a symptom of depression, hopelessness has increasingly been recognized as a powerful influence on a number of aspects of end-of-life decision making such as the desire for hastened death, suicidal ideation, requests for assisted suicide, and decisions to refuse life-sustaining interventions (Breitbart et al., 2000; Chochinov, Wilson, Enns, & Lander, 1998; Ganzini, Johnston, McFarland, Tolle, & Lee, 1998; Rosenfeld, 2004; see also chap. 6 by Gibson et al.). Several studies have identified hopelessness as the strongest predictor of desire for hastened death and suicidal ideation in terminally ill individuals, providing an independent contribution beyond that of clinical depression (Breitbart et al., 2000; Chochinov et al., 1998). In a study of terminally ill cancer patients, Breitbart and colleagues found that nearly 50% of their sample was neither depressed nor had high levels of hopelessness and, correspondingly, had no significant desire for hastened death. Among the handful of patients who were both depressed and hopeless, however, most (five of eight) had an elevated desire for hastened death. Furthermore, when either of these two conditions were present (i.e., depressed but not hopeless or hopeless but not depressed), roughly 25% had a high desire for hastened death, suggesting that depression and hopelessness represent independent and roughly comparable influences on desire for hastened death.

Studies of patients with amyotrophic lateral sclerosis (ALS) have demonstrated an even more powerful relationship between hopelessness and desire for hastened death or interest in physician-assisted suicide, finding that the effects of depression are overshadowed by hopelessness in this population (Ganzini et al., 1998; Rabkin, Wagner, & Del Bene, 2000). Given the nature of ALS, in which functional abilities gradually but inevitably deteriorate, feelings of hopelessness are not surprising as the disease progresses and functioning declines. Yet even in situations when hopelessness appears to be a relatively common phenomena (e.g., terminal illness with severe functional disability) most patients manage to sustain some form of hope as they confront death.

What Is Hopelessness?

Despite a growing awareness of the importance of hopelessness during the dying process, the construct itself has been poorly researched. Stotland (1969) first recognized hopelessness as a psychological phenomenon and differentiated hope and hopelessness as distinct constructs. According to Stotland's theory, hope entails a generally positive outlook for the future whereas hopelessness conveys an expectation that the future will be unpleasant. Although Stotland conceptualized hope and hopelessness as the two extremes along a single continuum, Nunn (1996) and others have argued against this formulation. Because one can acknowledge that there is little expectation for accomplishing important goals (i.e., the absence of hope) while simultaneously maintaining a generally positive outlook on one's future, the two (hope and hopelessness) can obviously co-occur. Hence, hope is not necessarily defined by the absence of hopelessness, nor is hopelessness merely the absence of hope (Tonge, James, & Hilliam, 1975).

Perhaps no situation highlights the distinctions between hope and hopelessness more clearly than terminal illness, in which one can acknowledge that there is no possibility of a "cure" yet continue to hope for one ("a miracle") nonetheless. Frankl (1986) described a related phenomenon, which he termed *tragic optimism*, as the maintenance of hope in the face of tragedy. Although terminal illness may not always be "tragic" there is no doubt that some terminally ill patients maintain a sense of optimism that seems to contradict objective reality. On the other hand, many patients who are faced with the loss of a hope for a cure subsequently give up hope for other goals that may be within their grasp (e.g., symptom control, meaningful contact with family). This conceptualization of hopelessness, and a greater understanding of what both hope and hopelessness mean in the context of terminal illness, has increasingly become the subject of research and discussion in the palliative care literature.

An important distinction many theorists have drawn pertains to the difference between hopelessness and pessimism. Whereas hopelessness is typically conceptualized as a "state" characteristic (i.e., a transient or situational cognitive style), pessimism refers a more long-standing personality characteristic (i.e., a "trait"). Pessimistic individuals may nevertheless remain hopeful about the future, despite their negative assessment of the likelihood that things will work out the way they want them to (i.e., "I *hope* that the medication will ease my pain but I don't *expect* it to help"). Likewise, the onset of hopelessness does not necessarily reflect an exacerbation of a long-standing pessimistic personality style. Many situational factors (e.g., learned helplessness, depression, terminal illness) may lead an individual to give up hope despite lifelong optimism.

Differentiating between denial and hope is also critical, particularly in the context of a terminal illness. Individuals who are in a state of denial regarding their terminal prognosis may nevertheless feel hopeless about their future. Likewise, acceptance of one's illness does not necessarily correspond to either retaining or giving up hope, it merely frames the context for the patient's hopes and goals. Although denial may seem beneficial at times, particularly when one is facing a terminal illness, empirical research has not supported this assumption. Chochinov and his colleagues (Chochinov, Tataryn, Wilson, Enns, & Lander, 2000) found that patients who had no awareness that their illness was in the terminal phase were three times more likely to be depressed than patients with complete or partial awareness. Unfortunately, these authors did not analyze the relationship between hopelessness and prognostic awareness.

Hopelessness and Medical Illness

The importance of hopelessness in medically ill populations is not limited to suicide and other manifestations of the desire for hastened death. Many researchers have linked hopelessness to the disease process, suggesting that hopelessness can directly affect the physical health of medically ill patients (see also chap. 6 by Gibson et al.). For example, a number of studies suggest that hopelessness may make patients more susceptible to illness, even after controlling for the effect of depression and other medical risk factors (e.g., Everson et al., 1996; Visintainer, Volpicelli, & Seligman, 1982). Hopelessness also appears to influence disease course negatively, in part by hindering patients' motivation to improve their health status. For example, Watson, Haviland, Greer, Davidson, and Bliss (1999) found that hopelessness was negatively associated with survival in a sample of cancer patients. Conversely, Scheier and colleagues (1989) found that optimism predicted higher levels of problem-focused coping, faster recovery, and better postsurgery quality of life in coronary bypass surgery patients. They suggested that patients who are extremely pessimistic are unlikely to use problem-solving coping strategies and thereby have poorer health outcomes. Thus, although many possible pathways exist between hopelessness, psychological well-being, and physical health, relatively little empirical research has attempted to explore the construct of hopelessness in the context of *terminal* illness and compare these findings to the existing empirical literature.

ASSESSMENT OF DEPRESSION AND HOPELESSNESS NEAR THE END OF LIFE

Assessment of depression and hopelessness near the end of life can be difficult for a number of reasons. First, patients may underreport their psychological distress because they worry they will be seen as "weak" or "bad" patients if they admit such symptoms to their families or doctors (Maguire, 1985). Second, as discussed earlier, the constructs of depression and hopelessness may differ in terminally ill populations compared with physically healthy samples for which assessment techniques have typically been developed. Third, physicians and other hospital staff may "normalize" symptoms of depression or hopelessness in terminally ill patients, attributing their symptoms to normal sadness or grief rather than recognizing the profound psychological changes that may occur (Passik et al., 1998). Given the complicated nature of assessing depression and hopelessness near the end of life, it is important that mental health professionals working with terminally ill people have both the clinical skills to distinguish between normal sadness and a depressive episode as well as an awareness of validated tools for measuring depression and hopelessness.

Clinical Assessment of Depression and Hopelessness

One well-known difficulty in diagnosing depression among medically ill patients is that many of the physical symptoms germane to depression can also be caused by the physical illness (Wilson, Chochinov, de Faye, & Breitbart, 2000). Distinguishing whether symptoms such as weight loss or decreased appetite, fatigue, sleep problems, and poor concentration are caused by depression, disease process, or somatic therapies (or a combination of these) can be an extremely difficult task for even an experienced clinician, yet this has important implications in terms of selecting appropriate interventions. Many clinicians simply ignore or avoid focusing on the "somatic" or "vegetative" symptoms of depression to minimize the confounding influence of the illness. Instead, "cognitive" symptoms of depression (e.g., feelings of guilt or worthlessness, anhedonia) take on heightened importance because these symptoms are less clearly influenced by illness.

Endicott (1984) proposed a formal system of symptom substitution to enable clinicians to differentiate depression from illness manifestations in severely ill patients by replacing somatic symptoms of depression with nonsomatic alternatives. Specifically, Endicott proposed that the four somatic symptoms of depression be replaced with additional cognitive–affective symptoms of depression as follows: (a) poor appetite and weight loss should be replaced by fearfulness or depressed appearance in body or face; (b) insomnia or hypersomnia should be replaced by social withdrawal or decreased talkativeness; (c) loss of energy or fatigue should be replaced with brooding, self-pity, and pessimism; and (d) diminished concentration should be replaced by failure to smile or be cheered up and the absence of a response to good news or funny situations. Although widely cited in the palliative care literature, these alternative criteria for depression have rarely been empirically studied, and the extent to which this model improves on the *Diagnostic and Statistical Manual of Mental Disorders* (*DSM–IV–TR*; American Psychiatric Association, 2000) criteria is unknown. Moreover, despite the intuitive appeal of Endicott's alternative diagnostic criteria, one study assessing the impact of this model on the diagnosis of depression found relatively little effect from symptom replacement (Chochinov et al., 1994).

Passik and his colleagues (2000) recommended a somewhat similar approach, but instead of proposing novel alternative symptoms, these authors simply focused more exclusively on cognitive symptoms of depression (e.g., anhedonia, hopelessness, worthlessness, and guilt) to minimize the confounding effects of illness. Anhedonia, defined as a loss of interest or pleasure in activities, has received the most attention of these cognitive symptoms as a potentially more useful indicator of depression in the medically ill. Loss of interest and pleasure, however, is also confounded by the functional decline that accompanies advanced illness. As physical limitations begin to restrict a patient's mobility, energy, and independent functioning, withdrawal from and loss of interest in certain activities is common. What is less common, at least among nondepressed patients, is the complete loss of interest and pleasure in all activities. Patients who are not depressed will typically refocus their interest on those activities that are less physically or mentally demanding without losing interest in activities altogether (Wilson et al., 2000). Visits from family or friends, watching favorite television programs or sporting events, or other less strenuous activities typically retain their appeal to terminally ill patients who are not severely depressed, and the failure to find pleasure in such activities is often indicative of a depressive disorder. In our clinical experience, severe anhedonia virtually always corresponds to a diagnosis of major depression and warrants aggressive intervention.

Chochinov, Wilson, Enns, and Lander (1997) evaluated the utility of a single question as a means for assessing depression by asking patients, "Have you been depressed most of the time for the past two weeks?" Chochinov and his colleagues were able to identify every depressed patient in their sample of terminally ill cancer patients on the basis of their response to this question. Although their criterion for "depression" was quite broad (either the presence of a major depressive episode or a "minor depression"), these results are still remarkable. This single question outperformed two alternative screening methods—a self-report measure of depression (the Beck Depression Inventory—Short Form; Beck & Beck, 1972) and a visual analog scale assessing overall psychological distress. These results highlight the need for clinicians working with the terminally ill to ask how the patient feels both emotionally and physically.

Unlike depression, the clinical assessment of hopelessness is far less well developed and no formal mechanisms have been recommended. Nonetheless, a number of issues have emerged in the growing literature on hopelessness near the end of life. The primary focus of this assessment pertains to the crucial distinction between a patient's realistic appraisal of her or his "hopeless" medical situation and a more pervasive feeling of hopelessness that extends beyond the prognosis. Many clinicians mistakenly assume that hope near the end of life is simply a function of prognosis; however, research and clinical observation has consistently demonstrated that hopelessness encompasses a much broader range of cognitions and expectations (e.g., Menon, Campbell, Ruskin, & Hebel, 2000). Assessment of hopelessness in terminally ill patients thus requires careful attention to their sense of hope (or hopelessness) about their personal relationships and sense of meaning or purpose in life. As an illness progresses, hopes often evolve such that patients develop more modest, time-limited aspirations, such as resolving interpersonal conflicts, making plans for after one's death, and physical comfort during the dying process. Therefore, assessment of hopelessness in terminally ill individuals requires first ascertaining what, if any, goals the patient has or has had recently and inquiring about his or her expectations for fulfilling these goals.

Another means of conceptualizing hopelessness at the end of life was suggested by Clarke and Kissane (2002), in their discussion of a "demoralization syndrome." These authors proposed the existence of demoralization as a syndrome that encompasses both depression and hopelessness, although the syndrome extends beyond these two facets. Clarke and Kissane described demoralization as "a clearly defined syndrome of existential distress occurring in patients suffering from mental or physical illness, specifically ones that threaten life or integrity of being" (p. 734). They suggested that demoralization is triggered by feeling unable to cope with a stressful situation or event that engenders a sense of hopelessness, helplessness, incompetence, isolation, and diminished self-esteem. When a person develops these feelings, it often fuels a sense of meaninglessness and existential despair. Indeed, although not studied by Clark and Kissane, a number of studies have highlighted the importance of existential despair and a loss of meaning as powerful correlates of hopelessness, depression, and desire for hastened death (e.g., McClain, Rosenfeld, & Breitbart, 2003; Nelson, Rosenfeld, Breitbart, & Galietta, 2002). Whether conceptualized as hopelessness, demoralization, existential despair, or a loss of meaning, all of these constructs reflect important (and related) clinical phenomena that can have a detrimental impact on patient quality of life near the end of life.

Empirical Measures of Depression and Hopelessness

A number of self-report and clinician-rated rating scales have been used to assess depression and hopelessness in terminally ill persons, each with its own benefits and drawbacks. Although these measures cannot generate a clinical diagnosis, self-report measures enable clinicians to screen a large number of patients in a rapid and reliable manner and initiate a discussion about the patient's mood and outlook toward the future. Thus, clinicians can focus their often limited time and attention on only those patients who reveal significant symptoms even when their own vocabulary for discussing psychological distress is limited.

One of the most widely used instruments for assessing depression in severely medically ill patients is the Hospital Anxiety and Depression Scale (HADS; Zigmond & Snaith, 1983). The HADS is a 14-item scale composed of two 7-item subscales measuring anxiety and depression. Unlike other self-report rating scales of depression (and anxiety), the authors of the HADS eliminated items reflective of "somatic" symptoms of psychological distress and instead focused primarily on cognitive–affective symptoms. Despite its frequent use and intuitive appeal, several studies have suggested that the

HADS Depression and Anxiety subscales, although conceptually distinct, are in fact highly overlapping (Carroll, Fielding, & Blashki, 1973; LeFevre, Devereux, Smith, Lawrie, & Cornbleet, 1999). Even more problematic, other studies have found that the HADS has relatively low accuracy rates (sensitivity and specificity) in identifying depression in terminally ill patients, suggesting that the routine use of this measure to identify patients in need of mental health consultation may be unwise (Lloyd-Williams, Friedman, & Rudd, 2001).

A number of other self-report instruments to identify depression have been widely used in both empirical research as well as clinical screening, including the Beck Depression Inventory (BDI; Beck, Ward, Mendelson, Mock, & Erbaugh, 1961) and the Zung Self-Rating Depression Scale (Z-SRDS; Zung, 1967). These measures have been used in numerous research studies of medically ill and occasionally of terminally ill populations, demonstrating a high degree of clinical and empirical utility despite the potential for confounding somatic–vegetative symptoms.[4] For example, Dugan, Passik, and their colleagues (Dugan et al., 1998) analyzed a large sample of ambulatory cancer patients who had been administered the Z-SRDS, finding considerable support for the utility of this scale in cancer populations. However, factor analysis of this measure indicated that the cognitive–affective items were the most sensitive portion of the Z-SRDS, providing the best indicator of clinically significant depressive symptoms (Passik et al., 2000). More recently, Lloyd-Williams, Friedman, and Rudd (1999) studied the utility of a brief (10-item) measure of depression that also eliminates somatic–vegetative symptoms of depression. They used the Edinburgh Postnatal Depression Scale (Cox, Holden, & Sagovsky, 1987), a scale originally designed for use in a postnatal population, with a sample of terminally ill patients. They found acceptable levels of sensitivity and specificity for detecting cases of depression in this study, but further research is clearly necessary before conclusions can be drawn regarding the utility of this measure.

A significant limitation of all these self-report measures is the difficulty in converting a symptom severity rating to a clinical diagnosis. Although various cutoff scores have been proposed for most of the measures, studies often generate conflicting data regarding the optimal cutoff scores and the assessment of "optimal" may differ depending on the study goals. For example, researchers or clinicians seeking to minimize "false negatives" (failing to identify depressed individuals) might apply a lower cutoff score, whereas clinicians seeking to preserve scarce mental health resources might elect to raise this threshold so as to minimize false positives (patients identified as depressed who are actually not). In short, it is often impossible to pinpoint a

---

[4]An abbreviated version of the BDI, the BDI Short Form (Beck & Beck, 1972) eliminated the somatic–vegetative symptoms for use with medically ill patients. However, empirical research has suggested that this modification has relatively little impact on the scale's characteristics or properties (e.g., Rosenfeld et al., 1996).

precise cutoff score that optimizes the classification of depression (i.e., minimizing *both* false positives and false negatives).

Fewer options are available to those clinicians seeking a measure of hopelessness for the terminally ill. The most widely used measure of hopelessness is the Hopelessness Scale (HS) developed by Beck and his colleagues (Beck, Weissman, Lester, & Trexler, 1974). This 20-item true–false measure was originally developed and validated in a psychiatric population (i.e., patients with depression) but has since been applied extensively to other populations, including terminally ill patients (e.g., Breitbart et al., 2000; Ganzini et al., 1998). There has unfortunately been a dearth of research evaluating the validity of this scale with medically ill populations, and a number of studies suggest that the utility of the HS may be weaker in nonclinical samples (Steed, 2001). Moreover, Abbey and colleagues (Abbey, Rosenfeld, Pessin, & Breitbart, in press) demonstrated that several HS items were of questionable utility when applied to a terminally ill sample. A number of items failed to discriminate between those who were hopeless and those who were not (i.e., low or zero item–total correlation). By eliminating these problematic items, Abbey et al. (in press) found that abbreviated versions of the HS were superior to the original scale, suggesting that the scale may need to be modified for use in a terminally ill population. Indeed, Abbey et al. (in press) found that a three-item version of the HS generated reliability and validity coefficients roughly comparable to the full 20-item scale.[5]

Another measure of hopelessness that may be useful with terminally ill patients is the Geriatric Scale of Hopelessness developed by Fry (1984). Although this scale has not been applied to a terminally ill population, a number of elements included in this measure are intuitively appealing and potentially more relevant than aspects of the HS. For example, Fry's measure tapped a number of aspects of hopelessness that were not included in the HS but may be important, such as feelings of lost personal and interpersonal worth, hopelessness related to one's lost spiritual faith, and feelings of nurturance and respect, and remembrance after death. Nevertheless, without further empirical analysis, the applicability and clinical utility of this measure is simply unknown. Likewise, a handful of research studies have used single-item methods for assessing hopelessness (e.g., Chochinov et al., 1998; Wilson, Scott, et al., 2000), but these investigators have not focused on the clinical utility of such assessment techniques and instead have focused solely on identifying correlates of hopelessness. Nevertheless, in the absence of validated measures of hopelessness specifically designed for use in the terminally ill, these measures may provide a reasonable starting point for clinicians interested in identifying patients with high levels of hopelessness.

---

[5]The items included in this abbreviated scale were Items 6 ("In the future, I expect to succeed in what concerns me the most"), 11 ("All I can see ahead of me is unpleasantness rather than pleasantness"), and 17 ("It's very unlikely that I will get any real satisfaction in the future").

TREATING DEPRESSION AND HOPELESSNESS
IN THE TERMINALLY ILL

Once severe depression or hopelessness has been identified in a terminally ill patient, ensuring a supportive clinician–patient relationship becomes paramount. Although many clinicians may be pessimistic about the prospects of helping a depressed individual who only has weeks or months to live, growing evidence suggests that mental health interventions can successfully alleviate some or all of the symptoms of depression and despair, even in patients with advanced disease (Block, 2000; see also chap. 6 by Gibson et al.). Nonetheless, clinicians must be aware of the unique challenges of working with terminally ill patients to optimize the chance for a successful outcome. For example, clinicians working with terminally ill patients must be particularly focused on maintaining or fostering a sense of hopefulness for the patient, without creating false hopes (e.g., the possibility of a cure). The clinician must balance respect for the patient's current emotional state with moving the patient's goals from prolongation of life to a hope for a peaceful death. Perhaps more than in any other clinical setting, maintaining regular contact with depressed terminally ill patients as they progress through the final stages of their illness is critical. This continuity ensures that patients will be reevaluated on a regular basis and reassures them that they will not be abandoned and that care will remain available throughout their terminal course.

Another crucial principle pertains to the clinician's responsiveness to patient-initiated discussions. It is essential to acknowledge the patient's distress and respond to her or him in a genuine manner, because patients are often quick to recognize a superficial or disingenuous response. Despite the seriousness of the patient's plight, it is not necessary for the clinician to appear overly solemn or emotionally restrained. Many dying patients are interested in discussing (and sometimes feel driven to discuss) their condition, yet find family members unwilling to do so. Hence, patients should be allowed to discuss death freely with the clinician maintaining an interested and interactive stance, rather than shying away from the "sensitive" topics.

Finally, to reduce emotional suffering near end of life, clinicians should have a low threshold for treating depression and hopelessness and use interventions judiciously to alleviate symptoms and improve quality of life (Block, 2000; Schwartz, Lander, & Chochinov, 2002). Appropriate interventions that not only target depressive symptoms but also focus on hope and meaning are especially useful in a terminally ill population. Depression in cancer patients is optimally managed by using a combination of interventions such as of supportive psychotherapy, cognitive–behavioral techniques, and antidepressant medication, each of which are discussed briefly in the following sections (Block, 2000; Maguire, Hopwood, Tarrier, & Howell, 1985).

Pharmacological Treatment of Depression

In general, pharmacotherapy is a mainstay for treating severe depression regardless of whether the patient is physically healthy or terminally ill (Massie & Holland, 1990). Yet the presence of a severe or terminal illness complicates the treatment process significantly, forcing considerations that are simply unnecessary in most physically healthy individuals. Factors such as prognosis (i.e., life expectancy) and the time frame, as well as ongoing physical symptoms and perceived vulnerability to side effects, all play important roles in determining the type of pharmacotherapy that may be most appropriate. These potential complications must be considered when prescribing medications from an ever-growing antidepressant arsenal (Schwartz et al., 2002). For example, a depressed patient who is expected to live for several months may be able to tolerate the 2 to 4 weeks often needed before a traditional antidepressant (e.g., selective serotonin reuptake inhibitor [SSRI]) begins to take effect; a depressed patient with less than a month to live may require a more rapidly acting intervention such as a psychostimulant, which is often effective within the first few days of treatment. Patients who are within hours or days of death and in acute emotional distress will likely benefit more from sedatives or narcotic analgesic infusions, interventions that, although not antidepressants, have an immediate calming effect (Pessin, Potash, & Breitbart, 2003).

Although there are a number of controlled studies demonstrating the efficacy of antidepressant drug treatment for depressive disorders in cancer and AIDS patients, only a few have focused on terminally ill patients (Massie & Holland, 1990; Popkin, Callies, & Mackenzie, 1985; Preskorn & Burke, 1992). Despite their apparent efficacy, a survey of antidepressant prescribing in the terminally ill found that out of 1,046 cancer patients, only 10% received antidepressants, 76% of whom did not receive them until the last 2 weeks of life (Lloyd-Williams, Friedman, & Rudd, 1999). Given the prevalence of depression in patients with advanced cancer and AIDS (roughly 20%), it is apparent that many depressed patients with advanced illness never receive appropriate pharmacological treatment, and others receive treatment only in the final weeks of life, often too late for an adequate response.

Because of the importance of a rapid treatment response in terminally ill populations, psychostimulants have become increasingly recognized as a preferred treatment in palliative care setting (Wilson et al., 2000). A number of psychostimulants are approved for use with patients with advanced medical illness, including methylphenidate, dextroamphetamine, pemoline, and modafinil, and have been shown to be effective in rapidly diminishing depressive symptoms, often within 2 to 3 days of initiating treatment (Burns & Eisendrath, 1994; Olin & Masand, 1996; Satel & Nelson, 1989). Psychostimulants are particularly helpful when a patient's clinical presentation includes a dysphoric mood, psychomotor slowing, and even mild cognitive impairment, because this class of medications has been effective in improving cognitive functioning and reducing fatigue (Fernandez et al., 1988). Even in relatively low doses, psychostimulants can increase appetite, promote a sense of overall well-being, and improve feelings of weakness and fatigue in cancer patients. In addition, stimulants have been shown to reduce sedation secondary to opioid analgesics, allowing patients to tolerate higher levels of analgesic medication than might otherwise be possible (Bruera, Chadwick, Brenneis, Hanson, & MacDonald, 1987). Unfortunately, psychostimulants are not without side effects, including nervousness, overstimulation, a mild increase in blood pressure and pulse rate, and tremor. In rare cases, dyskinesias or motor tics, and even paranoia or confusion can occur (Pessin et al., 2003).

Despite the appeal of psychostimulants, SSRIs are still the most common pharmacological intervention in patients with advanced or terminal illness (Wilson et al., 2000). This preference is likely related to several factors, including their demonstrated efficacy, relatively modest side-effect profile, and a low affinity for adrenergic, cholinergic, and histamine receptors, minimizing complications due to the complex medication regimens that many terminally ill patients have. The side effects that do occur are not typically severe and include loose stools, nausea, vomiting, insomnia, headaches, and sexual dysfunction, which can be unpleasant but not life threatening (Pessin et al., 2003). Unfortunately, SSRIs often require more than 2 to 4 weeks before significant improvement occurs, making them impractical for patients at the very end of life. This period may be even longer in patients with severe illness because they require a much lower starting dose and more gradual titration schedules than a physically healthy patient.

Psychotherapeutic Interventions for Depression and Hopelessness

For patients with cancer experiencing major depression, adjustment disorder, or dysthymia, a variety of psychosocial interventions have demonstrated efficacy (Newport & Nemeroff, 1998). Two types of psychotherapeutic interventions, cognitive–behavioral therapy and interpersonal therapy, have been especially helpful in reducing distress among cancer patients. Cognitive–behavioral interventions (CBT), such as relaxation and distraction with pleasant imagery, have been shown to decrease depressive symptoms in cancer patients with mild to moderate levels of depression (Newport & Nemeroff, 1998). A study by Donnelly and colleagues (2000) found that interpersonal psychotherapy (IPT) provided over the telephone resulted in significant decreases in psychological distress and improved coping in cancer patients.

Numerous outcome studies with physically healthy patients have demonstrated that empirically validated interventions such as IPT and CBT are as effective in treating depressive symptoms as antidepressant medications, and there is little reason to expect that terminally ill patients would respond differently (Hollon, Thase, & Markowitz, 2002). Despite the short-term nature of some psychological interventions (e.g., IPT, CBT), however, many terminally ill patients do not have sufficient time to wait for psychotherapeutic interventions to take effect. In cases when death is imminent, supportive psychotherapy may be the most useful approach to treating depression. Supportive psychotherapy with the dying patient consists of active listening with supportive verbal interventions and occasional interpretations, all of which can be highly reassuring for patients confronting death (Cassem, 1987). In addition, psychotherapeutic interventions that focus on eliciting concerns and conveying the potential for interpersonal connections, finding a sense of meaning, and reconciliation with friends and family, can enhance patient coping with death (Block, 2000). In a terminally ill population in which time considerations are paramount, however, psychotherapy in conjunction with pharmacological treatment may be the quickest, most effective, and therefore most appropriate intervention strategy to address patients' symptoms and distress near the end of life.

Although much less frequently studied, several psychotherapy approaches have demonstrated efficacy in reducing feelings of hopelessness. Hopelessness has been targeted as a measure of treatment outcome due to the strong association with suicidal ideation and behavior (Beck & Weishaar, 1990). In physically healthy samples, cognitive–behavioral therapy (Collins & Cutcliffe, 2003; Scott et al., 2000), problem-solving therapy (Townsend et al., 2001), and dialectical behavior therapy (Linehan, Armstrong, Suarez, Allmon, & Heard, 1991) have been shown to be especially effective at reducing hopelessness in suicidal patients. Although this literature does not address the treatment of hopelessness in terminally ill populations, it appears to be relevant for patients with significant suicidal ideation or desire for hastened death.

Several strategies to foster hope have been recommended by the American Academy of Hospice and Palliative Medicine based on research conducted by Herth (1990). Herth defined hope as the "inner power that facilitates transcendence of the present situation and moves people toward a new awareness and enrichment of being" (p. 1257). In pursuit of this goal, a number of strategies have been recommended, beginning with adequate symptom control (to enhance comfort and pain relief) and developing or resolving relationships with family and caregivers (to foster a sense of meaningful relationships and of being needed; Chochinov & Schwartz, 2002; Wilson et al., 2000). Interventions more directly focused on developing or maintaining a sense of hope include identifying feasible aims (to give a sense of direction and purpose), supporting spiritual and religious searching (to provide a sense of meaning), and helping the patient recognize personal attributes that have value (Breitbart & Heller, 2003). Finally, involving patients in treatment decisions may help maintain a sense of power and agency and encouraging patients to reminisce about their life and review uplifting memories can help reduce feelings of frustration and helplessness, and a lighthearted and even humorous approach (when appropriate, and after a sense of trust and respect has been established) can help patients maintain a positive outlook on their situation (Chochinov, 2002).

Although these and other clinical recommendations (e.g., Klausner et al., 1998; Parker-Oliver, 2002; Penson, 2000) have not been systematically analyzed, a number of structured individual and group psychotherapies have been designed specifically for palliative care settings, all of which target hopelessness as an essential component. For example, Breitbart and Greenstein developed a group intervention based on the work of Frankl (Breitbart, 2002; Greenstein & Breitbart, 2000). Called meaning-centered group psychotherapy (MCGP), this intervention is designed to reduce feelings of hopelessness and depression and to foster spiritual well-being by helping patients develop and sustain a sense of meaning in their lives (Breitbart, 2002). Although MCGP is currently part of an ongoing controlled investigation, preliminary data suggest that MCGP significantly decreases both hopelessness and desire for hastened death in terminally ill cancer patients.

Chochinov (2002) has proposed another model psychotherapeutic intervention for terminally ill patients that focuses specifically on maintaining a sense of hope and increasing a sense of meaning and purpose in life. This individualized intervention, termed Dignity Conserving Care, is designed to be performed at the bedside and does not require extensive, repeated "sessions" with the patient. Unfortunately, systematic data are not yet available regarding the efficacy of this intervention, despite the intuitive and practical appeal of the model. Nevertheless, the growing interest in depression and hopelessness near the end of life will continue to foster more and varied clinical interventions to identify feasible and appropriate methods.

SUMMARY

The detrimental impact of depression and hopelessness near the end of life has become increasingly recognized by mental health clinicians working in palliative care settings. Although countless techniques to recognize depression and hopelessness have been developed over the past several decades, few of these approaches have been applied to terminally ill populations. Indeed, the nature of hopelessness and symptoms of depression may differ for patients confronting death and plagued by severe physical symptoms, necessitating a modified approach to differentiate patients who need mental health intervention from those who are adequately coping with the dying process. Moreover, a growing number of clinical interventions have been proposed to help foster and maintain a sense of hope as death approaches, and these interventions hold considerable promise for palliative care settings. Yet despite this growing interest and empirical research, many gaps exist between the theoretical models that have been proposed and the empirical validation necessary before clear conclusions can be drawn. It is hoped that the growing interest and enthusiasm of mental health professionals working in palliative care settings will continue to facilitate these important goals.

REFERENCES

Abbey, J. G., Rosenfeld, B., Pessin, H., & Breitbart, W. (in press). Hopelessness at the end of life: An analysis of the Beck Hopelessness Scale. *British Journal of Health Psychology.*

American Psychiatric Association. (2000). *Diagnostic and statistical manual of mental disorders* (4th ed., text rev.). Washington, DC: American Psychiatric Press.

Beck, A. T., & Beck, R. W. (1972). Screening depressed patients in family practice: A rapid technic. *Post-Graduate Medicine, 52,* 81–85.

Beck, A. T., Ward, C. H., Mendelson, M., Mock, J., & Erbaugh, J. (1961). An inventory for measuring depression. *Archives of Internal Medicine, 154,* 2039–2047

Beck, A. T., & Weishaar, M. E. (1990). Suicide risk assessment and prediction. *Crisis, 11,* 22–30.

Beck, A. T., Weissman, A., Lester, D., & Trexler, L. (1974). The measurement of pessimism: The Beck Hopelessness Scale. *Journal of Consulting and Clinical Psychology, 42,* 861–865.

Block S. D. (2000). Assessing and managing depression in the terminally ill patient. *Annals of Internal Medicine, 132,* 209–218.

Breitbart, W. (2002). Spirituality and meaning in supportive care: Spirituality- and meaning-centered group psychotherapy interventions in advanced cancer. *Supportive Care and Cancer, 10,* 272–280.

Breitbart, W., & Heller, K. S. (2003). Reframing hope: Meaning-centered care for patients near the end of life. *Journal of Palliative Medicine, 6,* 979–988.

Breitbart, W., Passik, S. D., & Rosenfeld, B. (1999). Cancer, mind and spirit. In J. Wall & L. Melzak (Eds.), *Pain* (4th ed., pp. 1075–1112). London: Churchill-Livingston.

Breitbart, W., Rosenfeld, B., Pessin, H., Kaim, M., Funesti-Esch, J., Galietta, M., et al. (2000). Depression, hopelessness, and desire for hastened death in terminally ill patients with cancer. *Journal of the American Medical Association, 284,* 2907–2911.

Bruera, E., Chadwick, S., Brenneis, C., Hanson, J., & MacDonald, R. N. (1987). Methylphenidate associated with narcotics for the treatment of cancer pain. *Cancer Treatment Reporter, 71,* 67–70.

Burns, M. M., & Eisendrath, S. J. (1994). Dextroamphetamine treatment for depression in terminally ill patients. *Psychosomatics, 35,* 80–83.

Carroll, B., Fielding, J., & Blashki, T. (1973). Depression rating scales: A critical review. *Archives of General Psychiatry, 163,* 361–366.

Cassem, N. H. (1987). The dying patient. In T. P. Hackett & N. H. Cassem (Eds.), *Massachusetts General Hospital handbook of general hospital psychiatry* (pp. 332–352). Littleton, MA: PSG.

Chochinov, H. M. (2002). Dignity-conserving care—a new model for palliative care: Helping the patient feel valued. *Journal of the American Medical Association, 287,* 2253–2260.

Chochinov, H. M., & Schwartz, L. (2002). Depression and the will to live in terminally ill patients. In K. Foley & H. Hendin (Eds.), *The case against assisted suicide* (pp. 261–277). Baltimore: Johns Hopkins University Press.

Chochinov, H. M., Tataryn, D. J., Wilson, K. G., Enns, M., & Lander, S. (2000). Prognostic awareness and the terminally ill. *Psychosomatics, 41,* 500–504.

Chochinov, H. M., Wilson, K. G., Enns, M., & Lander, S. (1994). Prevalence of depression in the terminally ill: Effects of diagnostic criteria and symptom threshold judgments. *American Journal of Psychiatry, 51,* 537–540.

Chochinov, H. M., Wilson, K. G., Enns, M., & Lander, S. (1997). "Are you depressed?" Screening for depression in the terminally ill. *American Journal of Psychiatry, 154,* 674–676.

Chochinov, H. M., Wilson, K. G., Enns, M., & Lander, S. (1998). Depression, hopelessness, and suicidal ideation in the terminally ill. *Psychosomatics, 39,* 366–370.

Clarke, D. M., & Kissane, D. W. (2002). Demoralization: Its phenomenology and importance. *Australian and New Zealand Journal of Psychiatry, 36,* 733–742.

Collins, S., & Cutcliffe, J. R. (2003). Addressing hopelessness in people with suicidal ideation: Building upon the therapeutic relationship utilizing a cognitive behavioural approach. *Journal of Psychiatry and Mental Health Nursing, 10,* 175–185.

Cox, J., Holden, J., & Sagovsky, R. (1987). Detection of postnatal depression: Development of the 10-item Edinburgh Postnatal Depression Scale. *British Journal of Psychiatry, 150,* 782–786.

Donnelly, J. M., Kornblith, A. B., Fleishman, S., Zuckerman, E., Raptis, G., Hudis, C. A., et al. (2000). A pilot study of interpersonal psychotherapy by telephone with cancer patients and their partners. *Psychooncology, 9,* 44–56

Dugan, W., McDonald, M. V., Passik, S. D., Rosenfeld, B., Theobald, D., & Edgerton, S. (1998). Use of the Zung Self-Rating Depression Scale in cancer patients: Feasibility as a screening tool. *Psycho-oncology, 7,* 483–493.

Endicott, J. (1984). Measurement of depression in patients with cancer. *Cancer, 53,* 2243–2249.

Everson, S. A., Goldberg, D. E., Kaplan, G. A., Cohen, R. D., Pukkala, E., Tuomilehto, J., et al. (1996). Hopelessness and risk of mortality and incidence of myocardial infarction and cancer. *Psychosomatic Medicine, 58,* 113–121.

Fernandez, F., Adams, F., Levy, J. K., Holmes, V. F., Neidhart, M., & Mansell, P. W. (1988). Cognitive impairment due to AIDS-related complex and its response to psychostimulants. *Psychosomatics, 29,* 38–46.

Frankl, V. E. (1986). *The doctor and the soul*. New York: Vintage Books.

Fry, P. S. (1984). Development of a geriatric scale of hopelessness: Implications for counseling and intervention with the depressed elderly. *Journal of Counseling Psychology, 31*, 322–331.

Ganzini, L., Johnston, W., McFarland, B. H., Tolle, S. W., & Lee, M. A. (1998). Attitudes of patients with amyotrophic lateral sclerosis and their caregivers toward assisted suicide. *New England Journal of Medicine, 339*, 967–973.

Greenstein, M., & Breitbart, W. (2000). Cancer and the experience of meaning: A group psychotherapy program for people with cancer. *American Journal of Psychotherapy, 54*, 486–500.

Herth, K. (1990). Fostering hope in terminally ill people. *Journal of Advances in Nursing, 15*, 1250–1259.

Hollon, S. D., Thase, M. E., & Markowitz, J. C. (2002). Treatment and prevention of depression. *Psychological Science in the Public Interest, 3*, 39–77.

Klausner, E. J., Clarkin, J. F., Spielman, L., Pupo, C., Abrams, R., & Alexopoulos, G. S. (1998). Late-life depression and functional disability: The role of goal-focused group psychotherapy. *International Journal of Geriatric Psychiatry, 13*, 707–716.

LeFevre, P. L., Devereux, J., Smith, S., Lawrie, S. M., & Cornbleet, M. (1999). Screening for psychiatric illness in the palliative care inpatient setting: A comparison between the Hospital and Depression Scale and the General Health Questionnaire—12. *Palliative Medicine, 13*, 399–407.

Linehan, M. M., Armstrong, H. E., Suarez, A., Allmon, D., & Heard, H. L. (1991). Cognitive–behavioral treatment of chronically parasuicidal borderline patients. *Archives of General Psychiatry, 48*, 1060–1064.

Lloyd-Williams, M., Friedman, T., & Rudd, N. (1999). A survey of antidepressant prescribing in the terminally ill. *Palliative Medicine, 13*, 243–248.

Lloyd-Williams, M., Friedman, T., & Rudd, N. (2001). An analysis of the validity of the Hospital and Depression Scale as a screening tool in patients with advanced metastatic cancer. *Journal of Pain and Symptom Management, 22*, 990–996.

Maguire, P. (1985). Improving the detection of psychiatric problems in cancer patients. *Social Science and Medicine, 20*, 819–823.

Maguire, P., Hopwood, P., Tarrier, N., & Howell, T. (1985). Treatment of depression in cancer patients. *Acta Psychiatrica Scandica, 320*(Suppl.), 81–84.

Massie, M. J., & Holland, J. C. (1990). Depression and the cancer patient. *Journal of Clinical Psychiatry, 51*, 12–17.

McClain, C. S., Rosenfeld, B., & Breitbart, W. (2003). The influence of spirituality on end-of-life despair among terminally ill cancer patients. *Lancet, 361*, 1603–1607.

Menon, A. S., Campbell, D., Ruskin, P., & Hebel, J. R. (2000). Depression, hopelessness, and the desire for life-saving treatments among elderly medically ill veterans. *American Journal of Geriatric Psychiatry, 8*, 333–342.

Nelson, C. J., Rosenfeld, B., Breitbart, W., & Galietta, M. (2002). Spirituality, religion, and depression in the terminally ill. *Psychosomatics, 43*, 213–220.

Newport, D. J., & Nemeroff, C. B. (1998). Assessment and treatment of depression in the cancer patient. *Journal of Psychosomatic Research, 45,* 215–237.

Nunn, K. P. (1996). Personal hopefulness: A conceptual review of the relevance of the perceived future to psychiatry. *British Journal of Medical Psychology, 69,* 227–243.

Olin, J., & Masand, P. (1996). Psychostimulants for depression in hospitalized cancer patients. *Psychosomatics, 37,* 57–62.

Parker-Oliver, D. (2002). Redefining hope for the terminally ill. *American Journal of Hospice and Palliative Care, 19,* 115–120.

Passik, S. D., Dugan, W., McDonald, M. V., Rosenfeld, B., Theobald, D., & Edgerton, S. (1998). Oncologists' recognition of depression in their patients with cancer. *Journal of Clinical Oncology, 16,* 1594–1600.

Passik, S. D., Lundberg, J., Rosenfeld, B., Donaghy, K., Theobald, D., Heminger, E., et al. (2000). Factor analysis of the Zung Self-Rating Depression Scale in a large ambulatory sample of oncology patients. *Psychosomatics, 41,* 121–127.

Penson, J. (2000). A hope is not a promise: Fostering hope within palliative care. *International Journal of Palliative Nursing, 6,* 94–98.

Pessin, H., Potash, M., & Breitbart, W. (2003). Diagnosis, assessment, and treatment of depression in palliative care. In M. Lloyd-Williams (Ed.), *Psychosocial issues in palliative care* (pp. 81–103). New York: Oxford University Press.

Popkin, M. K., Callies, A. L., & Mackenzie, T. B. (1985). The outcome of antidepressant use in the medically ill. *Archives of General Psychiatry, 42,* 1160–1163.

Preskorn, S. H., & Burke, M. (1992). Somatic therapy for major depressive disorder: Selection of an antidepressant. *Journal of Clinical Psychiatry, 53*(Suppl.), 5–18.

Rabkin, J. G., Wagner, G. J., & Del Bene, M. (2000). Resilience and distress among amyotrophic lateral sclerosis patients and caregivers. *Psychosomatic Medicine, 62,* 271–279.

Rosenfeld, B. (1998). Psychological sequelae of HIV disease and HIV-associated neoplasms. In J. C. Holland & J. H. Rowland (Eds.), *Handbook of psychooncology* (2nd ed., pp. 861–897). New York: Oxford.

Rosenfeld, B. (2004). *Assisted suicide and the right to die: The interface of social science, public policy, and medical ethics.* Washington, DC: American Psychological Association.

Rosenfeld, B., Breitbart, W., McDonald, M.V., Passik, S., Thaler, H., & Portenoy, R. K. (1996). Pain in ambulatory AIDS patients—II: Impact of pain on psychological functioning and quality of life. *Pain, 68,* 323–328.

Satel, S. L., & Nelson, J. C. (1989). Stimulants in the treatment of depression: A critical overview. *Journal of Clinical Psychiatry, 50,* 241–249.

Scheier, M. F., Matthews, K. A., Owens, J. F., Magovern, G. J. Sr., Lefebvre, R. C., Abbott, R. A., et al. (1989). Dispositional optimism and recovery from coronary artery bypass surgery: The beneficial effects on physical and psychological well-being. *Journal of Personality and Social Psychology, 57,* 1024–1040.

Schwartz, L., Lander, M., & Chochinov, H. M. (2002). Current management of depression in cancer patients. *Oncology, 16,* 1102–1110.

Scott, J., Teasdale, J. D., Paykel, E. S., Johnson, A. L., Abbott, R., Hayhurst, H., et al. (2000). Effects of cognitive therapy on psychological symptoms and social functioning in residual depression. *British Journal of Psychiatry, 177,* 440–446.

Steed, L. (2001). Further validity and reliability evidence for Beck Hopelessness Scale scores in a nonclinical population. *Educational and Psychological Measurement, 61,* 303–316.

Stotland, E. (1969). *The psychology of hope.* San Francisco: Jossey-Bass.

Tonge, W. L., James, D. S., & Hilliam, S. M. (1975). Families without hope: A controlled study of 33 problem families. *British Journal of Psychiatry* (special publication no. 11). Ashford, Kent, England: Headley Bros. (for the Royal College of Psychiatrists)

Townsend, E., Hawton, K., Altman, D. G., Arensman, E., Gunnell, D., Hazell, P., et al. (2001). The efficacy of problem-solving treatments after deliberate self-harm: Meta-analysis of randomized controlled trials with respect to depression, hopelessness and improvement in problems. *Psychological Medicine, 6,* 979–988.

Visintainer, M. A., Volpicelli, J. R., & Seligman, M. E. P. (1982). Tumor rejection in rats after inescapable or escapable shock. *Science, 216,* 437–439.

Watson, M., Haviland, J. S., Greer, S., Davidson, J., & Bliss, J. M. (1999). Influence of psychological response on survival in breast cancer: A population-based cohort study. *Lancet, 354,* 404.

Wilson, K. G., Chochinov, H. M., de Faye, & Breitbart, W. (2000). Diagnosis and management of depression in palliative care. In H. M. Chochinov & W. Breitbart (Eds.), *Handbook of psychiatry in palliative medicine* (pp. 25–49) New York: Oxford University Press.

Wilson, K. G., Scott, J. F., Graham, I. D., Kozak, J. F., Chater, S., Viola, R. A., et al. (2000). Attitudes of terminally ill patients toward euthanasia and physician-assisted suicide. *Archives of Internal Medicine, 160,* 2454–2460.

Zigmond, A. S., & Snaith, R. P. (1983). The Hospital Anxiety and Depression Scale. *Acta Psychiatrica Scandinavica, 67,* 261–370.

Zung, W. (1967). Factors influencing the Self-Rating Depression Scale. *Archives of General Psychiatry, 16,* 543–547.

8

RESPONDING TO THE NEEDS OF CAREGIVERS NEAR THE END OF LIFE: ENHANCING BENEFITS AND MINIMIZING BURDENS

REBECCA S. ALLEN, WILLIAM E. HALEY, LUCINDA L. ROFF,
BETTINA SCHMID, AND ELIZABETH J. BERGMAN

Each of us will deal with the deaths of those we love as well as our own mortality. Yet we rarely consider the certainty of the end of life until confronted with the immediate needs of one we love who is dying. Patients with chronic, life-limiting illness are typically older adults, and often it is their family members who bear the responsibility of caring for them (Emanuel et al., 1999; Schulz, Beach, et al., 2001).

This chapter focuses on the experience and needs of family caregivers for individuals with chronic, life-limiting illnesses near the end of life. Our definition of family is inclusive of fictive kin but not court-appointed guardians or others without a personal relationship with the care recipient. First, we present an overview of issues facing family caregivers during palliative care. Next, we review family involvement in advance care planning and end-of-life treatment decision making. Then we present stress process models and the positive and negative impact of end-of-life caregiving among families. We next examine one means by which family caregivers cope with end-of-life caregiving stressors—religiousness and spirituality. Fifth, we provide an overview of interventions for family caregivers during the course of the care recipient's illness. Finally, we examine family caregivers' adjustment to bereavement. We conclude by providing suggestions for practice and research, as well as implications for public policy.

THE CONTEXT OF FAMILY CAREGIVING NEAR THE END OF LIFE

From the general literature on caregiving, it is well established that family caregiving can have serious negative effects on mental and physical health. Previous reviews demonstrate that extensive caregiving, such as that provided by families for relatives with dementia, increases rates of depression, anxiety, and guilt (Haley & Bailey, 1999; Pinquart & Sörenson, 2003). Family caregiving can also lead to a number of changes in physical health. The stress of caregiving has been shown to increase negative health behaviors in areas such as diet, exercise, and sleep (Gallant & Connell, 1998). Caregivers are also at increased risk for decreased immune system functioning and cardiovascular problems (Haley & Bailey, 1999). Highly strained caregivers studied in the Caregiver Health Effects Study had a 63% increase in mortality over noncaregivers and those caregivers who did not experience strain (Schulz & Beach, 1999).

Families choose to provide care for their loved ones for many reasons, including attachment, cultural expectations, and preferences for avoiding institutional care (Schulz, Gallagher-Thompson, Haley, & Czaja, 2000). Caregiver responsibilities vary, ranging from occasional assistance with instrumental activities of daily living (IADLs; e.g., financial management, medication management) to total responsibility for activities of daily living (ADLs) such as toileting or bathing. Although a large body of research looks at the impact of caregiving, little has focused on caregiving near the end of life. Family caregivers' involvement generally increases as the illness progresses, often reaching a point in which caregiving becomes an all-encompassing job near the patient's death (Haley, Allen, et al., 2002; Zuckerman & Wollner, 1999).

Emanuel's team (1999) interviewed 988 terminally ill adults and their caregivers in six sites in the United States to learn about the patterns of assistance to terminally ill patients. Often, family members were the exclusive providers of assistance. Haley, LaMonde, Han, Burton, and Schonwetter (2003) studied the caregivers of end-stage dementia and lung cancer patients and found that the cancer caregivers provided an average of approximately 100 hours of care each week.

Family members are also involved in many other aspects of care, including providing emotional support and symptom management. They are often asked to make reports of patients' symptoms, such as pain (Allen, Haley, Small, & McMillan, 2002), serving as a surrogate when the patient is either incapacitated or being sheltered by staff. The caregiver's report of a patient's pain by the family caregiver may not match that of the patient, however (Allen et al., 2002; Coates, Allen, Shuster, & Burgio, 2002).

Family caregivers often must assume responsibilities for which they have insufficient information, support, and training, given that they exert a meaningful influence on the nature of the patient's treatment (Zuckerman & Wollner, 1999). Zuckerman and Wollner noted that family caregivers fill several roles, including that of "negotiators of care systems." For example, family members are integrally involved in the initiation, discussion, and finalizing stage regarding the choice of hospice care (Chen, Haley, Robinson, & Schonwetter, 2003). By the same token, family members may actively discourage the use of hospice services, or the lack of a family caregiver may preclude provision of hospice care. In a survey of physicians (Weggel, 1999), family factors were cited as primary barriers to hospice referrals.

On the basis of this review, it is clear that family caregivers exert direct and indirect influence on treatment decisions and the nature of care throughout the course of life-limiting illness. Nonetheless, many state and federal laws regarding end-of-life decision making, such as the Patient Self-Determination Act passed in 1990 and instituted in 1991 (see Omnibus Budget Reconciliation Act, 1990), rely on the principle of autonomy—the concept that an individual has the right to determine the course of his or her medical care through end-of-life decisions. This discrepancy between public policy and the actual influence of family members on end-of-life care decisions must be taken into account in the practice of advance care planning and end-of-life treatment decision making (Allen & Shuster, 2002; King, Kim, & Conwell, 2000).

ADVANCE CARE PLANNING AND FAMILY DECISION MAKING

A number of institutions advocate advance care planning, and every state has passed legislation regarding this topic. Organizations such as the American Association of Retired Persons (AARP), American Bar Association (ABA), and the American Medical Association (AMA) have engaged in efforts to educate their own members and the general public about advance directives and to promote their use (AARP, ABA Commission on Legal Problems of the Elderly & AMA, 1995; AMA Council on Ethical and Judicial Affairs, 1998). Also, researchers are continuing to explore the factors that affect family decision making and interventions for increasing the effectiveness of advance directives. Although research is still inconclusive as to whether advance care planning and completion of advance directives aid in maintaining patient control over the dying process, there is some suggestion that at least advance care planning may ease the minds of patients, caregivers, and family members concerning end-of-life issues (Ditto et al., 2001).

Advance Directives and Informal Advance Care Planning

Although the use of advance directives has increased slightly, especially since the Patient Self-Determination Act, many people do not execute these legal documents (Shewchcuk, 1998). More often, families will opt for informal advance care planning. That is, they engage in discussions about end-of-life care, even if they do not follow through with legal documents. Unfortunately, many people choose not to address this issue and consequently have no plans for end-of-life care, leaving their family members with little information on which to base decisions when they are called on to serve as proxy decision makers. Factors that influence this planning process include culture, age, education, and health status (Phipps et al., 2003; Rosnick & Reynolds, 2003).

Although several studies have shown intraindividual treatment wishes to be relatively stable for 1 to 2 years (Ditto et al., 2003; Emanuel, Emanuel, Stoeckle, Hummel, & Barry, 1994), patient treatment preferences should be revisited within a family context periodically because declines in physical or psychological functioning may reduce individuals' interest in life-prolonging treatments. Also, family circumstances may change because of death, divorce, or other events, resulting in the need for revision of advance care plans. Individuals may not be aware of subtle changes in their treatment preferences (Gready et al., 2000) or may not be mindful of changes within the family system that would affect future medical care plans. Thus, many authors argue that effective advance care planning is an ongoing family process rather than a one-time, autonomous event (e.g., Allen & Shuster, 2002).

Discrepancies in Family Decision Making

As discussed later, proxy agreement studies generally show poor agreement between older adults and others regarding preferences for specific life-prolonging medical treatments (often proxy decisions are no better than chance). Studies of end-of-life medical decision making typically ask a participant (the "patient") and a family member such as a spouse or an adult child (the "proxy" or "surrogate") to imagine the patient in hypothetical scenarios involving various medical conditions, and they are given options for medical interventions to consider. The patient and proxy independently indicate their choices for the patient, and the responses of both parties are analyzed to determine the accuracy of the proxy in predicting the wishes of the patient.

Several studies found that proxies tend to be conservative in their decisions, that is, they have more overtreatment errors (opt for treatment that the patient does not want) rather than undertreatment errors (Ditto et al., 2001; Suhl, Simons, Reedy, & Garrick, 1994; Zweibel & Cassel, 1989). Others have found a bias among proxies to undertreat (Diamond, Jernigan, Moseley, Messina, & McKeown, 1989) or no significant difference in overtreatment versus undertreatment errors (Gerety, Chiodo, Kanten, Tuley, & Cornell, 1993; Sulmasy et al., 1998; Teno, Stevens, Spernak, & Lynn, 1998). This apparent inconsistency may be accounted for when the patient's cognitive and health status are considered. That is, the studies in which proxies made undertreatment errors involved patients who resided in nursing homes, implying impaired cognitive status and poor health. In contrast, the studies in which proxies made overtreatment errors involved relatively healthy patients drawn from the community and outpatient clinics.

Many researchers have found that agreement was highest for the most extreme (e.g., coma—no chance of recovery) and least extreme (e.g., current good health) scenarios (Ditto et al., 2001; Gerety et al., 1993; Sulmasy et al., 1998). This finding is consistent with the findings of research on stability of patient wishes in which participants' preferences also were more stable for the most and least extreme health scenarios (Gready et al., 2000). Many factors may contribute to treatment preference discrepancies between patients and proxies, including differences in how healthy and unhealthy individuals view illness and quality of life. Proxies may exhibit a projection bias in which they tend to make decisions based on their own treatment wishes from the vantage point of their relatively healthy state that are not correlated with the treatment wishes of the patient who is ill (Fagerlin, Ditto, Danks, Houts, & Smucker, 2001; Sulmasy et al., 1998).

Most studies on family decision making had a majority of female patients because they generally centered on older adults and women have a longer life expectancy than men. The studies that consisted of predominantly male patients typically recruited participants who had compromised health at the time of the study (e.g., residents of nursing homes, patients diagnosed with a serious illness; Gerety et al., 1993; Suhl et al., 1994; Sulmasy et al., 1998; Teno et al., 1998). However, sex of the patient or the surrogate has not emerged as a factor in the accuracy of substituted judgment. Regarding race and ethnicity, minority groups have generally not been adequately represented in this area of research. Most samples were predominantly Caucasian (ranging from 64% to 100% Caucasian). Two studies that examined race and ethnicity as a factor in accuracy of substituted judgment did not yield significant results (Phipps et al., 2003; D. P. Sulmasy, personal communication, October 5, 2001).

Providing care for a seriously ill loved one can be a precious final gift to the dying patient. Yet even as family members try to cope with stressors, they are expected to make sound decisions and to clearly communicate with professional care providers. How family members respond to the multifaceted demands and strains of caregiving depends on a number of factors including personal variables, cultural factors, social support, access to professional services such as hospice, and knowledge or experience in advance care planning and patient care.

STRESS PROCESS MODELS AND THE IMPACT OF FAMILY CAREGIVING ON LOVED ONES NEAR THE END OF LIFE

The broader caregiving literature demonstrates that the effects of caregiving are not uniform. Stress process models (Haley, Levine, Brown, & Bartolucci, 1987; Pearlin, Mullan, Semple, & Skaff, 1990; Schulz, Gallagher-Thompson, et al., 2000) suggest that it is overly simplistic to think that objective measures of patient impairment and caregiver strain alone determine the impact of caregiving. Caregivers also experience not only primary stressors related to the actual behaviors of coping, but also a variety of secondary stressors, such as role strain, financial strain, guilt, and family conflict (Pearlin et al., 1990). In addition, one must examine the interaction between these stressors, the caregiver's appraisal of these stressors, and the caregiver's coping resources. A variety of internal resources, including successful previous experience in coping with stress, the ability to find meaning in adversity, optimistic personality, and the use of problem-focused coping have been found to be beneficial to caregivers (Folkman, 2001; Haley & Bailey, 1999). In addition, external resources, such as social support and financial resources are advantageous in coping with caregiving.

A small but increasing body of research focuses on stress, coping, and adaptation in end-of-life caregivers. Emanuel and colleagues (1999) and Emanuel, Fairclough, Slutsman, and Emanuel (2000) conducted a national study that documents the high levels of assistance provided by family caregivers of terminally ill patients and the burdens experienced by families in the context of terminal illness. They showed that burden and depression are higher in family caregivers of patients with substantial care needs regardless of the specific terminal illness.

Schulz, Mendelsohn, et al. (2003) completed a study of the experiences of 217 caregivers for persons with end-stage dementia. These researchers found that more than half of caregivers reported feeling "on duty" 24 hours a day and that they had ended or reduced employment because of caregiving. Haley, LaMonde, Han, Narramore, and Schonwetter (2001) found that hospice caregivers for terminally ill patients with either lung cancer or dementia showed high rates of depression, lower life satisfaction, and poorer self-rated health than noncaregiving controls, with few differences in caregiver well-being across disease type.

Application of stress process models to end-of-life caregiving shows that additional stressors known to put caregivers at increased risk for depression include poor health and negative social interactions (Haley, LaMonde, et al., 2003). In addition, higher levels of social participation, larger social networks, and higher perceptions of the adequacy of social support can all be viewed as powerful resources for caregivers that reduce the risk of depression and increase life satisfaction (Haley, LaMonde, et al., 2003).

Haley, LaMonde, and colleagues (2001) found that many families report experiencing benefits from caregiving. Most caregivers do not provide care just because they feel obligated to do so and feel trapped in the role. Some caregivers feel that they are passing on a tradition of care and that by modeling caregiving, their children will be more likely to care for them if this becomes necessary. Some additional gains reported by caregivers include giving back to someone who has cared for them, satisfaction of knowing that their relative is getting excellent care, sense of personal growth, and gaining meaning and purpose in one's life.

RELIGIOUSNESS AND SPIRITUALITY AND END-OF-LIFE CAREGIVING

One means by which individuals cope with stress and experience meaning and purpose during caregiving is through religious participation and spirituality (Michael, Crowther, Schmid, & Allen, 2003). This sense of satisfaction and well-being can have important benefits for caregivers well after caregiving has ended (Carter, 1994; Michael et al., 2003).

Salience and Definitions of Religiousness and Spirituality

Approximately 95% of U.S. citizens say that they believe in God; 90% indicate that they pray; and at least two thirds report that they pray every day (Gallup & Lindsay, 1999). Not surprisingly, significant proportions of Americans report turning to religion and spirituality to deal with negative and stressful life situations (see Pargament, 1997, for a review; see also chap. 5 by Kaut). Thus, one might expect to see a number of studies that examine caregivers' use of religion and spirituality in dealing with the impending death of a loved one. However, only a few such studies exist (e.g., Mickley, Pargament, Brant, & Hipp, 1998; Rabins, Fitting, Eastham, & Zabora, 1990), and these suggest that end-of-life caregivers may use religion and spirituality to cope with their circumstances. Persons who are elderly, poorer, less well educated, African American, widowed, female, and more religious tend to turn most to religion as a source of coping with distressing life events (Pargament, 1997; Roff et al., 2004).

Scholars and the public at large make distinctions between the concepts of religiousness and spirituality (Michael et al., 2003; Shahabi et al, 2002). The distinctions typically used focus on religion and religiousness as social and organizational phenomena that are tied to institutions and fixed doctrines or creeds. Spirituality, by contrast, is seen as a more personal, emotional, and subjective domain that an individual can pursue in a solitary way without participation in a social body or adherence to a prescribed set of beliefs. Religiousness and spirituality are interrelated in that the quest is for the sacred, and each can foster the development of the other (Hill & Pargament, 2003; Michael et al., 2003). For many people, religious practice is the route to the sacred. For example, religious services, classes, and literature may encourage spiritual growth, and spiritual practices such as prayer or meditation are often salient aspects of religious services (Armstrong & Crowther, 2002).

Cultural Influences

It is unfortunate that research regarding the influence of religiousness and spirituality among diverse cultural, social, and economic groups within the end-of-life context of family caregiving is sorely inadequate. Most studies compare African American and White caregivers, and studies focus almost exclusively on Judeo-Christian spiritual traditions. Religious and spiritual orientation, gender, ethnic minority, sexual orientation, or disability status may significantly impact individual and family approaches to end-of-life care and decision making (Working Group on Assisted Suicide and End-of-Life Decisions, 2000). For example, persons of Chinese or Navajo descent may turn more to religion as a source of positive coping rather than engage in end-of-life planning discussions (Working Group on Assisted Suicide and End-of-Life Decisions, 2000).

African American caregivers rely more heavily on religious sources of support than do White caregivers (Armstrong & Crowther, 2002; Picot, Debanne, Namazi, & Wykle, 1997; Wykle & Segall, 1991). Picot and colleagues studied the relationship between religiosity and perceived rewards of African American and White caregivers of disabled elders. Prayer, self-rated religiosity, and comfort from religion were related to satisfaction with caregiving. Comfort from religion and prayer partially mediated the relationship between race and perceived caregiver rewards. In answer to a closed-ended question, both African American and White Alzheimer's disease caregivers indicated that they turned to religion or prayer as a method of coping (Wykle & Segal, 1991). A striking 80% of African American respondents, however, gave "prayer, faith and religion" as the response to a question regarding "the one special way" individuals coped with caring for their relative in comparison with 0% of the White caregivers. These findings suggest that interventions with African American end-of-life caregivers, and, potentially, other ethnic minority groups, must be especially sensitive to religious and spiritual concerns.

Positive and Negative Aspects of Religiousness and Spirituality

Most of the studies that report associations between religious or spiritual variables and caregiver outcomes find that higher or more positive aspects of religiousness and spirituality are associated with positive or desirable outcomes for caregivers (Crowther, Parker, Larimore, Achenbaum, & Koenig, 2002). Mickley et al. (1998) studied 92 hospice caregivers, assessing the relationships between their religious appraisals and their mental and spiritual health outcomes. Participants who saw their circumstances as part of God's plan or who reported gaining strength or understanding from God reported positive outcomes on mental and spiritual health measures. Religious appraisals contributed to participants' mental and spiritual outcomes over and above the effects of nonreligious appraisals.

In a study of 32 caregivers of patients with Alzheimer's disease and 30 caregivers of patients with metastatic cancer, Rabins and colleagues (1990) discovered that caregivers' self-reported strength of religious beliefs predicted their emotional well-being 2 years after initial interview. Davis, Nolen-Hoeksema, and Larson (1998) studied familial hospice caregivers while the patient was still living and at 1-, 6-, 13-, and 18-month follow-up. They found that making sense of the patients' death was predictive of caregivers' positive adjustment within the first year, whereas identifying positive growth and benefits were better predictors of positive caregiver adjustment at 13- and 18-month follow-up. In a study of 127 caregivers of disabled elders, Chang, Noonan, and Tennstedt (1998) found that caregivers who used religiousness or spirituality to help them cope reported better relationships with the care recipients which, in turn, were associated with less caregiver depression and role submersion.

Religious coping, however, may also have negative consequences for the caregiver. Caregivers who attribute their situations to the anger or abandonment of God or who see their caregiving role as a punishment from God might be expected to experience feelings of depression, guilt, or low self-worth. Shah, Snow, and Kunik (2001) studied 48 caregivers of Alzheimer's patients recruited through support groups. Nearly all (96%) described themselves as religious or spiritual. Participants reporting anger or distance from God or members of their religious group and those who questioned their faith had higher levels of depression and perceived burden. Mickley and colleagues (1998) also found that caregivers who perceived their circumstances as unfair punishment from God or as a result of God's having deserting them had low scores on mental and spiritual health measures. In a qualitative study of 45 caregivers of Alzheimer's disease patients (Smith & Harkness, 2002), 12 described negative experiences with their spiritual communities, and 24 described positive experiences, suggesting some caution might be exercised in relying on religious resources.

Health psychologists and other health care professionals should also be mindful that caregiver religiousness and spirituality has potential implications for the care recipient. Allen, DeLaine, et al. (2003) found that sponsors of nursing home residents with greater religiosity were less likely to have advance care plans for the resident than were those with less religiosity. Similarly, Guberman, Maheu, and Maille (1992) and Caffrey (1992) found relationships between religious beliefs and potential caregivers' motivations to provide care to older persons. Additional research is warranted to understand which client groups are most and least likely to use religious and spiritual resources and benefit from interventions that incorporate facilitation of meaning and purpose in dealing with the life-limiting illness and expected death of a loved one.

INTERVENTIONS FOR FAMILY CAREGIVERS

Many families and individuals with life-limiting illnesses have difficulty accepting the inevitable consequences of the disease, and diverse cultural, social, and economic groups require approaches to intervention that are respectful of differences in end-of-life care and decision making. Interventions that may require particular attention to issues of diversity include making advance care plans, seeking information about the benefits of palliative care, learning useful caregiving and communication skills, or engaging in meaningful activities to promote inter–generational ties and alleviate suffering. Health-related psychologists and other health care professionals must respect diversity and approach individuals and families with sensitivity when suggesting possible assessments, interventions, or programs (Haley, Larson, Kasl-Godley, Neimeyer, & Kwilosz, 2003).

Although we do not yet understand all of the factors that impact end-of-life decision making, either within an individual or in the context of family systems, intervention studies have been conducted targeting the use of advance directives and informal discussions to improve patient–proxy treatment preference agreement, which is reviewed in another chapter in this volume (see chap. 4 by Ditto). Instead, we briefly review some community-based, problem-solving interventions that target family caregivers for individuals with various stages of life-limiting illness.

The University of South Florida Team

At the University of South Florida, problem-solving skills training is used to teach hospice caregivers skills to cope with three common problem areas in community hospice care: (a) pain, (b) constipation, and (c) dyspnea (R01CA77307, S. McMillan, principal investigator [PI]). The intervention is described to participants using the acronym COPE and consists of the following components: (a) viewing problems from different perspectives to find new strategies to address the problem (Creativity); (b) positive but realistic attitude toward the problem-solving process (Optimism); (c) setting goals and thinking out steps to reach those goals (Planning); and (d) pursuit of useful information such as what caregivers need to know about the patient's condition, when to seek professional help, and what can be done by the caregiver to help the patient (Expert information). This problem-solving-based intervention is contrasted with an emotional support intervention and a usual treatment comparison condition. In the problem-solving skills intervention, a specific module was designed for each caregiver to learn assessment and problem-solving techniques useful in the management of the patient's pain, constipation, or dyspnea. Results are not yet available from this project.

The University of Alabama Team

This team has developed two interventions that combine problem-solving skills training with social support, meaning-centered therapeutic activity, or both. The Care Integration Team (CIT; K01AG00943, R. S. Allen, PI) focuses on caregivers of hospice patients and consists of four weekly home visits in comparison with a randomly matched minimal support control group. The problem-solving based intervention focuses on developing skills in four topic areas: (a) symptom management, (b) communication with hospice staff, (c) caregiver self-care, and (d) anticipatory grief. Treatment implementation measures are included in this study. Ten percent of intervention audiotapes are monitored to ensure adherence to the treatment protocol. Also, CIT has a caregiver training manual that serves as a guide to treatment components. Treatment receipt is measured through the length of contact between the interventionist and the family caregiver. Treatment enactment uses weekly tracking forms completed by the family caregiver to measure the usefulness of the skills learned and behavioral program developed for use by the caregiver in a certain problem area.

Developed to address some limitations of the CIT intervention, the Legacy intervention focuses on both the individual with life-limiting illness and the caregiver. It is geared toward positive coping and palliative rather than hospice care (1H79SM54569, R. S. Allen, PI; K01AG00943, R. S. Allen, PI). Thus, the patients do not qualify for hospice but are limited in the extent to which they can care for themselves. If a prognosis were given for their life expectancy, it would likely not exceed 2 to 3 years.

The Legacy intervention was designed to decrease the distress of palliative caregivers and care recipients through increasing perceptions of meaning in the context of an intergenerational activity. This is achieved through the joint development of the patient's "Personal Legacy" for future generations. The Legacy can take multiple forms: a family photo album, a family cookbook or scrapbook, audiotaped or videotaped stories of the older adult's life, or personal letters to younger family members. The intervention incorporates and expands on components of life review (Butler & Lewis, 1982; Haight & Burnside, 1993) and the Hospice Foundation of America's (2001) *A Guide for Recalling and Telling Your Life Story*. The intervention consists of three weekly, 1-hour to 90-minute sessions in which the caregiver and patient learn what a Legacy is, select a Legacy, obtain materials to create the project, and review their experience with members of the research team. A control group receives weekly 5-minute telephone calls and answers questions about spontaneous intergenerational activities.

The Legacy intervention is manualized, and interventionists must be certified to deliver the intervention to families. As in the CIT project, 10% of intervention audiotapes are evaluated for interventionists' adherence to research protocol in treatment delivery by an independent professional clinician not involved with the research project. Contact logs are used to document the content and length of all intervention sessions to measure receipt of treatment, including who initiates the contact and the purpose of the contact. For treatment enactment, interventionists working on the Legacy project note the extent to which a Legacy was completed by the family across the three sessions using a Likert-scale evaluation.

We believe that intervening with family caregivers during the provision of palliative care will ease the negative aspects of caregiving and facilitate positive aspects. We also think that improving the well-being of caregivers will result in improved quality of life for care recipients. By extension, it is possible that interventions during the provision of palliative care that improve the caregiving experience may also positively impact the caregiver's grieving process.

ADJUSTMENT TO BEREAVEMENT

Family caregivers respond to bereavement in a variety of ways, and caregiving experiences can significantly affect the course of bereavement. Although some bereaved caregivers experience a multitude of physical and emotional problems (e.g., depression, anxiety), most report only mild, acute distress. In fact, many caregivers adjust to bereavement in a positive manner, indicating physical and emotional improvement (Bonanno, 2004).

In most cases, death marks the end of an extended period of care provided almost exclusively by family members. While in the caregiver role, many family members must temporarily curtail other personal, social, and professional roles, or they must give them up entirely. They also must stand by as a loved one experiences a disability or chronic disease, many of which bring discomfort and pain. Naturally, then, death often brings the caregiver a sense of relief, from both the strain of providing care and the suffering of her or his loved one. Among spousal caregivers, relief is a common result of bereavement when the care-recipient had a severe illness, the relationship was characterized as high-stress, or the caregiver role was a strain (Schulz, Beach, et al., 2001).

Although most bereavement research identifies individuals only after the time of loss, there is increasing interest in understanding how the context of family caregiving may affect adjustment to bereavement. In a review, Schulz, Newsom, Fleissner, DeCamp, and Nieboer (1997) summarized the results of a number of studies, which indicated that caregiver and family issues significantly affect the adjustment to bereavement of family members. More specifically, stressful and difficult caregiving situations predicted stressful and difficult bereavement, marked by depression and low self-reported health and well-being. In addition, family tension and difficulty in providing care resulted in depression and greater family difficulty in coping with the loss.

The review by Schulz et al. (1997) also suggested that many caregivers experience some element of relief, or improvement of symptoms, when death leads to the cessation of caregiving. Schulz, Mendelsohn, et al. (2003) found that, among dementia caregivers, 72% reported the death of their relative to be somewhat or very much a relief. Schulz and colleagues (2003) also found that caregiver depression increased dramatically just after the death of the care recipient, but significantly declined over the first year. About 25% of bereaved caregivers, however, reported persistent depression and continued use of antidepressant medications for a sustained period after the death of their care recipient.

Utz, Carr, Nesse, and Wortman (2002) reported that social participation increased after the death of a spouse. Before the death, social participation was limited by the demands of providing care. In many cases, friends and relatives increase their level of support, at least temporarily, upon the death of a spouse. Many newly bereaved individuals seek out social opportunities. These researchers stated that efforts to identify those individuals who lack sufficient resources (e.g., children, people with no access to transportation) to seek opportunities for social contact independently are needed, because these individuals may be particularly at risk of increased isolation, depression, health deficits, and mortality.

Finally, adjustment to bereavement may vary across cultural contexts. Owen, Goode, and Haley (2001) found that White and African American caregivers differed in their reactions to the death of a relative with Alzheimer's disease. White caregivers were more likely than African Americans to report a sense of relief, whereas African American caregivers were more likely than White families to view this as a loss experience.

SUMMARY AND FUTURE DIRECTIONS

In this chapter, we have reviewed issues associated with family caregiving for individuals near the end of life in adulthood. Because of increased numbers of individuals living into very old age, greater research and clinical attention is being directed to end-of-life care. Of necessity, end-of-life issues such as advance care planning, family decision making, and the delivery of therapeutic interventions involve both individuals with life-limiting illnesses and their family members. We have attempted to provide a broad overview of these issues as well as positive and negative aspects of caregiving within stress process models, the use of religious and spiritual coping mechanisms, and issues that affect the adjustment to bereavement.

Because examination of family caregiving issues surrounding the end of life is in its infancy, many areas are yet in need of careful scientific inquiry. One glaring need concerns greater attention to diversity issues in the approach to end of life care and decision making. For example, few studies of patient–proxy agreement examine potential mediators of family decisions in diverse samples. Given racial and ethnic differences in preferences for life-prolonging medical treatments and need for information regarding end-of-life care (Working Group on Assisted Suicide and End-of-Life Decisions, 2000), it is imperative to investigate whether particular racial and ethnic groups have high or low concordance in treatment preference agreement. One potential mediator of agreement across racial and ethnic groups is reliance on religious and spiritual coping mechanisms. Knowledge of the issues that contribute to treatment preference agreement will inform the development of culturally sensitive interventions to improve the caregiving experience throughout the course of end-of-life care.

Regarding intervention research, one obvious need is the careful examination and measurement of treatment implementation to identify which specific aspects of interventions are related to improved outcomes among diverse family caregivers (Burgio, Corcoran, et al., 2001; Burgio, Fisher, Phillips, & Allen, 2003). Aspects of treatment delivery, treatment receipt, and treatment enactment have rarely been reported in the intervention research with palliative family caregivers conducted to date. Once the specific aspects of treatment that lead to better outcomes for family caregivers are identified, there is a need for translational research to disseminate effective treatments broadly into community contexts.

The caregiving context also deserves greater attention as a factor in determining bereavement outcomes. Caregivers who experience the death of the care recipient experience a complex combination of loss and relief. Family caregivers should be reassured that feelings of relief can be a normal part of the bereavement process (Schulz, Mendelsohn, et al., 2003). Nonetheless, it is important to address the needs of the significant number of family caregivers who do not experience a decrease in symptoms of depression or the need for antidepressant medication after the death of their loved one.

An immediate need in the realm of policy change has to do with funding for palliative care services. One possibility would be to expand hospice benefits to 1 year before mortality, as in Florida. This would be particularly beneficial for families whose loved ones live with noncancer life-limiting illnesses, such as dementia (Allen, Kwak, Lokken, & Haley, 2003). Investigation into predictors of 1-year mortality is needed to identify individuals and families who may benefit from palliative care services. Without question, these topics will continue to be a focus for research, service, and policy efforts in the coming decades.

REFERENCES

Allen, R. S., DeLaine, S. R., Chaplin, W. F., Marson, D. C., Bourgeois, M. S., Kijkstra, K., et al. (2003). Advance care planning in nursing homes: Correlates of capacity and possession of advance directives. *Gerontologist, 43,* 309–317.

Allen, R. S., Haley, W. E., Small, B. J., & McMillan, S. C. (2002). Pain reports by older hospice cancer patients and family caregivers: The role of cognitive functioning. *Gerontologist, 42,* 507–514.

Allen, R. S., Kwak, J., Lokken, K. L., & Haley, W. E. (2003). End of life issues in the context of Alzheimer's disease. *Alzheimer's Care Quarterly, 4,* 312–330.

Allen, R. S., & Shuster, J. L. (2002). The role of proxies in treatment decisions: Evaluating capacity to consent to end-of-life treatments. *Behavioral Sciences and the Law, 20,* 235–252.

American Association of Retired Persons, ABA Commission on Legal Problems of the Elderly, & American Medical Association. (1995). *Shape your health care future with health care advance directives.* Washington, DC: Authors. Retrieved March 10, 2004, from http://www.abanet.org/ftp/pub/aging/adb.doc

American Medical Association Council on Ethical and Judicial Affairs. (1998). Optimal use of orders not to intervene and advance directives. *Psychology, Public Policy, and Law, 4,* 668–675.

Armstrong, T., & Crowther, M. (2002). Spirituality among older African Americans. *Journal of Adult Development, 9,* 3–12.

Bonanno, G. A. (2004). Loss, trauma, and human resilience: Have we underestimated the human capacity to thrive after extremely aversive events? *American Psychologist, 59,* 20–28.

Burgio L. D., Corcoran M., Lichstein, K., Nichols, L., Czaja, S., Gallagher-Thompson, D., et al. (2001). Judging outcomes in psychosocial interventions for dementia caregivers: The problem of treatment implementation. *Gerontologist, 41,* 481–489.

Burgio, L. D., Fisher, S. E., Phillips, L. L., & Allen, R. S. (2003). Establishing treatment implementation in clinical research. *Alzheimer's Care Quarterly, 4,* 204–215.

Butler, R. N., & Lewis, M. I. (1982). *Aging and mental health.* St. Louis, MO: Mosby.

Caffrey, R. A. (1992). Caregiving to the elderly in northeast Thailand. *Journal of Cross-Cultural Gerontology, 7,* 117–134.

Carter, R. (1994). *Helping yourself help others: A book for caregivers.* New York: Times Books.

Chang, B., Noonan, A. E., & Tennstedt, S. L. (1998). The role of religion/spirituality in coping with caregiving for disabled elders. *Gerontologist, 38,* 463–470.

Chen, H., Haley, W. E., Robinson, B. E., & Schonwetter, R. S. (2003). Decisions for hospice care in patients with advanced cancer. *Journal of the American Geriatrics Society, 51*, 789–797.

Coates, A., Allen, R. S., Shuster, J. L., & Burgio, L. D. (2002, November). *Care integration team intervention during hospice care.* Poster presented at the Gerontological Society of America, Boston.

Crowther, M., Parker, M., Larimore, W., Achenbaum, A., & Koenig, H. G. (2002). Rowe and Kahn's model of successful aging revisited: Spirituality, the missing construct. *Gerontologist, 42*, 613–620.

Davis, C. G., Nolen-Hoeksema, S., & Larson, J. (1998). Making sense of loss and benefiting from the experience: Two construals of meaning. *Journal of Personality and Social Psychology, 75*, 561–574.

Diamond, E. L., Jernigan, J. A., Moseley, R. A., Messina, V., & McKeown, R. A. (1989). Decision-making ability and advance directive preferences in nursing home patients and proxies. *Gerontologist, 29*, 622–626.

Ditto, P. H., Danks, J. H., Smucker, W. D., Bookwala, J., Coppola, K. M., Dresser, R., et al. (2001). Advance directives as acts of communication: A randomized controlled trial. *Archives of Internal Medicine, 161*, 421–430.

Ditto, P. H., Smucker, W. D., Danks, J. H., Jacobson, J. A., Houts, R. M., Fagerlin, A., et al., (2003). Stability of older adults' preferences for life-sustaining medical treatment. *Health Psychology, 22*, 605–615.

Emanuel, E. J., Fairclough, D. L., Slutsman, J., Alpert, H., Baldwin, D., & Emanuel, L. L. (1999). Assistance from family members, friends, paid caregivers, and volunteers in the care of terminally ill patients. *New England Journal of Medicine, 341*, 956–963.

Emanuel, E. J., Fairclough, D. L., Slutsman, J., & Emanuel, L. L. (2000). Understanding economic and other burdens of terminal illness: The experience of patients and their caregivers. *Annals of Internal Medicine, 132*, 451–459.

Emanuel, L. L., Emanuel, E. J., Stoeckle, J. D., Hummel, L. R., & Barry, M. J. (1994). Advance directives. Stability of patients' treatment choices. *Archives of Internal Medicine, 154*, 209–217.

Fagerlin, A., Ditto, P. H., Danks, J. H., Houts, R. M., & Smucker, W. D. (2001). Projection in surrogate decisions about life-sustaining medical treatments. *Health Psychology, 20*, 166–175.

Folkman, S. (2001). Revised coping theory and the process of bereavement. In M. S. Stroebe, R. O. Hansson, W. Stroebe, & H. Schut (Eds.), *Handbook of bereavement research: Consequences, coping, and care* (pp. 563–584). Washington, DC: American Psychological Association.

Gallant, M. P., & Connell, C. M. (1998). The stress process among dementia spouse caregivers: Are caregivers at risk for negative health behavior changes? *Research on Aging, 20*, 267–297.

Gallup, G., Jr., & Lindsay, D. M. (1999). *Surveying the religious landscape: Trends in U.S. beliefs.* Harrisburg, PA: Morehouse.

Gerety, M. B., Chiodo, L. K., Kanten, D. N., Tuley, M. R., & Cornell, J. E. (1993). Medical treatment preferences of nursing home residents: Relationship to function and concordance with surrogate decision-makers. *Journal of the American Geriatrics Society, 41,* 953–960.

Gready, R. M., Ditto, P. H., Danks, J. H., Coppola, K. M., Lockhart, L. K., & Smucker, W. D. (2000). Actual and perceived stability of preferences for life-sustaining treatment. *Journal of Clinical Ethics, 11,* 334–346.

Guberman, N., Maheu, P., & Maille, C. (1992). Women as family caregivers: Why do they care? *Gerontologist, 32,* 607–617.

Haight, B., & Burnside, I. (1993). Reminiscence and life review: Explaining the differences. *Archives of Psychiatric Nursing, 7*(2), 91–98.

Haley, W. E., Allen, R. S., Reynolds, S., Chen, H., Burton, A., & Gallagher-Thompson, D. (2002). Family issues in end-of-life decision making and end-of-life care. *American Behavioral Scientist, 46,* 284–298.

Haley, W. E., & Bailey, S. (1999). Research on family caregiving in Alzheimer's disease: Implications for practice and policy. In B. Vellas & J. L. Fitten (Eds.), *Research and practice in Alzheimer's disease* (Vol. 2, pp. 321–332). Paris: Serdi.

Haley, W. E., LaMonde, L. A., Han, B., Burton, A. M., & Schonwetter, R. (2003). Predictors of depression and life satisfaction among spousal caregivers in hospice: Application of a stress process model. *Journal of Palliative Medicine, 6,* 215–224.

Haley, W. E., LaMonde, L. A., Han, B., Narramore, S., & Schonwetter, R. S. (2001). Family caregiving in hospice: Effects on psychological and health functioning among spousal caregivers of hospice patients with lung cancer or dementia. *Hospice Journal, 15,* 1–18.

Haley, W. E., Larson, D. G., Kasl-Godley, J., Neimeyer, R. A., & Kwilosz, D. M. (2003). Roles for psychologists in end-of-life care: Emerging models of practice. *Professional Psychology: Research and Practice, 34,* 626–633.

Haley, W. E., Levine, E. G., Brown, S. L., & Bartolucci, A. A. (1987). Stress, appraisal, coping, and social support as predictors of adaptational outcome among dementia caregivers. *Psychology and Aging, 2,* 323–330.

Hill, P. C., & Pargament, K. I. (2003). Advances in the conceptualization and measurement of religion and spirituality: Implications for physical and mental health research. *American Psychologist, 58,* 64–74.

Hospice Foundation of America. (2001). *A guide to recalling and telling your life story.* Washington, DC: Author.

King, D. A., Kim, S. Y., & Conwell, Y. (2000). Family matters: A social systems perspective on physician-assisted suicide and the older adult. *Psychology, Public Policy, and Law, 6,* 434–451.

Michael, S. T., Crowther, M., Schmid, B., & Allen, R. S. (2003). Widowhood and spirituality: Coping responses to bereavement. *Journal of Women and Aging, 15,* 145–165.

Mickley, J. R., Pargament, K. I., Brant, C. R., & Hipp, K. M. (1998). God and the search for meaning among hospice caregivers. *Hospice Journal, 13,* 1–17.

Omnibus Budget Reconciliation Act. Pub. L. No. 101-508, §§ 4206, 4751 (codified in 42 U.S.C., 1395cc(f) [Medicare] and 1396a(w) [Medicaid]) (1990).

Owen, J. E., Goode, K. T., & Haley, W. E. (2001). End-of-life care and reactions to death in African-American and White family caregivers of relatives with Alzheimer's disease. *Omega, 43*, 349–361.

Pargament, K. I. (1997). *The psychology of religion and coping: Theory, research, practice.* New York: Guilford Press.

Pearlin, L. I., Mullan, J. T., Semple, S. J., & Skaff, M. M. (1990). Caregiving and the stress process: An overview of concepts and their measures. *Gerontologist, 30*, 583–591.

Phipps, E., True, G., Harris, D., Chong, U., Tester, W., Chavin, S. I., et al. (2003). Approaching the end of life: Attitudes, preferences, and behaviors of African-American and White patients and their family caregivers. *Journal of Clinical Oncology, 21*, 549–554.

Picot, S. J., Debanne, S. M., Namazi, K. H., & Wykle, M. L. (1997). Religiosity and perceived rewards of Black and White caregivers. *Gerontologist, 37*, 89–101.

Pinquart, M., & Sörensen, S. (2003). Differences between caregivers and noncaregivers in psychological health and physical health: A meta-analysis. *Psychology and Aging, 18*, 250–267.

Rabins, P. V., Fitting, M. D., Eastham, J., & Zabora, J. (1990). Emotional adaptation over time in care-givers for chronically ill elderly people. *Age and Ageing, 19*, 185–190.

Roff, L. L., Burgio, L. D., Gitlin, L., Nichols, L., Chaplin, W., & Hardin, J. M. (2004). Positive aspects of Alzheimer's caregiving: The role of race. *Journal of Gerontology: Psychological Sciences, 59B*, P185–P190.

Rosnick, C. B., & Reynolds, S. L. (2003). Thinking ahead: Factors associated with executing advance directives. *Journal of Aging and Health, 15*, 409–429.

Schulz, R., & Beach, S. R. (1999). Caregiving as a risk factor for mortality: The Caregiver Health Effects Study. *Journal of the American Medical Association, 282*, 2215–2219.

Schulz, R., Beach, S. R., Lind, B., Martire, L. M., Zdaniuk, B., Hirsch, C., et al. (2001). Involvement in caregiving and adjustment to death of a spouse: Findings from the caregiver health effects study. *Journal of the American Medical Association, 285*, 3123–3129.

Schulz, R., Gallagher-Thompson, D., Haley, W. E., & Czaja, S. (2000). Understanding the interventions process: A theoretical/conceptual framework for intervention approaches to caregiving. In R. Schulz (Ed.), *Handbook on dementia caregiving* (pp. 33–60). New York: Springer Publishing Company.

Schulz, R., Mendelsohn, A. B., Haley, W. E., Mahoney, D., Allen, R. S., Zhang, S., et al. (2003). End of life care and the effects of bereavement among family caregivers of persons with dementia. *New England Journal of Medicine, 349*, 1936–1942.

Schulz, R., Newsom, J. T., Fleissner, K., DeCamp, A. R., & Nieboer, A. P. (1997). The effects of bereavement after family caregiving. *Aging and Mental Health, 1*, 269–282.

Shah, A. A., Snow, A. L., & Kunik, M. E. (2001). Spiritual and religions coping in caregivers of patients with Alzheimer's disease. *Clinical Gerontologist, 24*, 127–136.

Shahabi, L., Powell, L. H., Musick, M. A., Pargament, K. I., Thoresen, C. E., Williams, D., et al. (2002). Correlates of self-perceptions of spirituality in American adults. *Annals of Behavioral Medicine, 24*, 59–68.

Shewchcuk, T. R. (1998). Completing advance directives for health care decisions: Getting to yes. *Psychology, Public Policy, and Law, 4*, 703–718.

Smith, A. L., & Harkness, J. (2002). Spirituality and meaning: A qualitative inquiry with caregivers of Alzheimer's disease. *Journal of Family Psychotherapy, 13*, 87–108.

Suhl, J., Simons, P., Reedy, T., & Garrick, T. (1994). Myth of substituted judgment. Surrogate decision making regarding life support is unreliable. *Archives of Internal Medicine, 154*, 90–96.

Sulmasy, D. P., Terry, P. B., Weisman, C. S., Miller, D. J., Stallings, R. Y., Vettese, M. A., et al. (1998). The accuracy of substituted judgments in patients with terminal diagnoses. *Annals of Internal Medicine, 128*, 621–629.

Teno, J. M., Stevens, M., Spernak, S., & Lynn, J. (1998). Role of written advance directives in decision making: Insights from qualitative and quantitative data. *Journal of General Internal Medicine, 13*, 439–446.

Utz, R. L., Carr, D., Nesse, R., & Wortman, C. B. (2002). The effect of widowhood on older adults' social participation: An evaluation of activity, disengagement, and continuity theories. *Gerontologist, 42*, 522–533.

Weggel, J. M. (1999). Barriers to the physician's decision to offer hospice as an option for terminal care. *Wisconsin Medical Journal, 98*, 49–53.

Working Group on Assisted Suicide and End-of-Life Decisions. (2000). *Report to the Board of Directors.* Washington, DC: American Psychological Association.

Wykle, M. L., & Segal, M. (1991). A comparison of Black and White family caregivers' experiences with dementia. *Journal of the National Black Nurses Association, 5*, 29–41.

Zuckerman, C., & Wollner, D. (1999). End of life care and decision making: How far we have come, how far we have to go. *Hospice Journal, 14*, 85–107.

Zweibel, N. R., & Cassel, C. K. (1989). Treatment choices at the end of life: A comparison of decisions by older patients and their physician-selected proxies. *Gerontologist, 29*, 615–621.

9

INVOLVEMENT OF PSYCHOLOGISTS IN PSYCHOSOCIAL ASPECTS OF HOSPICE AND END-OF-LIFE CARE

STEPHEN R. CONNOR, JEFFREY LYCAN,
AND J. DONALD SCHUMACHER

Patients and families dealing with the reality of a life-threatening illness undergo one of life's most difficult emotional passages. As a result, psychological services can be valuable if provided in a manner that is in concert with expressed needs. The provision of such services to patients and families in hospice is the responsibility of an interdisciplinary team. These services have been delivered primarily by social workers who have been better prepared than psychologists to deliver multifaceted care in a community-based setting.

Yet a small number of psychologists have played an important role in the development of hospice care in the United States. These pioneers were willing to leave their offices and provide support in unconventional ways to dying patients and their families. These individuals have unfortunately been few and far between as hospice care has developed from a small grassroots movement to a multi-billion-dollar health care service over the past 25 years.

For psychologists to play a prominent role in end-of-life and hospice care, they will need to demonstrate expertise and flexibility in providing services. For example, a psychotherapist described visiting a hospice patient who said to her, "I don't need a therapist, why are you here?" She responded, "You probably don't need a psychotherapist, but I think you might want to talk with someone who has helped people with what you're going through a few hundred times." With that, the patient invited her in.

In this chapter, we inform the reader about the development of hospice care in the United States including its history, principles of care, common characteristics, services, and coverage. Then we address the challenges facing psychologists in this field, including theoretical and philosophical differences, lack of educational preparation, financial issues, and practical concerns. Finally, the chapter highlights opportunities for psychologists working with hospices including consultative services, direct patient and family care delivery, and grief counseling.

HISTORY OF HOSPICE CARE[1]

Hospice, often described as the gold standard for end-of-life care, is a model for individuals desiring to achieve a "good death." A holistic approach to care and a view of the patient and family as a unit are strengths of this model. The meaning of the word *hospice* can be traced back to the Latin word *hospitium* meaning "hospitality," and the French word *hospis*, meaning host, which forms the root for words such as *hospitality*, *hospital*, *hotel*, and *hospice*. The concept of hospice care can be traced as far back as fourth-century AD Rome.

More recently, Dame Cicely Saunders, a London physician, is credited with the development of the modern hospice movement. In 1963, Saunders introduced the idea of specialized care for the dying to the United States during a visit to Yale University. Saunders and Florence Wald, dean of the Yale School of Nursing, worked throughout the mid to late 1960s sharing experiences and developing programs that would become the foundation of the hospice philosophy in the United States. Another significant contributor during this time, Elisabeth Kübler-Ross (1969), wrote *On Death and Dying*, which proposed stages of dying. Perhaps more important, she identified three key issues:

1. All who are coping with dying are still alive and have unfinished needs that they may want to address.
2. We cannot be or become effective providers of care unless we listen actively to those who are coping with dying and identify with their needs.

---

[1]Much of the material in this section is adapted from the National Hospice and Palliative Care Organization's (NHPCO) "History of Hospice Care," which can be found at http://www.nhpco.org/i4a/pages/index.cfm?pageid=3285.

3. We need to learn from those who are dying and coping with dying to come to know ourselves better and to recognize the potential for living.

The first hospice program in the United States was established in New Haven, Connecticut, in 1971. The U.S. Department of Health, Education and Welfare described hospice as a model of humane care for terminally ill people that reduced cost and should receive consideration for federal support (Paradis, 1985). Demonstration projects were subsequently initiated at 26 hospices to assess cost-effectiveness of hospice care and determine what care a hospice should provide (Connor, 1998).

The 1980s brought major achievements in the form of financial support as Congress created a Medicare Hospice Benefit (Tax Equity and Fiscal Responsibility Act, 1982) and later made that support permanent. States also had the option of including hospice in their state Medicaid programs beginning in 1985, and hospice care became available to terminally ill nursing home residents (Omnibus Budget and Reconciliation Act [OBRA], 1985). Low payment rates initially kept hospices from seeking Medicare reimbursement; however, in the late 1980s Congress gave hospices a 20% increase in reimbursement and tied future increases to the hospital market basket index (OBRA, 1987). Finally, the Joint Commission on Accreditation of Healthcare Organizations initiated the first hospice accreditation program.

The growth of hospice continued into the 1990s beginning with the inclusion of hospice care in the Veteran's Benefit Package. The Civilian Health and Medical Program of the Uniformed Services (CHAMPUS) Hospice Benefit was implemented, and the hospice philosophy and services were becoming more accepted as part of the health care continuum.

The nineties also brought increased oversight, however, as the hospice community was placed under the scrutiny of "focused medical review." This came as a wake-up call to either improve documentation and certification procedures or be denied payment. The U.S. Office of the Inspector General announced that Operation Restore Trust would expand efforts to fight waste and abuse in Medicare and Medicaid to include hospice in five states (Office of the Inspector General, 1997). Later, Operation Restore Trust was expanded to include hospice in all 50 states. Operation Restore Trust eventually released a report on hospice that stated, "Overall, the Medicare hospice program seems to be working as intended."

Hospice entered the new century with a renewed sense of energy in the growing and developing end-of-life care movement. A 5% across-the-board rate increase was approved by Congress, and the U.S. Department of Health and Human Services released a report conducted as part of the Assistant Secretary for Planning and Evaluation study (ASPE; Gage, Miller, Mor, Jackson, & Harvell, 2000) outlining the significant contributions and cost savings created by using hospice care for terminally ill nursing home residents.

In addition, a Brown University study was released that supported the ASPE study results (Miller, Gozalo, & Mor, 2000).

Furthermore, Milliman USA published a national study reviewing the costs of hospice care and an actuarial evaluation of the Medicare Hospice Benefit (Cheung, Fitch, & Pyenson, 2001). The study supported the cost-effectiveness of hospice but raised the concern that inadequate reimbursement for hospice services would threaten the availability and quality of hospice care. More recently, a study published by Milliman USA concluded that hospices save Medicaid more than $282 million annually, approximately $7,000 per hospice beneficiary (Fitch & Pyenson, 2003). In addition, a study of patients with the most common terminal diagnoses found that most cohorts studied cost Medicare less and that as a group hospice patients actually showed longer survival (Pyenson, Connor, Fitch, & Kinzbrunner, 2004; however, see Campbell, Lynn, Lewis, & Shugarman, 2004).

In 2003, hospice care in the United States was being delivered from about 3,300 locations to approximately 950,000 patients and their families (National Hospice and Palliative Care Organization [NHPCO], 2004). Only half these patients were diagnosed with malignancies. The other half had diagnoses that included heart failure, obstructive lung disease, dementia, stroke, HIV/AIDS, or liver or kidney disease. The average length of service for a hospice patient in the United States in 2003 was 55 days, even though the benefit extends for 6 months (or more). As many as 7 of every 10 persons may be expected to need hospice and currently nearly 3 of 10 receive hospice care.

PRINCIPLES OF CARE AND COMMON CHARACTERISTICS

Hospice treats the whole person, addressing not only the physical needs of an individual, but also the psychosocial, spiritual, and emotional needs, by creating an environment that supports terminally ill individuals and their ability to live life to its fullest as they prepare for death (Beresford, 1993; Connor, 1998; Lattanzi-Licht, Mahoney, & Miller, 1998; Stoddard, 1992). The patient and family are considered to be the unit of care, and care planning is coordinated around their needs. The required interdisciplinary team, which includes a physician, registered nurse, social worker, and a counselor, work with other health care providers (often including chaplains, home health aides, volunteers, and therapists) to implement the plan of care collaboratively. The patient's attending physician often works together with the hospice team and orders all the care needs for the patient, while the hospice medical director oversees the care of all patients and supplements the services of the attending physicians.

Dying is an important part of life. Understanding this helps patients and families deal with the overwhelming burdens and movement from the crises that often precede death. In mainstream healthcare, dying is treated in a manner where individuals often make this journey in emotional and spiritual isolation. The goal of hospice is ultimately to help individuals meet end-of-life goals and desires in a comfortable and pain-free environment of their choosing.

Comfort care and symptom management are the focus of efforts to help patients and families obtain relief from the suffering and burdens of illness. Offering emotional, psychosocial, and spiritual support to the patient and family is imbedded in the philosophy of hospice. This differs from traditional health care that often continues curative therapies even when there is no longer a benefit provided (see also Kaut, chap. 5).

THE SERVICES

Today, 97% of hospices are Medicare certified (NHPCO, 2004) and must follow the Medicare Hospice Conditions of Participation (COPs; Centers for Medicare and Medicaid Services, 1994). The COPs and the National Hospice and Palliative Care Organization's Standards of Practice for Hospice Programs (NHPCO, 2000) define a basic level of services that a patient and family can expect to receive. In the hospice model, all team members' input has equal value. Team members provide perspectives on the care assessment, review, evaluation, and planning, depending on the issues, concerns, and goals of care. Hospice care is coordinated by a registered nurse who "case manages" with team members to implement symptom management, coordination of care, education, preparation, and support to the patient and family. This section highlights how services are provided to meet patient and family needs.

Counseling

Death has a profound psychological impact on the patient and family. Hospice staff will provide in-depth guidance, advice, and help in planning interventions for patients and families to address issues of ineffective coping. Counseling in hospice most often is associated with the team's social worker but is spread across the interdisciplinary team. Social workers focus on these needs by acting as the primary emotional support person, functioning as both counselor and guide through the dying process. Social workers also arrange community resources and provide support when difficult decisions regarding treatment choices, life support, and funeral and estate planning must be made. They also work with the patient and family to help resolve differing perspectives about needed care and wishes of the patient.

Spiritual Care and Bereavement Services

Spiritual care and bereavement services support the dying patient and family as the many issues surrounding death and dying, such as grief and loss, are sorted out. How meaning of life and transcendence are dealt with can significantly affect the response of all involved before death as well as the lives of the family following the patient's death. Spiritual care is much broader than just religious concerns and may extend into different philosophical or existential meanings surrounding life (see also Kaut, chap. 5). In fact, bereavement services are offered to families for at least 12 months following the death of their loved one in hospice care. Grief and supportive counseling begin before death in a variety of ways with group and individual sessions and written and verbal communications. The benefits of these services were supported in a recent study by Christakis and Iwashyna (2003), who found that widowed persons whose spouses were cared for in hospice were less likely to die in the year following death than those who were not cared for by hospice. Notably, hospice bereavement care, although required by Medicare Hospice regulation, is not a reimbursable service under Medicare and frequently is covered by charitable donations. Finally, hospices will also often offer grief and supportive counseling to the community at large.

Home Health Care

Home health aides are a critical component of the hospice team, providing personal services associated with activities of daily living, such as bathing, grooming, and positioning for patients too ill to complete this task. Aides also participate at times in some light housekeeping duties, chores, and errands, often spending more time with the patient and family than other team members and developing close bonds.

Supplemental Therapies

Hospices provide additional therapies (e.g., physical therapy) as needed to meet the patient's plan of care and goals of care that may help keep the patient at home, provide symptom relief, maintain strength, or assist with activities of daily living or other basic needs. Programs review the benefits and risks of providing these services carefully, considering the dying patient's control and dignity needs.

Volunteer Services

Volunteers founded hospice in the United States and are an integral part of the hospice care team; they play vital roles in helping people facing death. Volunteers work out of human concern, with an understanding of the hardships facing families dealing with these difficult situations and provide community links for the patient, family, and hospice. They spend time with the dying person, provide respite for the caregiver, run errands, conduct bereavement follow-up, provide practical assistance, and often become an important friend to the patient and family. Volunteers receive extensive training in working with dying patients and handling family interactions. Volunteers also help maintain hospice as a community service rather than just another health care provider; in 2003, volunteers provided 5% of all clinical staff hours.

COVERAGE

Before 1983, few insurers covered the cost of hospice care. In 1982, Congress added hospice to the Medicare program and since then Medicare has become the primary payer of services for hospice care, covering 80% of all hospice services provided in the United States (NHPCO, 2004). To be eligible for the hospice benefit, the beneficiary must be considered terminally ill with a prognosis of 6 months or less if the disease runs its normal course. The patient's attending physician and the hospice medical director must agree on the prognosis of the patient and certify the patient as being terminally ill; however, the patient may continue to receive hospice care longer than 6 months as long as she or he remains in a condition considered terminal.

Medicare will cover four levels of care: routine home care, respite care, continuous home care, and general inpatient care. Ninety-five percent of all hospice care provided is for routine home care (NHPCO, 2004), the benefit provided for the patient in a home setting (either a traditional family residence, nursing home, or assisted living facility). Respite care occurs when a patient is admitted to an inpatient unit for the purpose of giving the patient's caregiver up to 5 days of rest. Continuous home care is provided during times of crisis, and hospice can provide from 8 to 24 hours of mostly skilled care to bring symptoms under control and maintain the patient in his or her home setting instead of being transferred to an acute setting. The last level of care is general inpatient care, provided in a more acute environment, and is for the active management of uncontrolled symptoms and pain.

It is important for the beneficiary to understand all the additional services the Hospice Medicare Benefit provides compared with routine Medicare benefits. For the most part, hospice is covered in full, and individual financial resources can go toward other needs. A patient choosing the Medicare hospice benefit will receive all necessary care related to the terminal illness and can revoke the hospice benefit at any time. The benefit not only provides the patient with an interdisciplinary team of caregivers but also covers medications, durable medical equipment, and supplies needed to care for the patient through his or her terminal illness.

CHALLENGES FOR PSYCHOLOGY AND PSYCHOLOGISTS

Theoretical and Philosophical

The field of psychology includes a diverse collection of theoretical orientations and philosophies. Some of these approaches are useful in working with people who are dying and their families, and others are less so. In general, psychoanalytic and other long-term approaches to diagnosis and treatment are less appropriate for this population. Also, more strict behavioral approaches do not address the complex meaning-making inherent near the end of life.

The underpinnings of the hospice approach can be found in the philosophy of humanism. In essence, the belief is that all individuals have a right to determine how they want to be treated when facing a terminal illness. Dying persons will also use different coping strategies when facing the reality of impending death. Some will choose to avoid the reality of their condition, and others will seek to cope through mastery of all the facts of their situation. Hospice professionals seek to understand each person and to support his or her unique decisions about treatment and preferred style of coping in concert with how she or he has lived her or his life.

The notion of unconditional positive regard for the dying and their families and a focus on helping them to achieve as much actualization as desired arises out of concerns that dying patients in the parts of the health care system operating from the traditional medical treatment model are treated as impersonal objects with little to say about their care (Connor, 1998). The time of dying is a special period in the life cycle in which all individuals have a right to be treated with dignity and acceptance.

Hospice philosophy also values a family systems perspective. Patients are usually cared for by family members, and they make decisions about care in the context of their family, which is defined by emotional attachments more than by blood relationships. Some of the most important psychological tasks near the end of life involve resolution of relationships with significant people. Therefore, it is helpful to understand the patient's relational world because family of origin dynamics often determine how the person organizes the end-of-life experience.

For those who are able to face the reality of their impending death, the focus of remaining life often orients around a search for personal meaning. An understanding of the existential issues inherent in the dying experience is helpful. For example, Frankl's (1984) work on logotherapy and Yalom's (1980) work have been found to be useful (Greenstein & Breitbart, 2000).

Also, more recently, constructivist psychotherapy has been found to be helpful in assisting those seeking completion of their personal life narrative (Neimeyer & Mahoney, 1999).

In addition, because the dying process involves experiencing many losses leading up to personal death, therapists must have a clear understanding of loss and grief theory and practice (e.g., Rando, 2000; Worden, 2001). Current understanding of the research and its implications for clinical practice are summarized by Stroebe, Hansson, Stroebe, and Schut (2001).

Educational

Professional education in psychology does not necessarily prepare a psychologist clinically or personally for the kind of services needed in the hospice care setting (Working Group on Assisted Suicide and End-of-Life Decisions, 2000). There is little training in grief, mourning, and loss issues unless one chooses to pursue this area of specialization. Even with this area as a chosen specialty, finding appropriate training sites and supervision can be difficult. Few, if any, American Psychological Association-accredited training programs that focus on end-of-life care are available in the United States. As an example of the limitations in standard training, consider that many therapists believe the work of Elizabeth Kübler-Ross (1969) and the five stages of grieving she proposed is the most up-to-date way of understanding the dying and bereaved. In fact, the field of thanantology has much more recent research and training methods available, such as Rando's work on anticipatory mourning (Rando, 2000) and both Corr's and Worden's work on the tasks of grieving (Corr, Nabe, & Corr, 2002; Worden, 2001).

A prerequisite that is necessary but often not addressed is the need for the clinician to be aware of the many countertransference issues that arise in working with dying people (Katz & Genevay, 2002). Perhaps no other population confronts the psychologist with as common an experience. Death, after all, will also be the psychologist's end. It is a matter of bold fact that the therapist must be in touch with his or her own concerns about the process of dying before he or she walks in the room of a patient who will present such a confrontational mirror.

Financial

The use of psychologists in hospice care is limited by the current reimbursement system (Haley, Larson, Kasl-Godley, Neimeyer, & Kwilosz, 2003). Hospice providers are paid a set per diem rate for each day a patient is enrolled in hospice. All services delivered to a patient must be paid for out of this allotment. Core hospice services, which include the services of hospice physicians, nurses, social workers, and counselors (pastoral and dietary counselors are the ones specified), must be delivered by hospice employees. The services of psychologists are not mandated, and most counseling services can be provided by social workers who are already mandated. The hospice therefore has a disincentive to hire and pay a psychologist as a part of the core interdisciplinary team. As a result, services of psychologists have been viewed as an add-on or luxury item for financially pressed hospices.

All physicians are paid separately from the hospice's per diem payment. Therefore, the services of psychiatrists do not have the same payment disincentive as psychologists' services. Under Medicare, attending physicians bill Part B for their services. For all other consulting physicians, the hospice is permitted to pay for the care and can recover these costs through by billing Medicare separately from the per diem. This payment arrangement is not currently available for psychologists.

A psychologist who accepts Medicare Part B assignment and is treating a patient who enrolls in the Medicare Hospice Benefit may continue to treat and bill for that person if the condition he or she is treating is unrelated to the patient's terminal illness. Likewise, a patient may be referred to a psychologist for the treatment of a preexisting condition unrelated to the terminal illness outside the hospice benefit. Anecdotal reports, however, suggest that payment may be jeopardized for the psychologist because of assumptions that all psychological problems relate to the patient's terminal condition.

Practical

Psychologists are accustomed to clients who come to their offices and are motivated to receive psychological services. Hospice patients and families may be under psychological duress but may not identify themselves as needing services. They may react negatively to the suggestion that a psychologist could be helpful in coping with serious physical illness; however, health psychology is now playing a much more active role in the care of the medically ill, and therefore psychological care may be seen as more acceptable in the coming years.

Hospice patients are almost all too sick to come to clinic appointments. Any psychologists who wish to offer services to hospice patients must be prepared to provide the majority of their services to debilitated patients in home, nursing facility, assisted living facility, or hospital settings. These services will most often be provided on a short-term basis. As a result of all these issues, there is little room for the 50-minute hour in hospice practice.

OPPORTUNITIES

Consultative Services

Many of the psychologists who have been involved in hospice care have done so as consultants to the hospice program or team (Haley et al., 2003).

Having a psychologist at hospice weekly team meetings to discuss care planning and to be available for difficult cases can be a helpful resource in the care of dying patients and their families. Hospice personnel have been known to provide a "one size fits all" approach to psychosocial intervention. Supportive counseling usually means providing active listening and accurate empathy, which may not be enough for some people. Some patients experience serious psychological reactions in the time leading up to death, and hospice cares for many dysfunctional families, where more psychological expertise is needed.

Interventions should be targeted to meet patient and family needs and conditions. A competent psychologist can help to assess and inform hospice personnel about optimal treatment strategies and can be available to intervene in some of the more difficult cases. In fact, hospices can greatly benefit from the emerging depth of knowledge psychologists regarding the care of dying patients and their families (Haley et al., 2003; see also Kaut, chap. 5; Gibson, Breitbart, Tomarken, Kosinski, & Nelson, chap. 6; and Rosenfeld, Abbey, & Pessin, chap. 7).

Psychologists with competency in organizational development can also assist hospice programs in their own organizational health and growth. Hospices are undergoing enormous growth nationally. Increasing size necessitates new organizational structures and can be a painful process for groups of people who are comfortable with a smaller organizational dynamics where everyone knows everyone.

Hospice workers are some of the most compassionate and caring people in the health care system. Some also may have personal needs that can get in the way of healthy group dynamics and patient care. There are ways of reinventing organizations that are growing so that a sense of caring community can continue on a larger scale. If done carefully, with an ongoing sense of mission, hospices can avoid some of the problems inherent in growth. Managing these growth changes can be facilitated by a skilled organizational consultant who understands the challenges of organizational change.

Direct Patient Care Delivery

A psychologist interested in working collaboratively with a community hospice program can be successful, provided he or she can gain the respect of the hospice team (Haley et al., 2003). Many hospice workers began as volunteers who devoted their own time to helping meet the needs of dying patients. Demonstrating competency to the hospice team may mean offering to provide pro bono services for hospice patients and families. Psychologists could do this by offering to facilitate a bereavement support group for hospice family members. On the other hand, some hospices work with therapists to provide counseling on a sliding scale basis or a fixed low fee. Probably the most effective contribution would be a willingness to accompany a hospice worker on a home visit to a difficult patient or family and then demonstrate competency by helping to manage the problem the team is trying to address.

Hospices are particularly cautious about who cares for their patients and families. They would not want to introduce a professional in the home setting, even as a volunteer, without a strong belief that the person was competent to provide beneficial assistance. Thus, another way to demonstrate usefulness is to provide in-service training for the hospice staff on a topic relevant to care of the dying. Eventually, as the hospice team comes to appreciate the skills and contributions of a particular psychologist, it is more likely that his or her services would be used.

The goal of psychological therapy with a dying patient is not to uncover pathology or effect personality change but to seek closure and to remove barriers to effective coping (Shneidman, 1978). Uncovering unresolved issues with a patient who will not have the opportunity to work such issues through to resolution is unethical and not therapeutic. Near the end of life, the task at hand is to achieve self-determined life completion or closure (National Hospice Organization, Standards and Accreditation Committee, 1997). Not all dying patients will have the desire or ability to participate in this type of therapeutic activity. In fact, any long-term therapy with dying patients is a rarity, and, for the vast majority, it is contraindicated.

In addition, patients are not the only ones who may need psychological services in the hospice context. In many respects, family members are more in need of support (see also Allen, Haley, Roff, Schmid, & Bergman, chap. 8). Where reasonable and necessary, referral of family members to a psychologist for outpatient or in-home therapy during the patient's dying process may be appropriate and does not conflict with hospice claims billing.

After-Death Grief Counseling

Probably the largest need for psychologists working with hospices is in the care of family members who are having a difficult period of mourning. The great majority of family members cope well, with minimal need for intervention after a death (Haley et al., 2003). It can be expected, however, that a not insignificant percentage of hospice families will have problems adjusting during the bereavement period. Some experience a difficult adjustment and need more support than they can find through their own networks. Others may have severe grief symptoms, major affective disorders, or even pose a danger to themselves.

Psychotherapeutic services for these bereaved family members is underused and would be beneficial through reducing morbidity, mortality, and lost work time. The same issues apply here as those discussed earlier in that hospice personnel will be more inclined to make referrals for family members who need more than is provided through hospice bereavement education and support to clinicians whom they know to be skilled and competent in managing problems associated with grief, mourning, and loss.

RECOMMENDATIONS

Psychologists interested in end-of-life care will want to develop relationships with hospice providers in their communities. Hospices are increasingly providing care to a wide spectrum of individuals with life-threatening illnesses. Collaboration with hospices must entail a willingness to provide targeted services and an ability to demonstrate competence in the understanding and treatment of those experiencing grief and mourning.

Understanding the philosophical underpinnings and practical realities of care for dying people in the home setting is necessary, along with knowledge of how hospice care operates and the ability to be flexible in delivering services where they are needed. For the psychologist who is motivated to meet the needs of this population and the hospices that serve them, there are many opportunities for consultative services, individual and group therapy, organizational development assistance, and after-death grief therapy. This is also a field that can be personally rewarding to a therapist who is interested in life's meaning and in serving a population with great needs.

REFERENCES

Beresford, L. (1993). *The hospice handbook: A complete guide.* Boston: Little, Brown.

Campbell, D. E., Lynn, J., Louis, T. A., & Shugarman, L. R. (2004). Medicare program expenditures associated with hospice use. *Annals of Internal Medicine, 140,* 267–277.

Centers for Medicare and Medicaid Services. (1994). *Hospice conditions of participation (COPs).* Retrieved October 4, 2003, from http://www.access.gpo.gov/nara/cfr/waisidx_01/42cfr418_01.html

Cheung, L., Fitch, K., & Pyenson, B. (2001) *The cost of hospice care: An actuarial evaluation of the Medicare Hospice Benefit.* New York: Milliman. Retrieved October 4, 2003, from http://www.nhpco.org/files/public/TheCostsofHospiceCare.pdf

Christakis, N. A., & Iwashyna, T. J. (2003). The health impact of health care on families: A matched cohort study of hospice use by decedents and mortality outcomes in surviving widowed spouses. *Social Science and Medicine, 57,* 465–475.

Connor, S. R. (1998). *Hospice: Practice, pitfalls, and promise.* Philadelphia: Taylor & Francis.

Corr, C. A., Nabe, C. M., & Corr, D. (2002). *Death and dying, life and living.* Belmont, CA: Wadsworth.

Fitch, K., & Pyenson, B. (2003). *Value of hospice benefit to Medicaid programs.* Retrieved October 4, 2003, from http://www.nhpco.org/files/public/Milliman_Medicaid_Report.pdf

Frankl, V. E. (1984). *Man's search for meaning.* New York: Simon & Schuster.

Greenstein, M., & Breitbart, W. (2000). Cancer and the experience of meaning: A group psychotherapy program for people with cancer. *American Journal of Psychotherapy, 54,* 486–500.

Gage, B., Miller, S., Mor, V., Jackson, B., & Harvell, J. (2000). *Synthesis and analysis of Medicare's hospice benefit: Executive summary and recommendations.* Retrieved October 4, 2003, from http://aspe.hhs.gov/daltcp/reports/samhbes.htm

Haley, W. E., Larson, D. G., Kasl-Godley, J., Neimeyer, R. A., & Kwilosz, D. M. (2003). Roles for psychologists in end-of-life care: Emerging models of practice. *Professional Psychology: Research and Practice, 34,* 626–633.

Katz, R. S., & Genevay, B. (2002). Our patients, our families, ourselves: The impact of the professional's emotional responses on end-of-life care. *American Behavioral Scientist, 46,* 327–339.

Kübler-Ross, E. (1969). *On death and dying.* New York: Macmillan.

Lattanzi-Licht, M., Mahoney, J. J., & Miller, G. (1998). *The hospice choice: In pursuit of a peaceful death.* New York: Fireside.

Miller, S. S., Gozalo, P., & Mor, V. (2000). *Use of Medicare's hospice benefit by nursing facility residents.* Retrieved October 4, 2003, from http://aspe.hhs.gov/daltcp/reports/nufares.htm

National Hospice Organization, Standards and Accreditation Committee. (1997). *A pathway for patients and families facing terminal illness.* Alexandria, VA: Author.

National Hospice and Palliative Care Organization. (2000). *Standards of practice for hospice programs.* Alexandria, VA: Author.

National Hospice and Palliative Care Organization. (2004). *NHPCO facts and figures.* Retrieved September 21, 2004, from http://www.nhpco.org/i4a/pages/index.cfm?pageid=3362

Neimeyer, R. A., & Mahoney, M. (1999). *Constructivism in psychotherapy.* Washington, DC: American Psychological Association.

Office of Inspector General. (1997, January). *Operation Restore Trust review of hospice eligibility at the Visiting Nurse Association of Texas* (DHHS: Report No. A-06-96-00027). Washington, DC: Department of Health and Human Services.

Omnibus Budget Reconciliation Act. Pub. L. No. 99-272 (1985).

Omnibus Budget Reconciliation Act. Pub. L. No. 100-203 (1987).

Paradis, L. F. (1985). *Hospice handbook: A guide for managers and planners.* New York: Aspen.

Pyenson, B., Connor, S. R., Fitch, K., & Kinzbrunner, B. (2004). Medicare cost in matched and non-hospice cohorts. *Journal of Pain and Symptom Management, 28,* 200–210.

Rando, T. A.(2000). *Clinical dimensions of anticipatory mourning.* Champaign, IL: Research Press.

Shneidman, E. S. (1978). Some aspects of psychotherapy with dying persons. In C. A. Garfield (Ed.), *Psychosocial care of the dying patient* (pp. 202–218). New York: McGraw-Hill.

Stoddard, S. (1992). *The hospice movement: A better way of caring for the dying* (rev. ed.). New York: Vintage Books.

Stroebe, M. S., Hansson, R. O., Stroebe, W., & Schut, H. (2001). *Handbook of bereavement research: Consequences, coping, and care.* Washington, DC: American Psychological Association.

Tax Equity and Fiscal Responsibility Act. Pub. L. No. 97-248 (1982).

Worden, W. J. (2001). *Grief counseling and grief therapy: A handbook for the mental health practitioner* (3rd ed.). New York: Springer.

Working Group on Assisted Suicide and End-of-Life Decisions. (2000). *Report to the Board of Directors.* Washington, DC: American Psychological Association. Retrieved January 25, 2004, from http://www.apa.org/pi/aseolf.html

Yalom, I. D. (1980). *Existential psychotherapy.* New York: Basic Books.

10

RECOMMENDATIONS TO IMPROVE PSYCHOSOCIAL CARE NEAR THE END OF LIFE

DEAN BLEVINS AND JAMES L. WERTH JR.

As noted in every chapter of this volume, there has been tremendous progress in improving end-of-life care in recent decades. These advances in medicine and public health have created a situation in which life of very low quality may be maintained long past the cessation of the human body's natural ability to function—a situation for many that may be what Ditto (chap. 4) and others refer to as a "fate worse than death." Although this point is often made in discussions of self-determination and decision making near the end of life, it has also contributed to a rising concern over the need for personalization of care, responding to more than just the medical and biological aspects of life. There has been growing recognition of the importance of attending to this period of the life span among researchers, care providers, policymakers, and educators; much needs to be done, however, especially in considering the psychosocial issues that arise near the end of life.

This chapter highlights the needs and recommendations that have been discussed by the authors of the preceding chapters, those that crosscut the chapters, and concerns that may arise in the future. These points will be discussed for each of the major stakeholders important to end-of-life care:

educators, researchers, service providers, and policy makers. Prior to these reviews, however, it is important to consider the contributions of the principles and processes of translational or implementation research.

TRANSLATIONAL/IMPLEMENTATION RESEARCH

Translational/implementation research has developed significantly over the past decade as health services researchers and funding agencies have increasingly been explicitly concerned with the characteristics of interventions meant to improve the process and outcomes of health care delivery. In this vein, the Institute of Medicine (IOM; 2001) released a report titled *Crossing the Quality Chasm*, which emphasized the inappropriateness of targeting solely one stakeholder (e.g., providers) to influence health care system change. Any deficiency in care delivery is a systems-level problem and requires attention to various levels of the health care system. In addition to providers, it is important to consider consumers (i.e., patients and family); institutions (e.g., hospitals, hospices, nursing homes); support systems for institutions (e.g., payers such as insurance companies and Medicare); and regulatory factors at the local, state, and federal levels. Thus, as research establishing care practices and standards continues to develop, these must be considered within the entire U.S. health care system. The traditional approach to changing health care delivery has been limited to an overreliance on health care provider education and training, which is only one piece of the puzzle. The 2002 conference on which this book is based considered this interrelationship a critical element of discussing psychosocial issues near the end of life and therefore included the perspectives of every major discipline working in end-of-life care: medicine (especially psychiatry), social work, nursing, and spiritual providers, in addition to psychology. This representation was seen in both the presenters and conference attendees, and consequently across the chapters in this volume. Thus, the recommendations offered through the following sections are grouped by several major themes (i.e., education, research, care provision, and public policy) that concern the major stakeholders with the potential to influence or be affected by future attempts to improve psychosocial care near the end of life.

EDUCATION

Several national efforts have been initiated that are aimed at improving the knowledge of providers on the medical and psychosocial aspects of end-of-life care. Best known are the End of Life Nursing Education Consortium (ELNEC, http://www.aacn.nche.edu/ELNEC) and Education for Physicians in End-of-Life Care (EPEC, http://www.epec.net) programs for nurses and physicians, respectively. The Veterans Administration has also targeted medical providers with the Faculty Leaders Project (Office of Academic Affiliations, 2000), which has included curricula development at 30 sites across the United States. As Kaplan (Foreword, this volume) notes, programs have also been developed for social workers and spiritual–religious providers. Yet as several of this book's contributors note, no national programs have been developed for psychologists (see, e.g., Connor, Lycan, & Schumacher, chap. 9; Werth & Kleespies, chap. 3). Across the established programs, an emphasis has been placed on five areas considered critical for palliative care: (a) respecting patient goals, preferences, and choices; (b) comprehensive caring; (c) utilizing interdisciplinary teams; (d) respecting caregiver concerns; and (e) building systems and mechanisms of support (Last Acts, 1997).

Although there have been improvements in the educational resources available to some groups of providers, most of these materials narrowly target the physical symptoms that arise near the end of life (e.g., Office of Academic Affiliations, 2002). As a result, psychosocial issues receive the least amount of attention, minimizing their importance near the end of life and failing to equip providers with the skills necessary to offer appropriate care. Kaplan (Foreword) notes that attention to death and dying has only recently been included in the majority of medical textbooks, yet even that attention has been limited to a couple of pages at the most. The mental health literature has included several attempts to designate the specific content and issues critical to educating mental health providers (e.g., Werth, 1999; Werth, Gordon, & Johnson 2002; Working Group on Assisted Suicide and End-of-Life Decisions, 2000). For psychologists who provide services in the end-of-life arena, this has ethical implications in the form of professional competence (Werth & Kleespies, chap. 3). To assist providers with building the necessary foundation of knowledge, the preceding chapters have included such topics as advanced care planning, assessment and treatment of mental health issues, the importance of cultural and demographic characteristics, stress and coping, spirituality and existential concerns, the interactions of medical and physical health characteristics, caregiver issues, philosophies and approaches to end-of-life care, ethics, becoming involved in hospice care and on interdisciplinary times, and numerous others. An important point several of the contributors emphasized is that although these issues may be relevant to nonterminal people, they often require unique application for those facing the end of life. Thus, it is critical that any educational program build on existing knowledge while integrating new, specific information.

Similar to the EPEC and ELNEC programs, psychology needs to develop a discipline-specific curriculum that includes not only content knowledge, but also material on the current system of health care delivery in the United States, encouraging skills in communication and participation on interdisciplinary teams. It is critical to reemphasize a point made by Werth and Kleespies; Conner, Lycan, and Schumacher; and Kaplan in this volume:

although psychologists have much to offer individuals with terminal illnesses, they need to understand that, as representatives of a profession, they are latecomers to this area. They must learn how to become effective providers in settings and situations that are uncharacteristic of mainstream psychological treatment (see also Working Group on Assisted Suicide and End-of-Life Decisions, 2000).

In summary, education for professionals involved in end-of-life care has improved over the last several decades. Psychology has only recently begun making inroads into the established systems of care. Making further progress and becoming effective team members requires targeted graduate and postgraduate training and experience with people in end-of-life situations. This volume provides a review of a number of major psychosocial issues pertinent near the end of life, citing classic and contemporary resources across the chapters that can serve as an initial list to engage in further exploration of any of the topics discussed, including the development of educational curricula for psychologists aspiring to enhance their end-of-life competence (see also Kleespies, 2004; Rosenfeld, 2004; Working Group on Assisted Suicide and End-of-Life Decisions, 2000).

RESEARCH

An entire volume could be dedicated to the research needed to enhance understanding and the provision of psychosocial care near and at the end of life. Perhaps to a greater extent than the area of education, researchers have been very active in increasing an understanding of the psychosocial needs and the delivery process near the end of life. Much of this has been made possible by generous funding from such organizations as the Robert Wood Johnson Foundation and Open Society Institute and federal agencies such as the Agency for Healthcare Research and Quality (AHRQ) and National Institute for Nursing Research (NINR). All of the preceding chapters have highlighted areas of needed research. This section will summarize areas topically, beginning with broad theoretical and health services research questions and progressing to clinical and basic research issues.

Several contributors emphasized the changing nature of terminal care—that is, the increasing prevalence of chronic illnesses with a potentially terminal prognosis, such as AIDS, organ failure, and Alzheimer's disease. The recognition that individuals and families can benefit significantly from the hospice and palliative care approaches to end-of-life care has also raised questions of the appropriateness of existing care models. Should hospice care look and operate the same for patients in nursing homes or with noncancer diagnoses? As pointed out by Connor and his colleagues, hospice has been shown to improve the quality of life of dying persons and their significant others and reduce the costs associated with end-of-life care by avoiding inappropriate use of hospitalizations and emergency room visits. Nonetheless, there have been rampant difficulties for all stakeholders in such situations. Although the importance of considering the regulatory barriers to providing high-quality end-of-life care will be discussed below under the public policy section, it is appropriate in this section to highlight the need for demonstration projects experimenting with different approaches to providing hospice and palliative care services to the ever-broadening pool of individuals requesting such services (see also Field & Cassel, 1997). Psychologists have a unique opportunity in these projects not only to offer expertise on models of organizational change and collaboration but also to become involved in the delivery of services, becoming active members of care teams.

From a research perspective, it is critical that psychologists become involved on interdisciplinary and collaborative coalitions exploring questions about the delivery of services to people who are terminally ill. This requires working as equal partners with providers from numerous other disciplines, constructing care delivery models that not only address the needs of individuals and their family members but also are feasible and reimbursable given contemporary payers of health care (especially Medicare and Medicaid). This is a very different approach to research than what many research psychologists are accustomed to and requires skills in communication, negotiation, and group dynamics, in addition to an appreciation for the interaction of public health policy and the U.S. health care system as noted earlier.

Another area of research within which psychologists may lend particular expertise is in the development of new and appropriate methods of assessment for service needs near the end of life. The approach discussed by Kaut (chap. 5) is an ideal demonstration of how the unique contexts of care and needs of different individual–family–health care team units may lead to a system of monitoring that minimizes distress near the end of life. The need for improved methods of assessment was a theme that appeared in almost every chapter.

Gibson and colleagues (chap. 6) emphasized that there is much neglect of the psychosocial issues near the end of life. This can partially be attributed to the inexperience and discomfort of many providers, but a significant degree is the consequence of the nonuse and misuse of assessment instruments and approaches to care delivery. Although there have been some attempts to develop instruments that are appropriate for use with people who are terminally ill, a paucity of established methods jointly considers the multitude and complexity of issues near the end of life. Although attempts to develop measures of quality of life and patient and family member satisfaction with care capture a number of subjective areas that will be important to consider for individuals, the assessment of more basic symptom prevalence such as pain, delirium, anxiety, depression, and hopelessness must be further developed. The chapters by Gibson et al. (chap. 6), Rosenfeld et al. (chap. 7), and Allen et al. (chap. 8) each provide direction for such development (for a compendium of existing measures, see the *Toolkit of Measures of End-of-Life Care*: http://www.chcr.brown.edu/pcoc/toolkit.htm).

For example, Rosenfeld, Abbey, and Pessin highlighted the need to consider the differential relationships among depression, hopelessness, and pessimism on methods of coping and adjustment among persons with a terminal illness. A complicating factor in any attempts to do this, however, is that most assessments have been developed among physically healthy populations or people with nonterminal illnesses; thus, there remains the question of their appropriateness for use with those who are terminally ill. Although the use of validated assessment tools can be limited by medical issues near the end of life, the clinical interview approach suggested by Kaut may be an alternative, but the process and components of either form of assessment need to be empirically established.

Ditto provided an excellent review of the empirical literature pertaining to advanced care planning, questioning the wide adoption of such documents as living wills, given the lack of research attesting to their effectiveness at the end of life. The author specifically emphasized the poor agreement on the intended outcomes of advanced care planning, in addition to the lack of evidence demonstrating that they have (as least as they are currently used) resulted in improved treatment for people near the end of life. The assumptions of advance directives (e.g., communication, predicting future treatment desires) have not been validated by research. Thus, a critical task in this area is to determine whether these assumptions can be met and, if so, how current practices should be changed accordingly. Allen and colleagues summarized some of their current research efforts to increase the effectiveness of family communication around advance care planning and other end-of-life issues. In the absence of explorations such as these, it will not be possible to maximize self-determination near the end of life, except for those who retain the ability to make informed decisions for themselves and are equipped to advocate for their treatment preferences.

Parts of Stillion's chapter (chap. 1) and that by Blevins and Papadatou (chap. 2) emphasize the significant lack of knowledge regarding the influence of culture on end-of-life issues, although there is an awareness that cultural issues are important during the dying trajectory. There have been few attempts at transcultural research, with the existing work being limited by the use of convenience samples and varying definitions of the dimensions of culture. Blevins and Papadatou summarize a number of issues in need of theoretical development and future research, including exploration of how culture may influence the experience of dying and the grieving process, questioning existing approaches to understanding dying and death as progressing in stages or tasks to be achieved. Conducting transcultural and culturally sensitive research necessitates ambitious programs that are aimed at overcoming the logistical barriers to communication, cooperation, and conducting research across cultural subgroups. Finally, it is critical for researchers to keep in mind that culture refers to more than just ethnicity. Empirical investigations of age, disability–health status, cohort–generation, gender, spirituality and religion, and sexual orientation have been far and few between.

CARE PROVISION

Consistent with the perspective adopted throughout this volume, the provision of end-of-life care should be interdisciplinary. As Allen et al., Connor et al., Kaplan, and Werth and Kleespies point out, psychologists' roles in this process has been minimal to date. Some of this can be attributed to the lack of training for psychologists to contribute effectively to service delivery. It has also been the situation that the coverage of psychological treatment has been limited by the funding mechanisms for end-of-life care, as Connor and colleagues detail. Several chapter authors also emphasize that the delivery of care related to psychosocial issues among people who are terminally ill is very different from mainstream psychological practice. The combination of these factors, and the frequent barriers to collaboration between psychology and medicine have contributed to the poor inclusion of the expertise we can offer end-of-life care (for potential remedies to this, see, e.g., Connor, Egan, Kwilosz, Larson, & Reese, 2002; Hickman, 2002).

A number of factors have been highlighted across the chapters regarding the areas within which additional competency is required to provide effective care to the dying and their significant others. Developing a national training program as suggested earlier will increase the ability of psychologists to pursue postgraduate education in end-of-life care. The Veterans Administration has the largest program of postdoctoral fellowships in palliative care that is open to participation by clinical and counseling psychologists, which is an additional opportunity to acquire applied experience. It is important that such experiences be encouraged through other venues as well. We are aware of no psychology programs that specialize in training therapists for practice with people who are terminally ill, which is another potential avenue for the field to demonstrate its commitment to providing such care, especially in collaboration with other professionals. Thus, improving the provision of services to those who are terminally ill will require significant attention to graduate and postgraduate educational initiatives that involve the acquisition of content knowledge, the exploration of personal issues that may complicate the provision of care to people who are terminally ill and their loved ones, and applied experiential opportunities.

PUBLIC POLICY

Across all of the preceding discussions are issues that are relevant to public policy. An assumption throughout this section is that policies at the organizational level (e.g., of hospitals, nursing homes, hospices, etc.) are largely reactionary, responding to pressures of health care consumers; market forces; and local, state, and federal regulations requiring attention to the quality of care provided to persons near the end of life. Educational campaigns of providers and administrators of health care organizations on the effectiveness of attending to psychosocial issues may eventually invalidate this assumption, but at present there is a significant need for "top-down" direction to improve end-of-life care. Thus, the influence and importance of federal and state governments on the quality of care and the quality of life for persons with terminal illnesses cannot be overstated.

The single largest influence on improving care near the end of life was the initiation of the Medicare Hospice Benefit. Medicare has become the largest payer of hospice care for the terminally ill. However, the Medicare benefit and the process of utilization review are such that patients with noncancer diagnoses are discouraged from electing this service. Although the Centers for Medicare and Medicaid Services (CMS) through the Department Health and Human Services has clarified regulations over the years to minimize this situation, much work remains to be done (see Blevins & Deason-Howell, 2002, for a review).

Private insurance has often not been the focus of research and lobbying to improve the standards and available care for persons with terminal illnesses for at least three reasons. First, as noted especially in Stillion's chapter, the majority of persons who die are over 65 years of age and therefore eligible for Medicare. However, approximately a quarter of the population dies under the age of 65, and although Medicare covers those dying from renal failure, the remainder will be using private insurance, Medicaid, private funds, or some combination of these. Furthermore, several contributors highlighted how people often avoid the subject of dying and death until it is forced on them. This, in combination with the first point, creates a situation where the largest purchaser of private insurance (i.e., employers) are not motivated to be concerned about end-of-life care: Most working-age adults will not die until after they retire, and most employees, avoiding the subject of death, do not pressure employers to ensure end-of-life coverage in the insurance plans they purchase. As a result, private insurers either have not worked in payment systems that ensure adequate provision of services for the dying or, if they do have end-of-life policies (e.g., a policy mirroring Medicare's), they do not perceive a need to advertise it. Finally, the vast majority of persons with private insurance are under some form of managed care. It has been increasingly popular to criticize managed care companies of limiting access to appropriate care. Thus, private insurers, wishing not to give the appearance of this stereotype, will often not encourage the use of such services as hospice because of the frequent requirement that the enrollee have to agree to not seek further aggressive curative treatment. A significant challenge for the future is for the development of innovative approaches whereby private insurers can be brought into the process of providing end-of-life care similar to the manner in which Medicare has over the last several decades, but people must understand that hospice provides the highest quality end-of-life care if the point comes where curative treatment is no longer going to be effective. This is a place where psychologists, collaborating with members of the public health and medical communities, can enhance the understanding of all parties involved, assisting with educational outreach programs and inclusion of psychosocial issues in national health care quality improvement initiatives such as Healthy People 2010 (see http://www.healthypeople.gov).

Public policy is also critical when considering the appropriations process of Congress (i.e., the allocation of money to research-funding agencies). Agendas set forth by the president and the governmental agencies comprising the executive branch of the federal government can have a significant influence on the priorities for grant monies made available to researchers and providers attempting to understand psychosocial issues near the end of life and to develop and test innovative programs meant to improve the provision of services directly. Thus, the lobbying efforts of organizations such as Last Acts and the American Psychological Association, in addition to individual researchers, are extremely important and necessary in both the legislative and executive branches of government.

Individual policies regarding the provision of care near the end of life extend beyond just how health care is funded through Medicare and how grant funds are allocated. Ditto (chap. 4), in discussing advance directives, did an excellent job illustrating the sometimes poor connection between public policies and empirical evidence. Psychologists have an important opportunity to have an impact on such situations not only by conducting and disseminating more research, but also by collaborating with providers and policymakers to inform the lobbying efforts of others, ensuring appropriate interpretation and use of the published literature.

The legislative process of every state and the federal government is biased in that it is easier and more important to stop bad legislation than it is to pass legislation (good or bad). This characteristic has implications for the necessary perseverance of persons and agencies interested in improving end-of-life care through the political process. The outcomes of the legislative process are subject to many factors, only one of which is empirical knowledge. Others include the influence of powerful interest groups, policymakers' concerns about representing their constituents, and the process whereby laws are interpreted by the agencies that establish how the legislation will be carried out.

In addition, it must be emphasized that policymakers are ultimately concerned about the greatest good for the greatest number of people, not the process through which an individual person is treated. It is because of this difference in perspective between policymakers and providers that many misunderstandings may occur. Psychologists interested in having an impact on public policy need to be able to demonstrate the efficacy and effectiveness of whatever aspect of psychosocial care for which they wish to advocate. This is a critical point for psychologists who are conducting research if one of their motivating factors is influencing public policy. Interdisciplinary research teams will not only improve the quality of such work, they will also expand the available methodological approaches to answer questions that inherently cut across disciplines. Psychologists would be well served to consider the expertise of certain subspecialties within our own discipline (e.g., industrial and organizational psychology, gerontology) and the experience of disciplines that commonly work with large databases and use population-based survey research methods.

SUMMARY

Given the preponderance of literature attesting to the importance of psychosocial issues and their complicated interaction with the physical problems encountered by dying persons and their significant others, there is no doubt of the need for psychologists to become involved in providing care for terminally ill individuals and their loved ones. The purpose of this chapter was to provide an overview of the recommendations discussed by this book's contributors in the areas of education, research, care provision, and public policy. There is a significant need in each of these areas to enhance the ability and opportunities of psychologists if they are to become major players in offering their expertise near the end of life. We have only been able to discuss the highlights of these needs but have attempted to emphasize the recurrent themes across this volume's chapters. It will require a great deal of work, perseverance, and creativity for the discipline to continue to make progress in advancing the field and becoming acknowledged participants in the process of care provision. The direction provided by the participants of the first international conference on attending to psychosocial issues near the end of life, as contained in this volume, can serve as a reference mark from which the field can continue to move forward, maximizing the quality of care available and provided to dying persons and their significant others.

REFERENCES

Blevins, D., & Deason-Howell, L. M. (2002). End-of-life care in nursing homes: The interface of policy, research, and practice. *Behavioral Sciences and the Law, 20*, 271–286.

Connor, S. R., Egan, K. A., Kwilosz, D. M., Larson, D. G., & Reese, D. J. (2002). Interdisciplinary approaches to assisting when end-of-life care and decision-making. *American Behavioral Scientist, 46*, 340–356.

Field, M. J., & Cassel, C. K. (Eds.). (1997). *Approaching death: Improving care at the end of life*. Washington, DC: National Academy Press.

Hickman, S. E. (2002). Improving communication near the end of life. *American Behavioral Scientist, 46*, 252–267.

Institute of Medicine. (2001). *Crossing the quality chasm: A new health system for the 21st century*. Washington, DC: National Academy Press.

Kleespies, P. M. (2004). *Life and death decisions: Psychological and ethical considerations in end-of-life care*. Washington, DC: American Psychological Association.

Last Acts. (1997). *Precepts of palliative care*. Retrieved January 18, 2003, from http://wwwlastacts.org/docs/profprecepts.pdf

Office of Academic Affiliations. (2000, June). *VA Faculty Leaders Project for improved care at the end of life*. Retrieved May 10, 2003, from http://vaww.va.gov/oaa/flp/Compendium/Compendium2000.doc

Office of Academic Affiliations. (2002, February). *Hospice and palliative care services in the Department of Veterans Affairs: A report on the TAPC Project Survey*. Retrieved April 4, 2003, from http://vaww.va.gov/oaa/flp/TAPC_toolkit/TAPC_survey.doc

Rosenfeld, B. (2004). *Assisted suicide and the right to die: The interface of social science, public policy, and medical ethics*. Washington, DC: American Psychological Association.

Werth, J. L., Jr. (1999). When is a mental health professional competent to assess a person's decision to hasten death? *Ethics and Behavior, 9*, 141–157.

Werth, J. L., Jr., Gordon, J. R., & Johnson, R. R., Jr. (2002). Psychosocial issues near the end of life. *Aging and Mental Health, 6*, 402–412.

Working Group on Assisted Suicide and End-of-Life Decisions. (2000). *Report to the Board of Directors*. Washington, DC: American Psychological Association. Retrieved January 25, 2004, from http://www.apa.org/pi/aseolf.html

AUTHOR INDEX

Numbers in italics refer to listings in the reference sections.

Catania, J. A., 38, *48*
Centeno, C., 150, *157*
Center for the Advancement of Health, 32, *48*
Centers for Disease Control and Prevention, 14, 15, *24*
Centers for Medicare and Medicaid Services, *215*
Chabner, B., *84*
Chadwick, S., 175, *178*
Chambless, D. L., 65, *82*
Chang, B., 191, *197*
Chaplin, W., *200*
Chaplin, W. F., *197*
Charles, G., *109*
Chater, S., *182*
Chavin, S. I., *200*
Chen, H., 9, *83*, 185, *198, 199*
Cherny, N. I., 117–121, 124, 126, 127, *132*
Chesney, M., *109*
Chesney, M. A., *48*
Cheung, L., 206, *215*
Childress, J., 58, 67, 69, 73, 74, 77, *81*
Chiodo, L. K., 187, *199*
Chochinov, H. M., 6, 8, *10*, 36, *48*, 60, 66, *82*, 118, 121, 122, 126, 127, 129, 130, *132*, *134*, 138, 141, 146, 148, 151, *157*, *158*, 164–166, 168, 169, 172–174, 176, 177, *179*, *181*, *182*
Chong, U., *200*
Christakis, N. A., *50*, *54*, 68, *82*, 118, 119, 124, 126, 131, *134*, *135*, 208, *215*
Chung, P. M., 45, *53*
Cicirelli, V. G., 38, *48*
Cintron, A., 38, *48*
Clark, D., 38, *48*
Clarke, D. M., 170, *179*
Clarke, O., 77, 78, *82*
Clarkin, J. F., *180*
Clarridge, B. C., *82*
Claus, R. E., 79, *82*
Cleary, P., 77, *81*
Clinton, M., 45, *52*
Clipp, E. C., *54*, 112, 116, 118, 121, 126, 128, 130, *134*, *135*
Cloutier, V. M., *52*
Coates, A., 185, *198*
Coates, T. J., *48*
Cohen, C. B., *51*, *133*
Cohen, M. A., *156*
Cohen, R. D., *179*
Collette, L., *48*

Collier, A. C., *48*
Collins, S., 176, *179*
Comis, R., *159*
Committe on Bioethics, 68, *82*
Conant, K., *160*
Connell, C. M., 184, *198*
Connor, S. R., 7, 8, 62, *82*, 205, 206, 210, *215*, *216*, 225, 228
Conwell, Y., 185, *199*
Cook, M. R., 154, *159*
Cooke, M., 39, *48*
Coombs Lee, B., 72, *82*
Coppola, K. M., 17, *25*, *52*, 100, 103, *107*, *108*, *198*, *199*
Corbett, K. K., *51*
Corcoran, M., 196, *197*
Cornbleet, M., 171, *180*
Cornelison, A. H., 39, *48*
Cornell, J. E., 187, *199*
Corr, C. A., 32, *48*, 211, *215*
Corr, D., 32, *48*, 211, *215*
Cortez, J. D., *53*
Cote, T. R., 146, *158*
Cotter, L., *156*
Cottone, R. R., 79, *82*
Cox, J., 171, *179*
Coyle, N., 117, 120, *132*, 151, 153, *158*
Coyne, P., 9
Crawford, S. L., *49*
Crenner, C., *51*
Crisci, M. T., 38, *52*
Crocker, N., 68, *84*
Crowther, M., 189–191, *197*–*199*
Cruzan v. Director, Missouri Department of Health, 18, *24*, 90, 92, *107*
Crystal, S., *54*
Curnen, M. G. M., 59, *86*
Curtis, J. R., 39, *48*, 116, *134*
Cutcliffe, J. R., 176, *179*
Cuter, F., 145, *158*
Cuttini, M., *53*
Czaja, S., 184, *197*, *200*

Daaleman, T. P., 39, *48*, 131, *133*
Dacko, C., 105, *108*
Daiuto, A., *82*
Danis, M., *52*, 97, 100, *107*, *108*
Danks, J. H., *50*, *52*, 90, 99–101, 103, *107*, *108*, 187, *198*, *199*
Dannenberg, A. L., 146, *158*
Dash, J., 154, *160*
Davidson, J., 167, *182*

Davies, B., 66, 85
Davis, C. G., 191, *198*
Davis, R. B., *48*
de Faye, B. J., 6, *10*, 168, *182*
de Vonderweid, U., *53*
DeAngelis, L. M., *158*
Deason-Howell, L. M., 37, 38, *47*, 226, *228*
Debanne, S. M., 190, *200*
DeCamp, A. R., *200*
Deevey, S., 38, *48*
Del Bene, M., 165, *181*
DeLaine, S. R., 191, *197*
Delattre, J., *158*
Deliens, L., *52*
Delorit, M. A., *83*
Denicoff, K. D., 142, 150, *158*
Depaola, S. J., 38, *49*
Derogatis, L. R., 138, 139, 144, *158*, *159*
Devereux, J., 171, *180*
Diamond, E. L., 187, *198*
Dickens, B. M., *84*
Dickenson, D. L., 39, *49*
Ditto, P. H., *50*, *52*, 90, 94, 97–101, 103–106, *107*, *108*, 186, 187, *198*, *199*
Doka, K. J., *49*
Dominica, F., 32, *49*
Donnelly, J. M., *179*
Douglas, R., 39, *49*
Doukas, D. J., 5, 8, 91, *107*
Dresser, R., 70, 85, 92, 93, *107*, *198*
Driscoll, J., 38, *49*
Druley, J. A., 90, *107*
Dubovsky, S. L., 147, *158*
Duffy, S. A., 39, *50*
Dugan, W., 171, *179*, *181*
Dunn, D. S., 104, *109*
Durham, M. R., 28, *55*, 59, 87

Eastham, J., 189, *200*
Edgerton, S., *179*
Egan, K. A., 8, 62, 82, 225, *228*
Eisemann, M., *53*
Eisendrath, S. J., 174, *178*
Eiser, A. R., *107*
Eliason, G. T., 113, *133*
Ellenberg, L., 154, *160*
Elliott, C., 154, *159*
Elston, M. A., *55*
Emanuel, E. J., 72, 74, 82, 91, *107*, 111–113, 116–119, 121, 123, 124, 127, 128, 130, *133*, 183, 184, 186, 188, *198*

Emanuel, L. L., 74, 82, 91, 97, 104, 105, *107*, *108*, 111–113, 116–119, 121, 124, 127, 128, 130, *133*, 186, 188, *198*
Emmons, C. A., *84*
Endicott, J., 142, *158*, 168, *179*
Eng, C., *49*
Engelberg, R. A., 116, *134*
Enns, M., 60, 82, 138, *158*, 164–166, 169, *179*
Epps, C., Jr., *82*
Epstein, A., 77, *81*
Erbaugh, J., 171, *178*
Erikson, E., 21, *24*
Ersek, M., 39, *49*, 58, *82*
Esteban, A., 39, *49*
Ettelson, L. M., 91, *107*
Evans, A. T., *52*
Evans, S., *49*
Eversole, T., 61, 62, 80, *82*
Everson, S. A., 167, *179*
Exley, C., 119, 122, 129, *133*

Faber-Langendoen, K., *51*, *133*
Fagerlin, A., *52*, 99, 101, *107*, *108*, 187, *198*
Fainsinger, R., 151, *158*
Fairclough, D. L., 82, 121, *133*, 188, *198*
Fallowfield, L., 34, *49*
Farberman, R. K., 4, *8*
Farberow, N. L., 145, *158*
Farrell, K. R., 60, *83*
Farrenkopf, T., 60, 83, *87*
Farrenkopt, T., 6, *9*
Fassanellos, S., 142, *159*
Fatone, A., *134*
Feifel, H., 32, *49*
Fender, M., *47*
Fenn, D. S., 144, *159*
Fernandez, F., 151, 153, *156*, *158*, 175, *179*
Ferrando, S., *49*
Fetting, J., *158*
Field, M. J., 3, 8, 17, *24*, 60, 74, 83, 223, *229*
Fielding, J., 171, *179*
Fielding, R. G., 34, *49*
Fields, J., 103, *109*
Fink, C., 70, *87*
Fins, J. J., 118, 126, *133*
Finucane, T., 75, *83*
Fisher, C. B., 61, *83*
Fisher, S. E., 196, *197*
Fishman, B., *49*
Fitch, K., 206, *215*, *216*

Hanson, J., 150, *157, 175, 178*
Hansson, R. O., 7, *9,* 211, *217*
Haq, C., *52*
Hardin, J. M., *200*
Harkness, J., 191, *201*
Harper, M., 75, *83*
Harris, D., *200*
Harris, R., 100, *107*
Harrold, J., 7, *9*
Hart, G., 45, *52*
Hartwell, N., *160*
Harvath, T. A., *83*
Harvell, J., 205, *216*
Haughey, N., *160*
Haviland, J. S., 167, *182*
Hawkins, N. A., 106, *108*
Hawkshaw, M. J., 151, *160*
Hawton, K., *182*
Hayhurst, H., *182*
Hays, J. C., *50*
Hazell, P., *182*
Hazuda, H. P., *53*
Heard, H. L., 176, *180*
Heaton, R., *159*
Hebel, J. R., 169, *180*
Heck, R., 29, *47*
Hedberg, K., 72, *83, 86*
Heintz, R. T., 144, *159*
Heller, K. S., 38, *47, 176, 178*
Heminger, E., *181*
Hern, E. H., Jr., 29, 33, *50*
Herth, K., 176, *180*
Hickman, S. E., 63, 66, *83,* 225, *229*
Higginson, I. J., 39, 40, *51*
Hilgard, E., 154, *159*
Hill, P. C., 190, *199*
Hilliam, S. M., 166, *182*
Hines, S. C., 38, *50*
Hinkka, H., 40, *50*
Hipp, K. M., 189, *199*
Hirsch, C. S., *160*
Hirsch, D. A., 139, *161*
Hoare, C. H., 39, *50*
Hoffman, M. A., 112, *133*
Hogan, C., 12, *24*
Holden, J., 171, *179*
Holland, J. C., 138, 140–144, 150, *157, 159–
     161,* 174, *180*
Holley, J. L., 105, *108*
Hollon, S. D., 176, *180*
Holmes, D. S., 98, *108*
Holmes, V. F., 151, *158, 179*

Holt, L. L., 40, *50*
Holyoak, K., 98, *108*
Hopkins, D., 72, 83, *86*
Hopkins, S., *159*
Hopp, F. P., 39, *50*
Hopwood, P., 173, *180*
Horiuchi, B. Y., 29, 33, *47*
Hospice Foundation of America, 193, *199*
Houts, R. M., 39, *50,* 99, *107, 108,* 187, *198*
Howe, N., 22, 23, *26*
Howell, T., 173, *180*
Howen, C. W., 147, *159*
Hsu, M. A., *160*
Hu, L., 98, *108*
Hubbard, C., *54*
Hudis, C. A., *179*
Hughes, D., 69, *84*
Hummel, L. R., 186, *198*
Hung, J., 34, *49*
Huskamp, H., 7, *8*
Huzzard, L. L., *133*

Idler, E. L., *50*
In re Quinlan, A., 18, *24*
In re, L. W., *84*
Institute of Medicine, 44, *50,* 220, *229*
Irish, D. P., 58, *84*
Isingo, R., *53*
Iwashyna, T. J., 38, *50,* 208, *215*

Jackson, A., *83*
Jackson, B., 205, *216*
Jacobson, J. A., *50,* 100, 101, *107, 108, 198*
Jahnigen, D. W., *51*
Jamanka, A., *54*
James, D. S., 166, *182*
Jamison, S., 74, *84*
Jarrett, N., 45, *50*
Jay, S., 154, *159*
Jenkins, V., 34, *49*
Jernigan, J. A., 187, *198*
Johnson, A. L., *182*
Johnson, R. R., Jr., 6, *10,* 221, *229*
Johnson, T., 61, *84*
Johnston, W., 165, *180*
Jones, L., *55*

Kagawa-Singer, M., 38, *49, 50, 82,* 113, 122,
     127, *133*
Kahneman, D., 101, *109*
Kaim, M., *82, 157, 178*
Kanten, D. N., 187, *199*

Kaplan, G. A., *179*
Kaplan, R. M., 99, *109*
Karina, K., 139, *159*
Kasl, S. V., *50*
Kasl-Godley, J., *9*, *192*, *199*, *211*, *216*
Kastenbaum, R., 62, *84*
Kates, L. W., *51*, *133*
Katon, W., *159*
Katz, R. S., 60, 61, 83, *84*, 211, *216*
Kaut, K. P., 111–113, 115, 118, 122, 124, 125, *132*, *133*
Kavanaugh, J. J., 151, *158*
Kaye, J., 124, 131, *133*
Kayser-Jones, J., 37, 38, *50*
Kearney, M., 112, 116, 119, 121, 124, 126, 128, 131, *133*
Kellehear, A., 113, 131, *133*
Kellerman, J., 154, *159*
Kellokumpu-Lehtinen, P., *50*
Kelner, M., 116, *134*
Kendall, M., *52*
Kerridge, I., 16, *25*
Kiely, D. K., 40, *50*
Kijkstra, K., *197*
Kim, S. Y., *199*
Kinding, D., 15, *24*
King, D. A., 185, *199*
King, L., *84*
King, M., *55*
Kinzbrunner, B., 206, *216*
Kirchberg, T. M., 60, *84*
Kissane, D. W., 170, *179*
Kitchener, K. S., 58, 61, 62, 65, 79, 80, 81, 82, *84*
Klass, D., 45, *51*
Klausner, E. J., 177, *180*
Kleespies, P. M., 4–7, *9*, 60, 67–69, 72, 74, 78, *84*, 221, 222, *229*
Klein, D. F., 140, *161*
Kleinman, A., 44, *51*
Knapp, S., 61, *84*
Kochanek, K. D., 13, *25*
Koenig, B. A., 29, 49, *50*, *82*
Koenig, H. G., 122, 131, *133*, 191, *198*
Koffman, J., 39, 40, *51*
Koinuma, N., 34, *51*
Kopera-Frye, K., 112, *132*
Kornblith, A. B., *179*
Korzun, A. H., *159*
Kosmidis, H., 35, *53*
Kosunen, E., *50*
Koutsky, L., *159*

Kovacs, M., 145, *156*, *160*
Kovacs, P. J., 39, *51*
Kozak, J. F., *182*
Kraft, D., 104, *109*
Krakauer, E. L., 38, *51*, 71, *84*
Krotki, K. P., *53*
Kubler-Ross, E., *24*, 27, *51*, 116, 127, 129, *133*, *216*
Kunik, M. E., 191, *201*
Kutner, J. S., *51*
Kutner, L., 91, *108*
Kwak, J., 196, *197*
Kwilosz, D. M., *9*, 62, *82*, 192, *199*, 211, *216*, 225, 228
Kyung-hee, C., *48*

Lack, S. A., 138, *162*
Lafferty, W., *159*
Lammi, U.-K., *50*
LaMonde, L. A., 184, 188, 189, *199*
Lamont, E. B., 68, *82*
Lander, M., 166, 173, 174, *181*
Lander, S., 60, *82*, 138, *158*, 164, 165, 169, *179*
Lange, P., 148, *160*
LaPann, K., *53*
Larimore, W., 191, *198*
Larson, D. B., 40, *55*
Larson, D. G., *9*, 62, *82*, 116, 126, 127, 129, *133*, 191, 192, *199*, 211, *216*, 225, 228
Larson, J., *198*
Laruffa, G., *134*
Last Acts, 19, *24*, 28, 32, *51*, 221, 227, *229*
Lattanzi-Licht, M., 206, *216*
Laungani, P., 5, *9*, 28, 29, 31, 35, 37, *51–53*
Lavery, J. V., 72, *84*
Lawrie, S. M., 171, *180*
LeBaron, S., 154, *159*
Lee, M. A., 144, *159*, 165, *180*
Lefebvre, R. C., *181*
LeFevre, P. L., 171, *180*
Leichtentritt, R. D., 36, 39, 40, *51*
Leon, A. C., *160*
Leonard, C. V., 145, *158*
Lesko, L., 154, *160*
Lester, D., 172, *178*
Leventis, M., 113, *133*
Levine, E. G., 188, *199*
Levitt, M., *158*
Levy, J. K., *179*
Levy, M., 151, 153, 155, *160*

Pace, P., *156*
Pacquiao, D., 38, *53*
Pacquiao, D. F., *47*
Palmer, J. M., *52*
Pantilat, S. Z., 112, *134*
Papa, M. Z., *158*
Papadatou, D., 20, 26, 35, 39, 41, 45, *53, 54*
Paradis, L. F., 205, *216*
Pardo, C., *160*
Pargament, K. I., 189, 190, *199–201*
Parker, M., 191, *198*
Parker-Oliver, D., 177, *181*
Parkes, C. M., 29, *53*
Passik, S. D., 147, 148, *157, 159*, 164, 167, 171, *178, 179, 181*
Patient Self-Determination Act of 1990, 91, 104, 105, *109*
Patrick, D. L., *48*, 100, *107*, 116, 119, 122, 126, *134, 135*
Patterson, T., *159*
Pauker, S. G., 101, *108*
Paulson, D. S., 124, *134*
Paykel, E. S., *182*
Payne, S., 45, *50*
Payne, S. K., 7, *9*
Pearlin, L. I., 188, *200*
Pearlman, R. A., 72, *81*, 96, 97, 99, *108, 109*
Pellegrino, E. D., 70, *86*
Penley, W. C., *82*
Penman, D., 138, *157, 158*
Penson, J., 177, *181*
Penson, R., *84*
Perantie, D. C., 151, *161*
Pereira, D., *47*
Perkins, H. S., 39, *53*
Perry, M., *159*
Perry, S. W., 139, 152, 153, *161*
Pessin, H., *82*, 142, *157*, 174, 175, *178, 181*
Phillips, L. L., *197*
Phillips, R. S., *48*
Phipps, E., 186, 187, *200*
Piasetsky, S., *158*
Picot, S. J., 190, *200*
Pietsch, J. H., 5, 8, 28, 38, 42, *47*, 58, *82*
Pijnenborg, L., 72, *86*
Pinel, E. C., *108*
Pinquart, M., 184, *200*
Plows, C., *82*
Plumb, M. M., 142, 144, *161*
Popkin, M. K., 174, *181*
Portenoy, R. K., 151, 153, *158, 181*
Portera, L., *160*

Posner, J. B., *158*
Potash, M., 174, *181*
Powell, D., *156*
Powell, L. H., *201*
President's Commission for the Study of Ethical Problems in Medicine and Biomedical and Behavioral Research, 90, 92, 93, *109*
Preskorn, S. H., 174, *181*
Price, R. W., 152, 153, *156*
Prigerson, H. G., 66, *85*
Puchalski, C. M., 38, *53*
Pukkala, E., *179*
Pupo, C., *180*
Puustelli, A., *50*
Pyenson, B., 206, *215, 216*

Quesada, J. R., 142, *156*
Quill, T. E., 18, *25*, 68, *70–72, 84, 85*, 126, *134*

Rabins, P. V., 189, *200*
Rabkin, J. G., *49*, 165, *181*
Rabow, M. W., 112, *134*
Raghavan, K., 124, 131, *133*
Rando, T. A., 7, *9*, 66, *85*, 211, *216*
Rapkin, B. D., *133*
Raptis, G., *179*
Rault, R., 105, *108*
Rebagliato, M., 39, *53*
Redd, W. H., 155, *161*
Reedy, T., 187, *201*
Reese, D. J., 8, 62, *82*, 225, *228*
Retsas, A., 125, *135*
Rettig, K. D., 36, 39, 40, *51*
Reynolds, D., 145, *158*
Reynolds, S., *9, 83*, 186, *199*
Reynolds, S. L., *200*
Rhodes, L. A., 39, *48*
Rhymes, J. A., 29, *53*
Richter, J., 39, *53*
Robins, E., 144, *159*
Robinson, B. E., 185, *198*
Roche, V., 151, *161*
Rodgers, A. Y., 39, *51*
Roesler, M., *47*
Roff, L. L., *200*
Rogers, J. R., 62, 64, 65, *87*
Rosen, E. J., 6, *9*, 66, *85*
Rosenblatt, L., 60, *85*
Rosenfeld, B., 4, 7, *9*, 60, 67, 72, *82, 86*, 121, *134*, 142, 147, 148, *157, 159, 161*, 164, 165, 170, *178–181*, 222, *229*

Stewart, A. L., 118, 119, 122, *135*
Stiefel, F. C., 34, *48*, 142, 150, *161*
Stillion, J. M., 18, 20, *25*, *26*, 41, *54*
Stoddard, S., 206, *217*
Stoeckle, J. D., 91, *107*, 186, *198*
Stotland, E., 165, *182*
Strain, J. J., 140, *161*
Straker, N., 143, *160*
Strang, P., 40, *54*
Strang, S., *54*
Strauss, A., 27, 32, *49*
Strauss, W., 22, 23, *26*
Stroebe, M. S., 7, 9, 14, 26, 45, *54*, 211, *217*
Stroebe, W., 7, 9, 14, 26, 211, *217*
Strother, C. R., 22, *25*
Suarez, A., 176, *180*
Sue, D., 58, 86
Sue, D. W., 58, 86
Suhl, J., 187, *201*
Sullivan, A., 72, 86
Sullivan, M. C., 38, *54*
Sulmasy, D. P., 38, *54*, 70, 86, *135*, 187, *201*
Superintendent of Belchertown State School v. Saikewicz, 18, *26*
SUPPORT Principal Investigators, 18–19, *26*
Swallen, K. C., 15, *24*
Swartz, M., 68, *86*

Tanida, N., 40, *54*
Tanji, V. M., 29, *47*
Tardiff, K., *160*
Tarrier, N., 173, *180*
Tataryn, D. J., 166, *179*
Tatum, P., 38, *54*
Tax Equity and Fiscal Responsibility Act., 205, *217*
Taylor, A., 59, 86
Taylor, W. C., 101, *108*
Teasdale, J. D., *182*
Teetzel, H., 99, *109*
Temkin-Greener, H., 38, *54*
Tenenbaum, A. J., *54*
Tennstedt, S. L., 191, *197*
Teno, J. M., 119, *135*, 187, *201*
Ternestedt, B.-M., *54*
Terry, P. B., 105, *109*, *201*
Terzoli, E., 155, *161*
Tester, W., *200*
Texas Health and Safety Code, 76, 86
Thaler, H., *181*
Thase, M. E., 176, *180*
Theobald, D., *179*, *181*

Thibault, G., 68, 86
Thomas, J., 125, *135*
Thompson, A., *52*
Thoresen, C. E., *201*
Tierney, H., *160*
Tilden, V. P., 103, *109*
Tobin, D. R., 116, 126, 127, 129, *133*
Tolle, S. W., *50*, 103, *109*, 165, *180*
Tonge, W. L., 166, *182*
Tookman, A., *55*
Toombs, K., *55*
Toussaint, K. L., 28, *55*, 59, 87
Townsend, E., *182*
Townsend-Akpan, C., *52*
Tremblay, A., 150, 152, *157*
Trexler, L., 172, *178*
Triandis, H., 29, 31, *55*
Tross, S., 139, *159*, *161*
True, G., *200*
Truog, R., 75, 84, *86*
Trzepacz, P., 149, *162*
Tuley, M. R., 187, *199*
Tulsky, J. A., *54*, 134, *135*
Tuomilehto, J., *179*
Turner, H. A., *48*
Tversky, A., 101, *108*, *109*
Twycross, R. G., 138, *162*

Uhlmann, R. F., 96, *109*
Urassa, M., *53*
Utz, R. L., *201*

Vacco v. Quill, 70, 86
Van Brunt, D., 60, 85
van Delden, J., 72, 86
van der Maas, P., 72, 86
Van Ness, P. H., 40, *55*
VandeCreek, L., 39, *48*, 61, 84, 131, *133*
Vander Stichele, R. H., *52*
Varni, J., 154, *159*
Velin, R., *159*
Veterans Health Administration, 20, *26*
Vettese, M. A., *109*, *201*
Viola, R. A., *182*
Visintainer, M. A., 167, *182*
Volpicelli, J. R., 167, *182*

Waehler, C. A., 65, *86*
Wagner, G. J., 165, *181*
Walker, L., 90, *107*
Walkup, J., *54*
Wallace, J. I., 72, *81*

SUBJECT INDEX

Assessment relationship, 117–127
Assessment(s), 59–60, 111–132
    attitude of, 117, 127–129
    biological dimension in, 117–120
    of depression/hopelessness, 167–172
    developing methods of, 223–224
    issues/areas for, 117, 118
    model for, 113–127
    and preparing for good death, 127–132
    psychological dimension in, 120–122
    relationship in, 117–127
    spiritual dimension in, 123–127
Assistant Secretary for Planning and Evalu-
        ation study (ASPE), 205
Assisted death, 7, 72–74
Assisted suicide, 4, 72–74
Assisted Suicide Statement Work Group, 4
Asthenia, 155
Australia, 46
Authority, delegation of, 36
Autonomy, 32, 36, 73, 75, 185
Awareness, 33, 100

Baby boom generation, 22, 23
BCNU, 150
BDI (Beck Depression Inventory), 171
BDI Short Form, 171n
Beck Depression Inventory (BDI), 171
Behavioral interventions, 141–142, 155
Belief systems, 42, 112n., 113, 123–125, 189
Beneficence, 74
Benzodiazepine, 142
Bereavement
    anticipatory, 7, 66, 141, 211
    caregivers', 194–195
    cultural aspects of, 195
Bereavement research, 7
Bereavement services, 208
Bereavement support, 32–33
Bereavement support groups, 213
Best interest standard, 94n
Bias
    prediction, 102
    projection, 98
Biofeedback, 154
Biopsychosocial models of human behavior,
        114
    context of person's life in, 114–117
    framework for, 114, 115
Blacks, 15
Bleomycin, 150
Blood storage, 16

Body, needs of the, 119
Boundaries
    of competence, 58–59
    on relationships, 61–62
Brooding, 168
Brown University, 206
Burden
    of family caregivers, 188
    to others, 121, 143

California, 76
Cambodians, 42
Canada, 34
Cancer, 15
    and caregivers, 191
    and depression, 165, 171
    disclosure about, 34–35
    and mental health issues, 138–139
    and need for information, 34–35
Care, changing focus of, 31–33
Caregiver distress, 150
Caregiver Health Effects Study, 184
Caregivers/caregiving, 183–197
    and advance directives, 185–188
    benefits from, 189
    and bereavement, 194–195
    context of, 184–185
    extent of coverage provided by, 184–
        185
    gender differences in, 14
    health effects on, 184
    and hospice, 185
    interventions for, 192–194
    and religiousness/spirituality, 189–192
    stress of, 13
    stress process models related to, 188–189
Care Integration Team (CIT), 193, 194
Care provision, 225
Case managers, 207
Caucasians, 77, 187
Causes of death
    changes in, 15–16
CBT. See Cognitive–behavioral therapy
CDC (Centers for Disease Control and Pre-
        vention), 14
Centers for Disease Control and Prevention
        (CDC), 14
Centers for Medicare and Medicaid Services
        (CMS), 226
Central nervous system (CNS), 150
Cerebral hemorrhage, 15
Cerebrovascular diseases (stroke), 15

CHAMPUS (Civilian Health and Medical Program of the Uniformed Services), 205
Change(s)
    in causes of death, 15–16
    in health care, 16
    in hospice care, 213
    in public policy, 196
    in treatment preferences, 100
Chemotherapy, 16, 150, 155
Child development, 20–21
Children
    end-of-life issues for, 20–21
    in Greece, 35
China, 34, 42
Chronic conditions/disease, 15
    and assessments, 116
    changes in, 16
    in children, 21
    and suicide, 146
Chronic lower respiratory diseases, 15
Cigarette smoking, 14
Cis-platinum, 150
CIT. See Care Integration Team
Civic-mindedness, 22
Civilian Health and Medical Program of the Uniformed Services (CHAMPUS), 205
Claustrophobia, 140
Closure, 116, 214
CMS (Centers for Medicare and Medicaid Services), 226
CNS (central nervous system), 150
Cognitive–behavioral therapy (CBT), 143, 173, 175, 176
Cognitive coping strategies, 153
Cognitive disorder(s) in terminally ill individuals, 148–153
Cognitive psychology, 98
Cognitive symptoms of depression, 168
Cognitivism, 30–31
Cohort (term), 22, 41
Collaboration, 46, 223
Collectivism, 29–30
Comfortable dying, 17
Comfort care, 207
Communalism, 29–30
    "good death" in, 36
    and location of death, 37
    and need for information, 34–35
Communication
    advance directives as acts of, 92–95

in assessments, 122
and cultural differences, 45
cultural differences in, 34
with health professionals, 63
openness in, 32
and therapy issues, 66
Communication assumption, 94
Community, loss of, 72
Compassion, 73
Competence
    boundaries of, 58–59
    and depression, 73
    standard of, 58–61
    and substituted judgment, 93
Concerns, identifying, 126
Concrete operations stage, 21
Confidentiality, 63–65
Confusional states, 141, 145
Connectedness, need for, 124
Constructivist psychotherapy, 211
Consultation, 80, 212–213
Context of person's life, 114–117
Continuing professional education (CPE), 59
Continuity of contact, 173
Continuous home care, 209
Control issues, 62, 145
Conversation, 121–122
Cooperation with other professionals, 62–63
COPE (creativity, optimism, planning, expert information), 192–193
Coping strategies, 32–33, 210
COPs (Medicare Hospice Conditions of Participation), 207
Core values, 28–31
Corticosteroids, 142
Costs (of health services), 12, 123
Council on Ethical and Judicial Affairs (AMA), 77
Counseling services, 207
Countertransference, 60, 211
Couples therapy, 66
CPE (continuing professional education), 59
Critical Conditions, 19
Cross-cultural collaboration, 46
Crossing the Quality Chasm (IOM), 220
Culture(s), 27–46
    and assessments, 112n., 113
    and bereavement, 195
    and boundaries of competence, 58
    and changing focus of care, 31–33
    core value of, 29–31
    definition of, 28–29

and health care systems, 43–44

recommendations for advancing issues of, 44–45

and religious coping in caregivers, 190

research about, 224–225

research on specific, 37–43

similarities/differences between, 33–37

Death
child's understanding of, 20–21
moment of, 129–130
physical vs. social, 36
preparing for, 128

Death anxiety, 21, 60

Death awareness, 17–18, 32

Decision-making models, 79–80

Dehydration, 71–72

Delegating control, 105

Delegation of authority, 36

Delirium, 138–139, 149–153
AIDS-related, 147, 152–153
dementia vs., 149–151
management of, 151–152
and suicide, 144, 145, 147

Dementia, 149–153
delirium vs., 149–151
and family caregivers, 188, 195
HIV-related, 152–153
See Alzheimer's disease

Demoralization syndrome, 170

Denial, 166

Depression, 73, 138
assessment of, 167–172
clinical assessment of, 168–169
dying process compromised by, 163–164
empirical measures of, 170–172
in family caregivers, 188, 191, 195
pharmacotherapy for, 174–175
prevalence of, 164
psychotherapeutic interventions for, 175–177
and suicide, 144
in terminally ill individuals, 142–144
treatment of, 173–177

Destiny, 35

Determinism, 30

Dextroamphetamine, 174

Diabetes mellitus, 15

Diagnostic and Statistical Manual of Mental Disorders, Fourth Edition (DSM–IV), 148–149, 164n

DSM–III–R, 144

DSM–IV–TR, 168

Dialectical behavior therapy, 176

Diarrhea, 15

Dignity, need to maintain sense of, 36

Dignity Conserving Care, 129, 177

Diphtheria, 15

Direct patient care delivery, 213–214

Disability, 42, 75

Disclosures, 64–65

Discussion interventions, 103, 104

"Disease and treatment" living wills, 97, 103–104

Disintegration, fear of, 72

Dissociated somatization, 154

Dissociative imagery, 154

Distraction techniques, 142, 143, 175

Distress, patient's, 173

Distributive justice, 75, 77

Divine spirit, 30

DNR (do not resuscitate) orders, 76

Documentation
of consultation, 80
of preferences, 104

Documents, personal-control, 19–20

"Do no harm," 74

Do not resuscitate (DNR) orders, 76, 91

Double effect principle, 69–72

Drug interventions, 142

Durable powers of attorney for health care, 106

Duration of benefit, 78

Dying
and depression, 163–164
experience of, 129–130
as important part of life, 206–207
issues of, 204–205
psychosocial aspects of, 3
in United States, 19

EAC (ethics advisory committee), 69

Eastern cultures, 34

Edinburgh Postnatal Depression Scale, 171

Education, 45
about asthenia, 155
about personal control initiatives, 19
for psychologists, 211
recommendations for, 220–222

Education for Physicians on End-of-Life Care (EPEC), 45, 220

Elderly persons
gender differences in number of, 14
number of, 12

paraneoplastic syndrome in, 150
ELNEC (End of Life Nursing Education Consortium), 45, 220
Embolism, 15
Emotion, 103
Emotionalism, 30–31
Empathy, 213
Empirically supported treatment, 65
Employment, family caregivers and, 188
End-of-life decisions, 64
End-of-life insurance coverage, 226
End-of-life issues, 11–24
    for adults, 4
    APA's commitment to, 4
    for children/adolescents, 7, 20–21
    generational perspective on, 22–23
    and health care changes, 16
    and life expectancy, 11–16
    and location/timing of death, 16–17
    and personal control initiatives, 19–20
    and psychologists, 3
    and social movements in 20th century,
        17–19
End of Life Nursing Education Consortium
    (ELNEC), 45, 220
Enteritis, 15
EPEC, 45, 220
Eskimos, 15
Estate wills, 105
*Ethical Principles of Psychologists and Code of
    Conduct* (APA), 5, 57–67
Ethics advisory committee (EAC), 69
Ethics Code. *See Ethical Principles of Psychologists and Code of Conduct*
Ethics/ethical issues, 57–81
    and changing focus of care, 31–32
    of competence, 58–61
    decision-making model for, 79–80
    for dying persons/loved ones/professional care providers, 67–79
    of hastening death, 67–74
    and health care changes, 16
    in human relations, 61–63
    of privacy/confidentiality, 63–65
    of prolonging life, 74–79
    for psychologists, 57–67
    with therapy, 65–66
Ethnicity, 14–15
    and culture research, 41–42
    nationality vs., 41, 42
    See Culture
Euthanasia, 71

Existential despair, 170
Existentialism, 113, 124
Exley, C., 129
Experience
    of dying, 129–130
    with illness, 101
"Expert" caregivers, 32
"Expert" information, 193
Expressivism, 32
Extended family, 37

Family
    definition of, 183
    discussion with, 104
    and "good death," 36
    and hospice movement, 17
    and location of death, 37
    and openness, 32
    and palliative care, 18
    psychological services for, 214
    as surrogate decision makers, 69
Family systems perspective, 210
Family therapy, 66
Fear
    of disintegration, 72
    of isolation, 140
Fearfulness, 168
Feeding tubes, 18
Filipinos, 42
Financial challenges
    with end-of-life care, 7, 12
    for psychological services, 211–212
Finland, 34
Fluid and electrolyte balance, 151
Fluorouracil, 150
Focused medical review, 205
Free will, 30
French-speaking countries of Europe, 34
"Function and outcome" living wills, 97
Funding
    hospice, 209–210, 212, 226–227
    for palliative care, 196
    of physicians, 212
    of research, 227
Futility of treatment, 74–76

Gay men, 43, 139
Gender differences
    and culture research, 43
    and family decision making, 187
    in life expectancy, 13–14
General inpatient care, 209

Hospital Anxiety and Depression Scale (HADS), 170–171
"Hospitalization dip," 101
Houston Bioethics Network, 75
Humanism, 210
Human relations, 61–63
Hyperactive delirium, 152
Hypnosis, 153, 154

ICUs (intensive-care units), 78
Idealism, 23
Ideologism, 31
Imagery techniques, 142, 154
Incompetence, 64
India, 30
Individualism, 29
Indonesia, 30
Industrialized societies, 30, 31
Infant mortality, 16
Influenza, 15
Informal advance care planning, 186
Information
    expert, 193
    need for, 34–35, 126, 141
Informed consent to therapy, 65–66
Inpatient care, 209
In-service training, 214
Institute of Medicine (IOM), 220
Institutionalized death, 17
Institutional review committees, 76
Instructional advance directives, 91, 94, 96–98
Insurance coverage, 209–210, 226–227
Integrated care, 128
Integrity of the practice of medicine, 75
Intensive-care units (ICUs), 78
Interactive video, 104
Interconnectedness, 30
Interdependence, 30
Interdisciplinary teams, 206, 223, 228
International Psycho-Oncology Society, 34
Interpersonal prediction, 95
Interpersonal psychotherapy (IPT), 175
Interventions for family caregivers, 192–194
Intrapersonal prediction, 95
IOM (Institute of Medicine), 220
IPT (interpersonal psychotherapy), 175
Isolation
    and AIDS/suicide, 147
    sense of, 141
    and suicide, 145, 146
Israel, 36, 42

Italy, 12, 13, 42

Japan, 42
    cancer-disclosure rates, 34
    life expectancy in, 11–13
Jews, 36
Joint Commission on Accreditation of Healthcare Organizations, 205
Joint replacements, 16

Kaposi's sarcoma (KS), 147
Karma, Law of, 30, 35
Kidney dialysis, 16
Kidney disease, 15, 16
Kidney transplants, 77
Knowledge of issues, 118–119
KS (Kaposi's sarcoma), 147

Last Acts, 4, 19, 32, 227
Last Acts Partnership, 4, 19
Learning from dying, 205
Legacy intervention, 193–194
Levorphanol, 150
Life expectancy, 11–16
    and causes of death, 15–16
    and ethnicity, 14–15
    and gender, 13–14
    implications of increasing, 12–13
    and location/timing of death, 16–17
Life history, 124–125
Life review, 193
Life span development, 130
Life-sustaining treatment, 67–69, 144
Likelihood of benefit, 78
Limits of confidentiality, 63–64
Listening, active, 143, 176, 204, 213
Listening skills, 140, 148
Living alone, 14
Living wills
    as advance directive, 19
    development of, 90, 91
    disease-and-treatment, 97
    function-and-outcome, 97
    issues with, 102–106
    See advance directives
Location of death, 16–17, 36–37
Loss
    of community, 72
    finding meaning in the wake of, 7
    of loved one, 33
Loss and grief theory, 211
Lower respiratory diseases, 15

Lung cancer, 14

Magical thinking, 21
Major depression
    and cancer/AIDS, 164
    diagnosis of, 142–143
    and pain, 139
    prevalence of, 138
    and suicide, 144
Malignant tumors, 15
Managed care, 226
Marital status, 14
Materialism, 30
Meaning
    and hopelessness, 177
    loss of, 170
    need to attribute, 35–36
    search for, 113, 210
    and spirituality, 125
Meaning-centered group psychotherapy
    (MCGP), 177
Meaning-centered psychotherapy, 143–144
Meaning in the wake of loss, 7
Medicaid, 23, 91, 205, 206, 226
Medical utility, 77
Medicare
    and advance directives, 91
    and baby boom generation, 23
    enrollees/expenditures of, 12
    hospice conditions of participation
        (COPs), 207
    and hospice funding, 17, 205, 206, 209–
        210, 212, 226–227
    Part B, 212
    and time frame of terminal illness, 69
Memorial Sloan-Kettering Cancer Center
    (MSKCC), 144, 146, 147
Memories, 125, 177
Mental clarity, 141
Mental health issue(s) for terminally ill in-
        dividuals, 137–156
    anxiety as, 139–142
    cognitive disorders as, 148–153
    depression as, 142–144
    and physical symptoms, 153–155
    prevalence of, 138–139
    suicide as, 144–148
Meperidine, 150
Methotrexate, 150
Methylphenidate, 174
Migration, 42
Millennial generation, 23

Milliman USA, 206
Minor depression, 164
Modafinil, 174
Moment of death, 129–130
Morphine sulfate, 150
Mourning. See Bereavement
Multicomponent cognitive–behavioral inter-
        ventions, 154
Multiple relationships, 61–62
Mutual consideration, 30
Mutual releases, 63

Narcotic analgesics, 139, 150, 174
National Center for Health Statistics
    (NCHS), 14
National Hospice and Palliative Care Orga-
    nization (NHPCO), 45, 207
National identity, 37, 41
National Institute for Nursing Research
    (NINR), 222
Nationality, 37, 41, 42
National Vital Statistics Reports, 14
Nature-of-treatment decisions, 100
NCHS (National Center for Health Statis-
    tics), 14
Needs
    hierarchy of human, 113, 119
    unfinished, 204
    universal, 33–37
Nephritis, 15
Nephrosis (kidney disease), 15
Nephrotic syndrome, 15
Netherlands, 72
Neuroleptics, 148, 151–152
NHPCO (National Hospice and Palliative
    Care Organization), 45, 207
Nigeria, 42
NINR (National Institute for Nursing Re-
    search), 222
Nonmaleficence, 74
North America, palliative care movement in,
    32
Nursing home residents, 205
Nursing staff, 150
Nutrition, 151

OBRA (Omnibus Budget and Reconciliation
    Act), 205
Olanzapine, 152
"Old old," 12
Omnibus Budget and Reconciliation Act
    (OBRA), 205

Openness, 32
Open Society Institute, 222
Operation Restore Trust, 205
Opioid analgesics, 70
Opioid-induced nausea, 155
Optimism, 167
Oregon, 72, 74
Oregon Death with Dignity Act, 72
Organic mental disorders, 138–139. *See also*
    Delirium
    in AIDS, 152–153
    and suicide, 145
Organ transplants, 16, 76–79
Outpatient settings, 139
Overtreatment errors, 186–187

Pain
    and mental health issues, 139, 153, 154
    and suicidal ideation, 146
    and suicide, 145
Pain control, 17, 18, 20, 127
Palliative care, 18, 225
Palliative terminal sedation, 71
Pancreatic cancer, 142
Paraneoplastic syndrome, 150
Paratyphoid fever, 15
Parenteral neuroleptics, 152
Partnership for Caring, 4, 19
Passive termination of life, 90
Pastoral counseling, 143
Patient participation, 32
Patient Self-Determination Act (1990), 91,
    185, 186
Patient's rights, 18
Pay, ability to, 78
Pemoline, 174
Penicillin, 16
Periodic review of directives, 186
Personal control initiatives, 19–20
Personal growth, 130
Personal issues (of professionals), 60–61
Personal legacy, 193
Personal life narrative, 211
Personal story, 35–36
Pessimism
    and depression, 168
    and health outcomes, 167
    hopelessness vs., 166
Pharmacotherapy, 153, 174–175
Philippines, 34
Physical distress, 119
Physical symptoms, control of, 3

Physician-assisted suicide, 43, 70–71
Physicians
    Medicare funding of, 212
    predictive accuracy of, 103–104
    protection from legal action for, 18
Pneumonia, 15
Policy changes, 196
Postterminal phase of grief, 33
Power of attorney, 19, 64
Pragmatism, 31
Prayer, 189
Premature withdrawal (of caregivers), 146
Preoperational stage, 21
Present, act of being, 122
Privacy, 63–65
Private insurance, 226–227
Problem-solving therapy, 176
Pro bono services, 213
Procarbazine, 150
Process directives, 106
Professionals
    communication with, 63, 104
    cooperation with other, 62–63
    ethical issues for, 67–79
    and living wills, 104
    personal issues of, 60–61
Prognosis, suicide and, 145
Project Grace, 19
Projection bias, 98, 187
Prolonging-life decisions, 74–79
Protests, 23
Proxy advance directives, 91, 106, 186–187
Psychiatric hospitalization, 148
Psychiatrists, 212
Psychological services
    consultative opportunities for, 212–213
    direct patient care delivery opportuni-
        ties for, 213–214
    educational challenges facing, 211
    financial challenges facing, 211–212
    grief counseling opportunities for, 214–
        215
    need for, 203–204
    practical challenges facing, 212
    theoretical/philosophical challenges fac-
        ing, 210–211
Psychologists, 212
    educational recommendations for, 221–
        222
    and end-of-life issues, 3
    ethical issues for, 57–67
Psychopharmacological interventions, 143

Suicide among terminally ill individuals, 144–148
    and AIDS, 146–147
    management of, 147–148
SUPPORT. *See* Study to Understand Prognoses and Preferences for Outcomes and Risks of Treatments
Supportive psychotherapy, 140–141, 143, 173, 176
Support systems, 148
Surgical procedures, 16
Surrogate decision makers, 69
    accuracy of, 96–99
    and proxy advance directives, 91
    reducing burden of, 105
    substituted judgment of, 93–95
Susceptibility to illness, 167
Sweden, 11–13, 145
Symptom control, 143, 146, 176, 207
Symptom substitution system, 168

Talkativeness, decreased, 168
Task-orientation, 31
"Tasks," 32–33
Tax Equity and Fiscal Responsibility Act (TEFRA), 17, 205
Technology
    and allocation of resources, 76
    and changes in health care, 16–17
    end-of-life-scenario simulation with, 104
    and quantity of human life, 89–90
TEFRA. *See* Tax Equity and Fiscal Responsibility Act
Terminal dehydration, 71–72
Terminal illness (term), 68–69
Terminal sedation, 71
Texas, 76
Theory development, 44–45
Therapy, 65–66
Third-party requests for services, 62
Thrombosis, 15
Time
    in cognitivism cultures, 30
    to prepare for death, 12, 15–16
Time frame
    and assessments, 128
    of terminal illness, 68–69
Timing of death, 16–17
Toolkit for Measures of End-of-Life Care, 59
Tragic optimism, 166
Training, 45, 211, 225

Transcultural research, 46
Transformational imagery, 154
Transfusions, 16
Translational/implementation research, 220
Truth telling, 32
Tuberculosis, 15
Typhoid, 15

Understanding of death (in child development), 20–21
Undertreatment errors, 187
Unfinished needs, 204
United Kingdom, 12, 13, 42
United States
    cancer-disclosure rates, 34
    life expectancy in, 11, 13
    number of older adults in, 12
    Congress, 205, 209, 227
    Department of Health, Education, and Welfare, 205
    Department of Health and Human Services, 226
    Department of Veterans Affairs Training and Program Assessment for Palliative Care, 45
    Medicare program. *See* Medicare
    Office of the Inspector General, 205
    Supreme Court, 18, 70–71
Universal needs, 33–37
    to attribute meaning, 35–36
    for care/support, 36–37
    for information, 34–35
    to maintain sense of dignity, 36
University of Alabama, 193–194
University of South Florida, 192–193
Urgency of need, 78

Verbal statements, 91
Veterans Administration, 221, 225
Veteran's Benefit Package, 205
Vinblastine, 150
Vincristine, 150
Virtual reality, 104
Vitamins, 151
Voluntary euthanasia, 72–74
Volunteer services, 208–209

Weight loss, 154–155
Western cultures, 32, 34
Widows/widowers, 14
Wills, estate, 105
"Wishless," 95n

Withdrawal of food and water, 18
Withdrawal of treatment, withholding vs., 68
Worthlessness, 142

Xers generation, 23

Yale School of Nursing, 204

Zung Self-Rating Depression Scale (Z-SRDS), 171
Zyprexa, 152

ABOUT THE EDITORS

James L. Werth Jr. received his PhD in counseling psychology from Auburn University in 1995 and his master's of legal studies from the University of Nebraska—Lincoln in 1999. As the 1999–2000 American Psychological Association William A. Bailey AIDS Policy Congressional Fellow, he worked on aging and end-of-life issues in the office of U.S. Senator Ron Wyden (Democrat–OR). He has been an assistant professor in the Department of Psychology at the University of Akron since August 2000; he is also the pro bono psychologist for the local HIV services organization where he provides counseling and supervises graduate students. He has authored or coauthored more than 50 articles and book chapters, edited or coedited 5 special journal issues, and written or edited 3 books on end-of-life matters and HIV disease. He is the only person to have served on all of the American Psychological Association's major end-of-life workgroups and was one of two psychologists invited to speak at a congressional briefing, "Promoting Quality Care Near the End of Life: What Policymakers Need to Know." Finally, he has coordinated amicus curiae briefs on mental health issues near the end of life for the U.S. Supreme Court, Ninth Circuit Court of Appeals, and the Florida Supreme Court.

Dean Blevins received his PhD in psychology from the University of Akron, in addition to degrees in political science and education. After finishing his doctoral work, he completed a 2-year fellowship in health services research and pursued a master's degree in public health. He is currently a career development awardee in the Veterans Health Affairs Merit Review Entry Program in Little Rock, Arkansas. He holds positions as a research health scientist with the Central Arkansas Veterans Healthcare System's Center for Mental Healthcare and Outcomes Research; an assistant professor at the University of Arkansas for Medical Sciences, College of Medicine, Department of Psychiatry; and a program evaluator for the South Central Mental Illness Research, Education, and Clinical Care Center. His research program focuses on improving mental health care through translational and implementation research related to end-of-life care. He is additionally a consultant in patient outcomes assessment and program evaluation, working in numerous health care settings, including state agencies for long-term care, community and private mental health providers, HIV/AIDS community-based organizations, nursing homes, and hospices. He has published or has in press numerous manuscripts and has given more than 50 professional talks on death and dying, aging, public policy, and mental health care in various settings around the country.